TENDING THE STUDENT BODY

Youth, Health, and the Modern University

In the early twentieth century, university administrators and educators regarded bodily health as a marker of an individual's moral and mental strength and as a measure of national vitality. Beset by social anxieties about the physical and moral health of their students, they introduced compulsory health services and physical education programs in order to shape their students' character. *Tending the Student Body* examines the development of these health programs at Canadian universities and the transformation of their goals over the first half of the twentieth century from fostering moral character to promoting individualism, self-realization, and mental health.

Drawing on extensive records from Canadian universities, Catherine Gidney examines the gender and class dynamics of these programs, their relationship to changes in medical and intellectual thought, and their contribution to ideas about the nature and fulfilment of the self. Her research will be of interest to historians of medicine, gender, sport, and higher education.

CATHERINE GIDNEY is an adjunct professor in the Department of History at St. Thomas University.

Tending the Student Body

*Youth, Health, and the
Modern University*

CATHERINE GIDNEY

UNIVERSITY OF TORONTO PRESS
Toronto Buffalo London

© University of Toronto Press 2015
Toronto Buffalo London
www.utppublishing.com
Printed in the U.S.A.

ISBN 978-1-4426-4787-9 (cloth)
ISBN 978-1-4426-1596-0 (paper)

Library and Archives Canada Cataloguing in Publication

Gidney, Catherine (Catherine Anne), 1969–, author
Tending the student body : youth, health, and the modern university / Catherine Gidney.

Includes bibliographical references and index.
ISBN 978-1-4426-4787-9 (bound). ISBN 978-1-4426-1596-0 (pbk.)

1. College students – Health and hygiene – Canada – History – 20th century.
2. College students – Medical care – Canada – History – 20th century.
3. Youth – Health and hygiene – Canada – History – 20th century.
4. Youth – Medical care – Canada – History – 20th century.
5. Universities and colleges – Health promotion services –
Canada – History – 20th century.   I. Title.

LB3499.C3G53 2015   378.1'971   C2014-905276-6

University of Toronto Press acknowledges the financial assistance to its publishing
program of the Canada Council for the Arts and the Ontario Arts Council, an agency of
the Government of Ontario.

 Canada Council   Conseil des Arts
for the Arts   du Canada

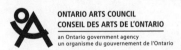

University of Toronto Press acknowledges the financial support of the Government of
Canada through the Canada Book Fund for its publishing activities.

This book has been published with the help of a grant from the Federation for the
Humanities and Social Sciences, through the Awards to Scholarly Publications
Program, using funds provided by the Social Sciences and Humanities
Research Council of Canada.

Contents

Illustrations

Acknowledgments

This book would not have been possible without the help of a number of people. I would like to thank the archival staff at the Division des archives de l'Université de Montréal, the Division des archives de l'Université Laval, the Esther Clark Wright Archives at Acadia University, the Dalhousie University Archives, the Mount Allison University Archives, McGill University Archives, St. Francis Xavier University Archives, University of Alberta Archives, the University of British Columbia Archives, the former United Church of Canada/Victoria University Archives, the University of Manitoba Archives, the University of Toronto Archives, and the University of Western Ontario Archives. Marnee Gamble at the University of Toronto Archives, David Mawhinney at Mount Allison University Archives, and Bruce Kidd all took time out of their busy schedules to help me locate relevant photographs. The research for this project would not have been undertaken without post-doctoral fellowships from Associated Medical Services, Inc. (Hannah Institute), and the Social Sciences and Humanities Research Council of Canada, as well as a research grant from the New Brunswick and Atlantic Studies Research and Development Centre at St. Thomas University. I am also grateful for the institutional support provided by the history departments at the University of Waterloo and St. Thomas University, and especially the help of Margie Reed at the latter institution.

Portions of the book first appeared in "Institutional Responses to Communicable Diseases at Victoria College, University of Toronto, 1900–1940," *Canadian Bulletin of Medical History* 24, 2 (2007): 265–90, and "The Athletics–Physical Education Dichotomy Revisited: The Case of the University of Toronto, 1900–1940," *Sport History Review* 37 (2006): 130–49. My thanks to these journals for allowing me to use this material.

Much of chapter 5 is reprinted with permission of the publisher from my contribution to *Feminist History in Canada: New Essays on Women, Gender, Work, and Nation*, edited by Catherine Carstairs and Nancy Janovicek © University of British Columbia Press 2013. All rights reserved by the Publisher.

Conversations often spur ideas. It was in the midst of a discussion with Lara Campbell about material I had found at the Victoria University Archives, and as a result of her enthusiastic response, that I sacrificed an extended afternoon in her company in order to scurry back to the archives to quickly gather the information that became the basis of this project. Her generosity of spirit is a constant source of inspiration. Wendy Mitchinson, Pat Harrigan, and Paul Axelrod have provided much-appreciated support and encouragement for the project. Bill Westfall and the late Cathy James kindly provided me with a quiet home base in Toronto from which to delve more fully into the research and to which I could always count on returning after a day's work for wonderful nourishment and lively conversation. Over the years a number of academics have offered insightful feedback on various parts or all of the text: Lara Campbell, Bruce Curtis, Michael Dawson, R.D. Gidney, Cathy James, Wyn Millar, Wendy Mitchinson, Ian Nicholson, Marguerite Van Die, Carey Watt, and the anonymous reviewers of the manuscript. Len Husband ably guided the project through the publication process.

Family and friends have sustained me through the years it has taken to complete this project. I consider myself fortunate to have the friendship of colleagues and their families at St. Thomas University. My book club of feisty and intelligent women is always inspiring. Michael Boudreau, Karen Commander, Elif Dalkir, Peta Fussell, Bonnie Huskins, Fran Lipsett, Nicole Perry, Lisa Todd, Julia Torrie, Jacob Sweezey, and John Umbach provided both encouragement and much-needed distraction. In addition to being a good friend, Kimberly Sauvé looked after my children with compassion and empathy so that I could write the history of other youth. Mal and Rita Dawson ferried me around for endless years so that I could get to my research. My parents, as always, continue to provide intellectual and moral support. My two lovely daughters, Alexandra and Emma, remind me that life is full of joy. I dedicate this book to Michael Dawson. His support is inestimable and, of course, I owe him one.

Freddy Beach, February 2014

TENDING THE STUDENT BODY

Youth, Health, and the Modern University

Introduction

In November 1931, Dr Edna Guest presented her report on the health of women residents to the dean of women at Victoria College, University of Toronto. As usual, her report provided a summary of student health, grading students in such categories as "feet," "thyroids," "spine," "eyes," "tonsils," "menstruation," and in an attempt to assess their level of rest, "holidays." While Guest found many of the women to be in relatively poor health on entering university, she happily recorded that with supervision and instruction, their health was much improved by their senior year. As well as providing medical care for the students, Guest was responsible for the medical inspection of the residences, including the evaluation of rooms for proper light, desk space, ventilation, draughts, and overcrowding. At the end of her report, she also acknowledged the advances made over the course of her ten-year employment at Victoria, noting the establishment of "a health centre which not only cares for our students when they are ill, but is an educational health centre." Indeed, she argued for the need for gymnasium work to correct defects and train students in leisure time as well as health lectures to teach otherwise ignorant girls "the anatomy and general mechanism of the normal, healthy human being ..." After all, she continued, "Do they need Latin in their curriculum so much more than they need a direct health course?"[1]

In general, students today assume access to some type of health facility in order to be treated for such things as viruses, bacterial infections, sprains, and abrasions. They can draw on specialized and trained counsellors for academic, career, personal, or mental health issues. And they can exercise in often state-of-the-art gymnasium facilities. Students assume they are free to seek out such services as they need. They expect a high level of privacy in treatment and take for granted that health services and the various options for physical activity are differentiated from other aspects of campus life.

As Guest's report indicates, the origins of such programs lie in the first half of the twentieth century. Yet unlike in the present, when health care and physical activity are treated as services provided to students by the university, Guest's report points to the way in which in the past many health experts and educators believed the university to be a place of training for bodies as much as for minds. They perceived the nineteenth-century adage of *mens sana in corpore sano* – a sound mind in a sound body – as not only relevant to the modern university, but perhaps even crucial in order to ward off elements of decay and degeneracy endemic to modern civilization.[2] The longevity of this belief can be readily seen at Mount Allison University where, in 1961, administrators saw fit to approve the placement of the motto over the entranceway of their newly created athletics building.[3] For many educators, bodily health was a visible marker of an individual's mental strength and moral fortitude as well as an indicator of the future stability, and virility, of the nation. With access to those they believed would become the future leaders of the nation, and possessed of the latest knowledge and expertise, educators and health professionals understood the university as a key site in the salvation of society.

As a result, at the turn of the twentieth century, university administrators began instituting a variety of health programs integrated into all aspects of students' lives. They began to hire a host of experts – dieticians, nurses, doctors, and physical educators – to supervise students' health. They gradually instituted compulsory medical examinations and physical training, and often compulsory health lectures, for students. And they set up infirmaries, access to a doctor through the year, and in some cases by the 1920s provided hospitalization insurance. Health experts and educators saw their role as identifying and separating the contagious; grading students and providing advice on physical exercise; and inspecting and pronouncing on proper living conditions, dining, clothing, and behaviour. They took it, too, as their responsibility to teach students how to live in the best way possible. In tackling these tasks, doctors, deans, physical instructors – all largely working outside the academic stream of the university – played an influential role in the process of character formation, a central goal of the early-twentieth-century Canadian university.

The belief in the need for such programs did not originate in Canadian universities but, rather, arose from broad North American, British,

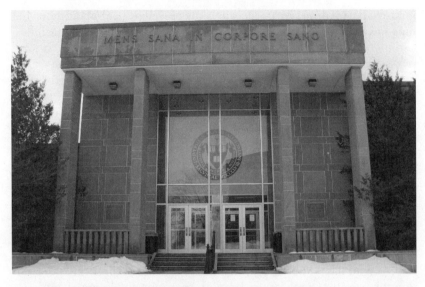

0.1 Mount Allison University Athletic Centre. Note the motto: *mens sana in corpore sano*. Photo by C. Gidney.

and European concerns in the late nineteenth century about youth and the nature of modern society. Growing anxiety about student health developed within the context of changing economic and social conditions caused by industrialization, urbanization, mass immigration, and the emancipation of women as well as the reactions to these conditions resulting in the social gospel, moral reform, eugenic, mental hygiene, and public health movements. Between the 1880s and 1920s, health experts and concerned citizens created and employed a variety of voluntary and state agencies to temper the effects of modernity, to soothe concerns about the fragmentation of society, and to enact transformative change. The development of physical training and health services on university campuses emerged as one response to the perceived negative effects of a rapidly changing society.

The belief in the importance of physical training can most directly be traced to a transatlantic trend of increased public interest in organized sport and athletics that had developed gradually over the course of the nineteenth century but gained impetus in the 1880s. In Canada, historians attribute this development to a number of factors: the new values of industrial capitalism, greater leisure time as well as fears about how that time was being spent, municipal provision of athletic fields and facilities, and increasing support by social reformers and Protestant churches for morally uplifting amusements.[4] Sport and athletics also became widely perceived as valuable training for national militaristic and imperial aims as well as for an Anglo-Christian cultural vision keen to spread civilization throughout the British Empire.[5]

Part of the emphasis on sports arose from changes within the British public school system, changes which helped reshape Canadian attitudes. In the mid-nineteenth century, headmasters and writers such as Thomas Arnold and Thomas Hughes began to promote team sports as a way of cultivating gentlemanly virtues and Christian manliness. In the international context, historians have traced the rise of athleticism within educational facilities as a means of imparting such values as discipline, order, moral and physical courage, and the leadership necessary for the duties of nation and Empire. Imperialism demanded a fit and virile citizenry. J.A. Mangan has demonstrated that British private schools, and by extension the private schools of the Dominions, promoted imperial aims and Anglo-Protestant ideals through the "Games Ethic."[6]

This emphasis on manliness was also reinforced in the late nineteenth century by both religious and secular emphases. Within mainline churches, one strand of thought, as embodied in Canada in Ralph Connor's novels, and in the United States through the persona of Billy Sunday, popularized the notion of a "muscular Christianity," an attempt to emphasize Christ as manly and robust over what was seen as an increasingly feminized, pietistic church.[7] Secular corollaries emerged in the psychology of Stanley Hall and the personality of Teddy Roosevelt, both of whom, as Gail Bederman points out, rejected the feminized domesticity of the late nineteenth century in favour of a virile and tough masculinity.[8]

Fear of effeminacy in young men, church leaders' concerns over the declining church membership among urban male youth, and the desire to maintain appropriate social outlets for both girls and boys led to the creation in the late nineteenth century of a variety of youth organizations such as the Boy Scouts, Girl Guides, Boys' Brigade, Canadian Girls in Training, YMCA, and YWCA. As leisure time and access to leisure activities increased, church leaders and moral and social reformers worried about the proper use of spare hours and set about to create opportunities for youth, and other members of society, to engage in activities that would improve the body and mind. These organizations helped reshape

the vision of sport from an immoral activity to one appropriate for respectable Christian youth.[9]

This cult of athleticism was matched by a growing enthusiasm in the
nineteenth century for gymnastics and physical culture. Beginning in
the late eighteenth and early nineteenth centuries, physical educators
in Germany and Sweden began developing systems of physical culture
aimed at individual and national regeneration. These systems spread
to both Britain and the United States and from there into Canada. By
the 1890s, the Swedish system in particular had gained hold in England
and was taught in female schools of physical training and private girls'
schools. By the early years of the twentieth century, Swedish gymnastics
had become incorporated into the British education system.[10] Meanwhile, in the United States, some leading educators had begun to in-
corporate gymnastics into boys' schools and universities as early as the
1820s. Concerned about female frailty, advocates of women's health began encouraging women to engage in moderate exercise, with calisthenics appearing in some girls' schools and women's colleges by the 1830s.[11]
In the second half of the nineteenth century, American educators, drawing on European influences, began developing their own homegrown
variations of physical culture, which would become influential throughout North America. Though still in piecemeal form, by the turn of the
century, physical culture had gained influence in Canada, incorporated,
for example, in girls' private schools and ladies' colleges, in normal
school courses, and in the Strathcona Trust program, which encouraged
the implementation of military drill in schools.[12]

The interest of educators, church leaders, and moral reformers in
physical training and athletics as a means of shaping youth occurred amid
growing concerns about individual and societal health. In the nineteenth
century, a variety of movements linking good health to morality – through,
for example, dietary regimes, exercise programs, or temperance – swept
across the United States.[13] At the same time, increasing urbanization and
the resultant health consequences sparked the emergence of a strong
public health movement that focused North Americans' attention on improved private and public sanitary conditions.[14]

The beginning of mass schooling also led health experts and educators to turn to the school as a means of identifying the ill and containing
the spread of disease. In the late nineteenth and early twentieth centuries, educators and health reformers began to worry about children's
long hours at desks in unhealthy school rooms which were unclean and
had poor ventilation, lighting, and heating, and improper furniture – all

of which could lead to "school disease," a newly emerging catchall for such things as eyestrain, poor posture, and spinal curvature. They also worried about schools as potential sites for the spread of contagious diseases.[15] In addition, educators and health reformers sought to improve the classroom and playground, to make schooling more practical and relevant to students' needs and the needs of modern industrial society, and to mitigate some of the effects of modernization such as poverty and ill health. Such concerns led them to advocate, and led school authorities to sanction, a range of medical and health initiatives such as physical exercise, medical examinations, inspection of school buildings and grounds, the implementation of health curricula, and the introduction of vaccination.[16]

Attention to school health emerged at the same time as the development of theories articulated by experts, but widely embraced by the public, of childhood and adolescence as particularly volatile life stages requiring guidance and supervision. One of the earliest and most famous child psychologists, G. Stanley Hall, helped to develop and disseminate the notion of normal adolescence as a period of internal turmoil and stress, resulting in external manifestations that could be either extremely negative or positive, depending on the nature of the guidance.[17] Schools, then, became a central site through which experts could gain access to, and help shape, youth.

Anxieties over the development of youth, and the health of Anglo-American citizens more generally, were given impetus by new concerns and developments in the early decades of the twentieth century. Recruitment during the South African War and the First World War highlighted the poor health of male citizens, increasing fears about the weakening of the male body due to industrial society and a feminized religion.[18] Declining birth rates among the white middle-class Anglo-American population, combined with rising levels of immigration from outside that population, led to fears about race suicide.[19] The growth of white-collar work, a by-product of industrialization and urbanization, led to concern about the sedentary nature of modern life and its eviscerating effects on the body.[20]

University educators absorbed, and helped articulate, many of these societal anxieties. While many set their sights on rectifying social ills in the population at large, some turned their attention to their own student body. This book examines the implementation of health programs as well as the ideals behind them. It focuses on the period roughly from the turn of the century, when some university administrators in Canada established the first programs in physical training, to the 1960s, at which point most universities provided some form of health service and many had developed formal, centralized, and bureaucratized departments.

I argue that concern about student health led to the creation of new sites through which administrators could exert their moral vision of the university and shape the student body. Physicians, physical educators, deans of men and women, administrators, and some faculty all helped introduce a variety of health services and physical education programs. By mid-century, practitioners in both of those areas had begun to develop their own priorities and to work towards the specialization and disciplinary credibility of their own fields. Institutional changes occurred at the same time as ideological shifts. While in the early part of the century health experts and educators focused on environmental causes of disease, in the interwar years they turned their attention to the eradication of tuberculosis, and by the postwar years began to focus on mental health. That reorientation matched a shift away from educators' emphasis on developing character and towards the creation of individual personality and the potential for self-realization. While student health became part of a new and growing area within universities, namely student services, the belief in the importance of physical training faltered for a host of reasons, not least of which was that it became unhinged from its nineteenth-century ideological roots. In the process, the entire university community helped create, and adapted to, new ideas about the nature and fulfilment of the self.

At a basic descriptive level, then, I seek to answer a number of questions: What programs did universities institute? When and how did they establish them? While administrators spent the early decades of the twentieth century developing health provisions, by the late 1960s and early 1970s, many of the elements of the physical education programs had been dismantled while health services had become unrecognizable. How did that process occur and why did support for some aspects of the programs disappear and not for others?

In answering those questions, I hope to contribute to our growing understanding of the ways in which universities underwent fundamental institutional change in the twentieth century. A number of historians have examined the development of the modern university in this period, which was marked by an increasing adherence to the ideals of research and utility, the specialization of knowledge, and the growing prominence and influence of the social and applied sciences.[21] Drawing on beliefs about the power of scientific investigation to improve the individual and society, health experts not only carved out areas of expertise within this context but gained credibility from this intellectual turn. Pouring resources into health and physical education facilities, essentially a non-academic sphere of the university, marks the beginning of what would become a trend in the second half of the twentieth century towards the development of the new field of student affairs or student services.

At the same time, such questions will help illuminate transformations in medical practice. At the beginning of the period, physicians could offer patients few solutions to their ailments. By the end of the period, much of the structure for modern medicine was in place, as were the beginnings of universal health care. Yet the process of that transformation is still little known. This book thus offers some insight into the nature of the change within the context of the university – the way in which programs were set up, the types of medical treatment provided, the solutions (and lack thereof) to medical problems, the shift from sanitary science to bacteriology, the bureaucratization of medical services, and the expansion of health provisions.

Central to that transformation is the rise of medical expertise. Historians have explored this topic in some depth, from the growth of the medical profession to the influence of medical authorities in fields such as child rearing, child development, sexuality, and marriage preparation, among others.[22] Here, I examine the way in which medical expertise gained influence within the university and in particular the methods by which one sub-field built upon another. In addition, the book contributes in a modest and partial way to our understanding of citizens' growing support for the health policies and practices that became integrated into the modern welfare state. Historians have begun to illuminate the way in which citizens both demanded, and assumed a right to, welfare provisions.[23] Within the university, educators and medical experts established health systems and taught students the importance of these systems, while students in turn demanded the extension of health provisions. In doing so, administrators, physicians, physical educators, and students all added to the growing expectations of access to publicly funded health care.

While the establishment of health programs had institutional consequences – for both the development of the university and of medical services – much of the primary aim of establishing them focused on the contribution educators could make to the process of character formation. A central aim of the book, then, is to examine the ideological rationales for such programs and what they tell us about the nature and culture of university life. Equally, I ask what their disappearance and transformation reveal about institutional and cultural change.

Historians have examined the way in which, both in the classroom and through extra-curricular activities, educators aimed to shape the minds, morals, and spiritual development of students in order to produce students who would be able to both contribute to and help reproduce the social, cultural, and economic fabric of society.[24] In doing so, they have generally overlooked the way in which administrators and health experts drew on new ideas about health to reinforce and bolster their beliefs about morality, intellectual vigour, and citizenship.[25] In this book, then, I focus on how ideas about health intersected with those of morality in the process of character formation.

At the same time, ideas about the nature, aims, and purpose of individual formation were never static. The beliefs of moral and social reformers, eugenicists, and early health experts remained powerful shaping forces well into the twentieth century. But new ideas in the fields of psychology, psychiatry, adolescent behaviour, and educational theory began to reshape the language employed to understand individual growth and the values associated with citizenship. Central to this process was the shift from character to personality – an issue that forms the core of the second part of the book. Historical sociologists and philosophers have argued that the belief in the realization of the self as a key component necessary for the development of individual identity has become a central feature of late modern society.[26] The broadening scope and influence of psychology, both as an academic discipline and a field, contributed much to this process.[27] In this book, I do not examine psychology itself but rather how educators and health professionals took up the ideas of psychologists – particularly the concept of personality – and how that process gradually helped reshape beliefs about the self as well as educators' overall mission of student formation. While creating better citizens remained a common refrain among university educators, the nature and meaning of citizenship underwent fundamental change.

In tracing this shift from the ideal of character to that of personality, this book examines the process of middle-class youth formation. Studies of twentieth-century moral and social reform efforts have tended to focus on beliefs about, and actions towards, those groups that did not conform or were perceived as not conforming to reformers' own middle-class Anglo-Celtic values.[28] Yet as we'll see, health experts' vision of citizenship was one that encompassed all elements of Canadian society. Their critique of individuals extended to those who were middle class or aspiring to join it.

Indeed, many health experts would come to see the university constituency as a key group in need of advice and training. Through the period
under consideration, university students constituted an intellectual elite –
in the 1930s, just under 3 per cent of youth aged twenty to twenty-four
attended a post-secondary institution, a rate that had reached only 8
per cent by 1961. Their background was largely middle class. The bulk
of university students originated from professional and managerial families, though some came from the upper echelons of society and small
numbers had fathers who could be classed as skilled, semi-skilled, or
unskilled workers.[29] Yet educators did not assume that students were
immune to the ravages of ill health. Class did not necessarily protect
one from epidemic disease or genetic predispositions. Moreover, while
some students drew on family resources and attended university without economic worry, others came from families who skimped and saved
to send their children to university; and in other cases students worked,
often as teachers, for several years prior to enrolment in order to be
able to afford the cost of a university education. In some cases, economic downturns jeopardized students' continued enrolment.[30] Thus
educators perceived university students to be in need of health care
provisions.

In addition, despite the fact that university-age students were generally
between the ages of eighteen and twenty-two, administrators and experts
usually treated them as if they were in an extended phase of adolescence.
While studies of youth often take the teens as an end point, educators,
and students themselves, adhered to a belief that students were not yet
fully formed adults. Indeed, the aim of their education was to finish off
that process.[31] As a result, despite the ages and backgrounds of the students, university administrators and health experts did not assume that
they possessed the modern health knowledge necessary to succeed in
life, nor in many respects did they have confidence that students were
able to seek out that knowledge on their own.

Health experts also perceived students as an important constituency
because of their future role in society. The small numbers of students
who worked or were enrolled in universities belie the increasing social,
cultural, and economic importance of these institutions. Indeed, during
the period under consideration, these would be transformed from small
liberal arts institutions with some professional faculties into multiversities providing the major source of professional training, scientific and
medical research, and technical knowledge. Those students who entered
the university portals would become a significant source for the next
generation of professionals, politicians, civil servants, social workers,

managers, artists, and community leaders. Graduates would take the values and ideals learned in university with them into the home, workplace, and community.

If the age and class of university students affected educators' beliefs about the need to provide health services to them, so too did their ideas about gender. Influenced by nineteenth-century notions of gender formation, educators aimed to create boys and girls who, respectively, embodied the ideals of manliness and womanhood. Ideas about health and the shape of the body came to inform the process of character formation. Physical training was very much a part of helping to create, define, and reinforce gendered practices.[32] This study contributes to an existing literature on the role physical education played in defining gendered ideals in the nineteenth and early twentieth centuries and extends that research into a later period.[33] It focuses not only on students, but also in particular on the female experts who lived under many of the same constraints they imposed. It thus examines the possibilities opened up to female professionals, as well as their limits, by the implementation of health care and physical education programs on university campuses. It also suggests that the tracked institutional and ideological changes can tell us something about women's changing place on campus.

In order to provide regional, religious, linguistic, and institutional diversity, I have mined a variety of university archival holdings across Canada.[34] Because of the richness of the sources at Victoria College, University of Toronto, in the first four decades of the twentieth century, that institution plays a particularly prominent part in the story. Not surprisingly, programs were strongest at institutions with better finances and established athletic facilities. They also appeared earliest at denominational colleges where the aim of creating moral citizens was more prominent. Yet the significance of the programs lies in the fact that they spread to many institutions and that even where they were never fully, or even extensively, implemented, administrators voiced their belief in the need for such programs. This is not a comprehensive history of physical culture and athletics, of the growth of student health services, or even of the development of either of these at any one particular institution, though certainly some of the chronology and institutional growth is recorded. Each of these could be usefully studied on its own. Rather I am interested in what these areas reveal about the changing ideals of student formation as well as the nature of the university itself. Equally, I raise questions about how the structure of universities and professional culture shaped the areas of physical culture and health services and the students for whom these programs were intended.

The study is divided into two parts. The first section focuses on the creation of a system of student health and its ideological underpinnings from approximately the turn of the century to the 1940s. The second section focuses on both the expansion of health provisions and the ideological and practical changes occurring within universities from the 1930s to the 1960s. The concluding chapter draws together the overall argument, highlighting the aims and purpose of university authorities and medical experts in developing student health programs and pointing to the long-lasting, and often unintended, consequences of these programs.

1

Institutional Development of Student Health Programs

In the nineteenth century, college and university administrators paid some attention to the health of their students and the safety of their buildings. College authorities often needed to convince parents that their children and young adults would return from their course of study unharmed. This was particularly true at residential institutions which, if not legally, at least morally, assumed responsibility for the care of students. Small and cash-strapped, most colleges and universities depended on student tuition for financial viability. As a result, promotional pamphlets and college calendars often emphasized the healthy environment or location of the institution. Some administrators created classes in calisthenics for young women, hired gymnastics instructors for young men, and engaged nurses for students living in residence.[1] Such health provisions might not only reassure parents about sending their children to a residential college, but also alert them to the progressive nature of the institution. After all, parents wanted to ensure that their children would be not only physically and morally safe, but also improved through access to the most progressive education, and educational facilities, possible.

Those services, however, were not universal and, even where implemented, tended to be limited in nature. Their aim was to attract and retain students as much as to ensure student health. By the 1930s and 1940s, however, many universities provided some type of health service, and required a physical examination and physical training. Moreover, at least some educators had come to perceive bodily health to be a crucial component in the role of the university in shaping students' character. This chapter examines the reasons why physical examinations and physical culture gained an increasing foothold on Canadian campuses; it also delineates the nature of that process.

Creating Health Programs

Concern about female student health began to intensify in the late nine-teenth century. As women gained entrance to institutions of higher edu-cation, they faced a barrage of criticism about their physical and mental capacity to study, as well as about the effects of this education, especially on their reproductive functions. In Britain and North America, oppo-nents of women's education argued that mental strain led to nervous disorders and reproductive failure, as energy was drawn from the repro-ductive system to the brain. Proponents argued that supervised physical activity would counter this problem by maintaining a proper balance between physical and mental exertion. The arguments of the opponents proved forceful enough that administrators in American women's col-leges quickly turned to programs in physical culture, often overseen by female physicians, as a means to protect women's health and defend women's access to higher education.[2]

Anxieties about women's ability to combine intense study with good health in general, and reproductive health in particular, remained prominent within Canadian universities in the early decades of the century. A 1909–10 resolution by the committee of management of the women's residence at Victoria College, Toronto, stated, "It has been deemed advisable to require henceforth of those entering residence a medical certificate – from the house physician stating that the student is physically able to undertake a prolonged course of study. This has been done in the Royal Victoria College, [McGill University], Montreal, and with good results."[3] Such concerns would continue to circulate within medical discourse well into the 1930s.[4] As a result, many universities built residences for their female students – a home away from home which could provide not just physical shelter and convenience but protection and guidance.[5] Health facilities became a key feature, with many women's residences providing a nurse and small infirmary, access to a doctor, and a dietician to oversee the kitchen. Administrators usu-ally required of students that they either obtain a medical certificate from a family physician prior to admission or present themselves for an on-campus medical examination during the first few weeks of the school term. At some institutions, they also organized classes in phys-ical culture, ranging from a half hour every day to one or two hours a week.[6]

Administrators' concern about student health extended to men, but for different reasons. Educators recognized that male student culture was periodically rowdy and violent and could lead to the destruction of property and personal injury. They worried in particular about men engaged in athletics. By the end of the nineteenth century, American universities had become important sites in the development of athletic facilities and the growth of team sports. Yet the excessiveness of American college sport, particularly the game of football, dismayed many university authorities, faculty members, and alumnae. In the early years of the twentieth century, some faculty and administrators voiced strong concerns about the brutality of football, which had led to athletic injuries and even a number of deaths; its elevation above the academic purposes of the university; and its increasing commercialism.[7]

Canadian educators and students alike worried about this American influence on their own institutions.[8] In the midst of the American furor over athletics, administrators at the University of Toronto re-examined their own policy regarding athletes. In 1906, the university underwent a process of institutional reform, aimed primarily at administrative reorganization. By coincidence, during that year two rugby players died, one of whom had a pre-existing condition and whose death, authorities subsequently came to believe, could have been avoided if the student had had a medical exam and been prevented from playing. This, along with the leadership of the Rev. D. Bruce Macdonald, chairman of the board of governors and a strong supporter of college athletics, led reformers to include in their recommendations regarding general university reforms a proposal for the appointment of a physical director who held an M.D. and who could undertake medical examinations and prescribe proper exercise. As a result of the recommendation, university administrators created the position of physical director in 1907, at which point medical examinations became compulsory for male students engaged in athletics. The university appointed a medical examiner for female athletes in 1912.[9]

Concern for male athletes was not limited to the University of Toronto. McGill, vying for athletic bragging rights over Toronto, was equally concerned about its athletes. Indeed, it hired a physical director for male students in 1858 and one for women in 1889. In hiring R. Tait McKenzie in the 1890s, the university early on committed itself to employing an instructor in gymnastics who also had medical training. By 1911–12, administrators had instituted a physical exam not just for athletes but for all entering students. By 1921, it had consolidated all activity in the School of Physical Education, under the directorship of A.S. Lamb, who would become a leader in national and international amateur sport.[10]

Similarly, Queen's University, with its own strong athletic tradition, established compulsory physical education and medical examinations for first-year students in 1912.[11]

The onset of the First World War reinforced concerns about the fitness of youth. Students and faculty at the University of Toronto, for example, raised alarm over reports about the significant number of unfit young Canadian men and argued that the war demonstrated the need to maintain a healthy male citizenry.[12] A number of universities instituted military training for men. At the University of Toronto, McGill University, and the University of British Columbia, this was accompanied by compulsory medical exams which determined the fitness of men for military drill and relegated the unfit to physical training.[13] Some institutions also created voluntary programs for women, while a few instituted compulsory service.[14] Universities such as Toronto, Western Ontario, McGill, and Acadia, which established compulsory programs in military drill or physical training during the war, continued with compulsory physical education programs at war's end – some for only a few years but others for many decades.[15]

During the interwar years, other institutions began to require similar programs. Administrative records provide little clue as to why they did so. Certainly, by the 1920s, there was a clear trend in leading North American universities towards such programs. Canadian administrators' concerns about student health also formed part of a broader transatlantic dialogue. In Britain, anxieties over student fitness and health ignited during the interwar years in relation to the country's civic universities. After the First World War, the government established a University Grants Committee (UGC) in order to funnel state aid more effectively to British universities. That committee raised concerns about facilities for students, particularly to accommodate the growing number of poorer students, and about the intellectual, moral, and physical fitness of these students to take up their role as citizens.[16] In the 1930s, the UGC provided funding for gymnasiums and pools, while a number of universities set up health centres and insurance schemes. Yet anxieties about student health continued, with the Social and Preventive Medicine Committee of the Royal College of Physicians advocating compulsory medical exams and supervision in 1946, and the Institute of Social Medicine at Oxford University undertaking several student health surveys in the immediate post-war period.[17] Concern was also raised during this period at several meetings of the Congress of the Universities of the British Empire. A handful of Canadian administrators and physical educators took part in those conferences. Representatives from Toronto and McGill provided details of their programs and the rationales behind them. Administrators from other universities returned home enthusiastic about such programs. For example, in 1936, President Carleton Stanley of Dalhousie University acted as chairman of the session on "Physical Education in the Universities" at that year's congress. A year later, that institution established a compulsory program.

Though the reasons behind their implementation remain obscure, there can be no doubt that health and physical training programs appeared at various institutions. For example, by at least 1920, the University of Saskatchewan required students to engage in physical exercise; a daily medical clinic was established by 1928, and a physical examination was instituted in 1938. McMaster instituted compulsory gymnasium classes for women in the early 1920s and both physical education classes and a physical examination for all first- and second-year students in 1930–1. By 1924–5, administrators at Dalhousie required students to submit to a medical exam by the staff of the university's public health clinic. In 1931–2, they established the Dalhousie Students' Health Service. Physical training became compulsory there in 1937–8. Similar provisions developed elsewhere.[18]

The Second World War brought renewed concerns about the fitness of the nation's youth.[19] In September 1940, university administrators, meeting at the National Council of Canadian Universities, overwhelmingly agreed to comply with demands from the federal government that military drill be compulsory for all male students.[20] Some administrators also instituted such programs for women.[21] The 1940s and early 1950s witnessed the extension of health programs as well as the establishment of health services on those campuses where they did not already exist. Although the University of Alberta had instituted compulsory military training and established a medical services fund during the First World War, by 1918 only the latter remained in place. Administrators reinstituted compulsory training during the Second World War, along with a compulsory medical exam for all new students; both of these remained in place for new students after the war.[22] Prior to the war only first- and second-year students at McGill required a medical examination. By 1945 authorities expected all students to undergo a yearly examination.[23] Health services developed in a similar way at UBC. By 1925, when the university moved to Point Grey Reserve, students received some basic medical attention through the provincial health department. Because the university was established on unorganized territory under the jurisdiction of the provincial government, the provincial health officer appointed a medical health officer for the Reserve. By 1927, the provincial health officer had added a public health nurse, permitting the operation of a permanent office on campus. By at least 1932, new students had to report to the university health service for an examination. During the 1945–6 school year, UBC required all first- and second-year students to participate in a physical activity program for two hours each week.[24] While the University of Manitoba struggled financially to provide equivalent services to those at UBC or the University of Alberta, by 1952 it too required all students entering the university from grade 11 to take one year of physical education.[25]

In the first half of the century, then, administrators at a number of universities instituted physical culture and medical examinations as a compulsory part of university entrance and graduation. The adoption of such programs was often piecemeal, occurring for particular groups such as female residents or athletes, prior to their extension to the whole student body. It depended, too, on institutional finances. Yet by the 1940s and 1950s, a clear pattern had developed whereby administrators recognized the need for, and attempted to implement, some type of physical education and health service program in order to care for the student body.

The Medical Examination

As students made their way to campus each fall, the first aspect of these health programs that they encountered was the medical examination. For most students attending university in the early decades of the century, this would likely have been their first experience with such a process. In the late nineteenth century, medical examinations became incorporated into life insurance policy requirements. They would become part of the selection process for workers by some larger corporations in the early decades of the twentieth century, for parts of the civil service in the Second World War, and for school teachers during the 1940s and 1950s.[26] In these early decades, then, a physical examination was still a relatively new medical procedure for most North Americans.

In universities, medical officers scheduled physical examinations for both male and female students over the course of a few weeks in the early part of the fall term. Students either made appointments for their examinations or simply appeared during hours set by the medical staff. In the first few decades of the twentieth century, the medical officer usually performed all of the examinations, aided only by a nurse. As administrators required compulsory medical examinations for all students, larger staffs became necessary. For example, in the early 1920s, the University of Toronto Health Service required eight to nine physicians, along with a number of specialists, to perform the medical examinations for the male students alone.[27]

As medical staff undertook a greater number of examinations, they found it increasingly difficult to ensure that all students appeared before them in a timely manner. Beginning in the 1920s and 1930s, but continuing into the post-war years, many universities instituted fines and threatened students with suspension if they failed to turn up for their exams. In the late 1940s, for example, university administrators at McGill imposed a fine of five dollars on students who failed to show up at the appointed time and an additional five dollars if they failed to appear by the beginning of November, and thereafter threatened suspension.[28]

The examination itself took anywhere from fifteen to twenty-five minutes. When the medical officer alone performed the bulk of the examination, the time allocated tended to be shorter. Marion Hilliard, the attending physician at Victoria College's women's residence in the 1930s, dedicated fifteen minutes to each student. The health service personnel at Dalhousie University limited the number of examinations to three per hour. At Macdonald College, McGill University, where health officials divided the examination into segments, each woman received more time: ten minutes for weight and measurement, five minutes for examination by a college physician, and ten minutes for a consultation with a staff member.[29]

Medical officers attempted to maintain a sense of decorum for female students. While in the 1920s, male students at Toronto appeared before the examining physician completely nude, women did not. In 1923, Dr Edith Gordon, the medical adviser for female students at the University of Toronto wrote to the president of the university, Robert Falconer, that during the examination "the student is asked to remove all clothing and to put on a one piece examination robe. This preserves the sense of modesty of the student ..."[30] In the 1930s, Dr Edna Guest described the examination process at Victoria College, University of Toronto. She wrote,

> Miss Phelps has this year, as usual, weighed and measured each of our one hundred and eighty two girls in dressing-gown, vest and bloomers only, and has recorded measurements together with the girls' past illnesses, etc. on

her chart. She has then sent each one in to me with her card, when [*sic*] I
have examined her from head to toe in bloomers only, noting any defects
of posture, of shoulders, of hips, of spine, of feet, etc., her teeth, tonsils,
heart, etc.[31]

It should be noted, however, that although doctors abided by commonly
held notions of female propriety, neither female nor male students
would have experienced any great degree of privacy while standing one
behind the other in various states of undress.

At colleges where administrators had instituted physical training, the
main purposes of the medical exams were to direct students into appropriate exercise programs and to identify those who required special corrective exercises. Beginning at the turn of the century and continuing
into the 1930s, physicians focused on taking a medical history and performing an external examination. As in American universities, medical
examiners also gave significant attention to the study of anthropometry –
the gathering and comparison of measurements of various body parts.[32]
In 1895, the physical director at McGill University, R. Tait McKenzie,
drew up the first medical examination card. McKenzie emphasized the
importance of recording a brief medical history, listening to the heart
and lungs, and taking extended anthropometric measurements.[33] In the
first two decades of the twentieth century, health officials at the wom-
en's residence at Victoria College filled out two medical cards. The first
included measurements of the neck, waist, hip, calf, upper arm (with
biceps contracted and then relaxed), forearm (with hand closed and
then open), chest (during expansion and then contraction), shoulder
to hip (left side and right side), and weight. The second, titled "Gymnasium Card," provided a medical history highlighting information such
as childhood diseases, later illnesses, current complaints (acute and
chronic), and had room for the medical officer to note any "physical
defects," make general remarks, and recommend any special exercises.
By 1930, these cards had been pared down, though they contained much
of the same information.[34]

Few records exist as to the exact nature of the medical examination.
By the mid-nineteenth century, doctors had access to diagnostic tools
such as the stethoscope, the ophthalmoscope, and the laryngoscope,
and by the end of the century, the thermometer and instruments for
blood pressure. By the very early twentieth century, there were standardized examinations, such as eye and IQ tests, and basic charts, such as
weight-height tables.[35] Prior to the First World War, medical examinations seem to have focused primarily on a visual, external examination.

By the 1920s and 1930s, physicians had also begun to probe for internal disease and abnormalities. In the interwar years, common lab work in small hospitals included "measurements of sugar and urea, the Wasserman test for syphilis, analysis of urine for protein, sugar and ketones, and analysis of gastric fluid."[36] This type of activity was common particularly at larger universities which had the facilities and staff to perform laboratory work, had a connection to a local hospital, or where the medical service formed part of a pre-existing clinic. At Dalhousie University in the early 1930s, for example, the physical included not only testing for blood pressure, sight and hearing, an examination of the throat and teeth, and an examination of the heart and lungs, but also urinalysis.[37] In the 1920s and 1930s, universities also began to require vaccinations against communicable diseases and, by the 1940s, regular testing for tuberculosis.

The purpose of the medical examination was twofold: to prevent contagion and ensure the health of students. In the late nineteenth century, some American universities, particularly elite ones, instituted compulsory medical examinations as part of their admissions process in order to eliminate the unfit.[38] In general, this seems to have been less the case in Canada, where students received their medical examination after admission. Administrators did, however, prevent students found carrying disease from continuing their programs. It was common practice to immediately send a student with active tuberculosis either home or directly to a sanatorium. Unvaccinated students might also be denied admission. In 1936, for example, authorities at McGill University refused to admit "a conscientious objector to vaccination" until "he complied with the regulation."[39] On occasion, a physician might deem a student to be in too poor health to continue with their studies. In 1929, Edna Guest reported,

> During our examination we found one girl in such poor physical condition that, after much thought and a thorough discussion of the student's health with the Dean, it was decided to recommend that she should not attempt a college course at present. We recommend that the girl be put under the care of a specialist at once, in an effort to restore her to sufficiently good health to help her make a useful, happy citizen of herself. It probably never will be wise for her to attempt a college course.[40]

In some cases, health officials might also alert administrators and faculty to a non-infectious but potentially "problematic" student. The policy at McGill was as follows: "In cases of infectious conditions, in which the student might be a menace, medical opinion should be respected, but in cases involving distraction, e.g., tic, epilepsy, etc., recommendations should be forwarded to the faculty concerned for its decision."[41]

Evidence of refusal of entry to university is, however, rare. Indeed, J.C. Simpson, head of the department of biology and embryology at McGill University, noted to an international audience at the 1926 Congress of the Universities of the British Empire that the compulsory medical occurred after entrance to university, so there is no "feeling on the part of the student that he may be kept out of the University because he is unfit."[42] Much more common was the use of medical examinations to categorize students according to fitness. The medical examiner at the University of Toronto noted in 1908–9 that, after performing over 600 examinations, he had rejected few students as unfit for athletics. He continued, "Quite a number, however, needed proper directing, and quite a number had to take some precautionary measures."[43]

During the First World War, medical officers' ratings of students, particularly those of men, often followed general military categorizations. At Toronto in 1919, the physical director graded students as fit for frontline service; fit for secondary service, such as in the army medical or service corps; fit only for service at home; or unfit for service.[44] After the war, physicians at Toronto and McGill used slightly modified categories: "A. Fit for all forms of physical exercise, B. Fit for a limited number of forms, C. Fit for Gymnasium work only, D. Fit for remedial Gymnasium work, or temporarily unfit, E. Unfit for any form of physical exercise." The latter system remained in place at Toronto well into the 1950s.[45]

Care during the Year

After the initial examination, students' access to a medical officer differed according to institution. Physicians might keep tabs on individual students about whom they were particularly concerned. Of her work at Victoria College in the early 1930s, Dr Guest wrote, "We are trying to have a clinic each week to check up on those students who are not up to standard either generally, or in some one field. The different types which will return are in the following grouping – (1) heart conditions (2) menstrual disorders (3) students that are underweight (4) those who have shown some maladjustment, such as insomnia."[46] Guest also provided the dean of women with a special list of students who required additional surveillance.[47] Similarly, the 1931 minutes of the McGill Committee on Health Service noted that they provided students whose weight ranged 10 per cent below or 15 per cent above normal with charts on which to record their monthly weight. The students then had to periodically report back to the health service.[48]

In addition to follow-up practices, sometimes students also had access to a physician if they became ill. This tended to be particularly true for students in residence. Yet some university health services also provided this service. At McGill, the university physician held a clinic each weekday which provided general practitioner's services. Unlike at other institutions, the physician also saw sick students in their homes if necessary, averaging two to four visits a week.[49] Similarly, at the University of Alberta a physician was available part time.[50] In general, however, while medical officers did some consultation work and provided some basic first aid, their services did not include major or ongoing treatment.[51] For example, if medical staff at McGill in the early 1920s discovered that a student had a physical abnormality, they then expected the student "to apply to his physician for such remedial measures as his case may require."[52] Similarly, the medical officer at UBC provided some first aid but usually referred students to a family physician.[53]

In at least some cases, this was due to opposition by local doctors to university health services on the grounds that such programs created unfair competition. In the United States, college administrators often encountered anger from local physicians who opposed both the notion that students required their own physicians and the contract practice employed by many colleges.[54] The first attempts, in the early 1930s, by the University of Western Ontario to employ physicians to care for students ran into opposition from local family physicians.[55] In Toronto, administrators sought to avoid angering local doctors by sending city students to be treated by their family physicians. At Victoria College, the university had a policy of allowing the college physician to treat out-of-town residence students who did not have a family physician in Toronto.[56] The University of Toronto health service would not even treat these students, instead directing them to local physicians recommended by the students' family physicians.[57]

Although university physicians often did not provide extensive treatment, many universities did offer some direct care through an infirmary. Because administrators believed female students to be in greater need of medical supervision than men, infirmaries tended to be established first in women's residences. In older colleges, administrators either converted rooms into makeshift infirmaries or, where funding permitted, refurbished an area within the building for this purpose. Residences built slightly later, such as in the 1920s, often included infirmaries in the architectural plans. As a result, the quality of infirmaries differed quite significantly by institution. For example, in the women's residence at Victoria College, built in 1903, the infirmary consisted of two single rooms.[58] As the physician complained, this resulted in an unsuitable situation whereby the nurse often had "to do all the treatments in the corridor during the term" and "take the girls into her own room for a private talk with them."[59] In 1904, the alumnae society of Mount Allison University refurbished the third floor of the Ladies' College as an infirmary, with one main room and two side rooms, one for infectious cases and the other for the nurse.[60] In contrast, at Shirreff Hall, the women's residence at Dalhousie University, built in 1923, the infirmary consisted of one large and two small wards, a nurse's quarters, a diet kitchen, and bathrooms, all contained in a separate wing isolated from the rest of the building.[61] Some residences had no space for an infirmary. In these cases, administrators often purchased or rented a separate building.[62]

Whether infirmaries were housed in a residence or in a separate facility, administrators intended them to be used by students with minor illnesses requiring only a couple of days, or at most a week, of bed care.[63]

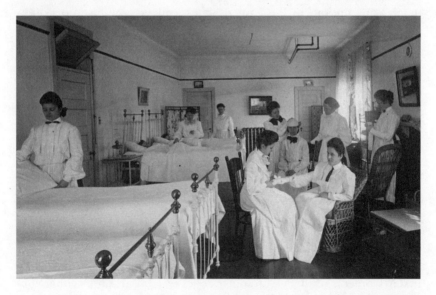

1.1 Mount Allison Ladies' College Hospital, 1909. Mt. Allison University Archives, Ref. 2007.07/332.

Most infirmaries contained only two to four beds and had limited capacity for isolation cases. At institutions such as Toronto, where there was a permanent physician, students gained access to an infirmary after reporting to the physician.[64] At other places, such as the University of Alberta, where there was only a part-time physician, the infirmary acted as a clearing house – where nurses assessed the nature and seriousness of student illness before calling in the physician.[65]

Some institutions provided students with access to not only a physician and infirmary, but also extended services. In the mid-1920s, the Students Representative Council at the University of Saskatchewan created an accident and sickness benefit fund which helped defray the costs of both sports injuries and serious illnesses. Students paid three dollars, and after the first five dollars expended could receive coverage up to one hundred and fifty dollars.[66] More commonly, universities provided a more defined form of hospital coverage. The University of Alberta had one of the earliest and most advanced hospitalization schemes. During the First World War, with the introduction of compulsory military drill and medical examinations, staff at the university set up a medical services fund. The fund allowed students to have free medical treatment in the case of illness or accident, and covered the cost of minor operations, hospitalization for thirty days, hospital charges, nursing care, medicine, and ambulance and physicians' fees.[67]

McGill University helped cover some of the cost of student hospitalization. In 1921, administrators there authorized payment for up to seven days hospitalization. By 1941, they covered "half the public ward rates for hospitalization, out-patient consultants, and laboratory examinations up to a maximum of $125.00 in any one Session."[68] Medical staff referred "special cases" – students faced with financial constraints – to one of the local hospital clinics, where they received consultant services and lab tests at minimal cost.[69] In the 1930s, the department of physical education at the University of Western Ontario covered up to twenty-five dollars' worth of hospital expenses for select cases of students suffering from serious illness.[70] It is unclear when the University of Toronto set up equivalent provisions, but by 1942 its health service paid for diagnostic X-rays, anaesthetists' and surgeons' fees, operating room fees, and the cost of hospitalization at a rate of up to two dollars per day for a maximum of thirty days.[71] In 1947, Dalhousie University provided some hospitalization coverage for five days, including "medical and surgical attendance, medicines, dressings, laboratory tests and x-rays."[72]

Despite these benefits, hospitalization schemes still left many services uncovered. The University of Alberta is a good example here. Despite their extended program, students remained responsible for a number of items: cost beyond a public ward, special nursing, specialist consultations, specialist fees for operations or treatment, operating-room fees, X-ray diagnosis and treatment, and physiotherapy. The fund did not cover pre-existing illnesses, such as chronic or hereditary diseases, or medical conditions that had been left untreated. Nor did it cover accidents or illnesses resulting from what administrators considered irresponsible or immoral behaviour, such as hazing, the contraction of venereal disease, or alcoholism.[73] By the late 1940s, this category included drug addiction and "pregnancy or any condition relating thereto."[74]

Paying for Student Health Programs

Students paid for some of the cost of both health services and physical training, often as part of incidental fees collected with tuition. In the early decades of the twentieth century, students usually paid two dollars towards the medical service. This cost crept up to around four or five dollars in the interwar years. During the 1940s and 1950s, fees ranged from five dollars to eight dollars.[75] Students also paid for some of their own physical training. At the University of Toronto, fees ranged anywhere from two to thirteen dollars, helping to defray the cost of hiring instructors and maintaining facilities.[76] Students also ended up paying for a variety of additional services. In 1941, women at Victoria College not only paid a three-dollar fee for the medical examination, but also an additional fifteen dollars to help cover the cost of providing medical and nursing care. Administrators charged male students using the infirmary, who had already paid seven dollars for access to the attending physician and upkeep of the infirmary, an additional dollar fifty a day to cover meals, laundry, and medication.[77] Similarly, at University College, students who took ill in residence or in their lodging rooms had access to a physician for a fee of one dollar during the day and two dollars at night.[78] In addition, if the physical examination revealed evidence of disease, students might also be required to assume the cost of further tests. For example, in the 1930s, administrators at University College required female students to have an intracutaneous tuberculin skin test. A student who tested positive then had to pay for a chest X-ray, the next step in the process of determining if a student had active tuberculosis.[79]

Student fees never covered everything. For example, universities often provided the capital outlay for establishing and maintaining an infirmary and provided ongoing grants to support nursing services.[80] In addition, administrators often relied quite heavily on the generosity of doctors, specialists, and hospital staff, who donated their time. During her stint as physician at Victoria College in the late 1920s and early 1930s, Edna Guest received five dollars per student for the fall examinations. However, during the rest of the year, she attended to students at the college for free. Guest wrote the dean of women that she did this in part "because I was very interested in seeing – or trying to offer to every girl of Victoria, health education."[81] But she also felt that her arrangements with the residence placed her in an awkward position when it came to demanding payment from students. In 1926 she stated, "It is impossible for me to collect fees privately from the girls for when I go to see one, I end up seeing three – four or five, – probably 2 or 3 of these are not ill enough to charge, but if one is charged all must be charged or there is discontent." In addition, Guest noted, "the nurse is constantly seeking general advice from me for the girls."[82] Despite her complaints, the situation remained much the same in the early 1930s.[83]

Administrators also relied on the voluntary services of individual faculty members who acted as consultants, performed medical and dental examinations, did laboratory work such as urinalysis, read chest X-rays, or attended to athletic injuries. The University of Alberta is a good case in point. Administrators there expected members of the faculties of medicine, dentistry, and pharmacy to take on the task of physical examinations and other related health care functions in addition to their regular duties. When the university initiated its medical services fund in 1915, the medical director, Dr Moshier, a full professor, provided his services free. Several years later, Dr Gray, who ran his own large practice and received a small allowance as a lecturer in surgery at the university, became director without further compensation. In 1918, the fund committee noted that Gray should be given an honorarium. While the fund, created from a yearly two-dollar student fee which was re-invested annually, was "healthy" and such an honorarium could have been paid, the committee noted that no provisions had been made for paying the director when the fund was set up.[84]

This type of activity may well have been seen as a form of war service. The University of Alberta's medical services fund, had, after all, been set up at the beginning of the First World War and formed part of the larger system of compulsory military drill and examination during that period. Yet the problem of remuneration for medical care continued well beyond the war years. By the 1940s, some physicians were expressing discontent over the lack of remuneration for their services. While the University of Alberta now paid the director of medical services and the infirmary physician on a part-time basis, each received only a small honorarium for the physical examinations of first-year students – work which, they argued, in fact required three full days and cut significantly into time allocated to their own private practices.[85] The university medical officer at McGill University complained that his time was "supposed to be divided on the basis of two-fifths for health service, and three-fifths for the Department of Public Health and Preventive Medicine." But he found that, during the college year, that division was reversed.[86]

While administrators often relied on the services of individual physicians or members of their own medical faculty, they also drew on the resources that could be provided by various university departments. The medical adviser of women at the University of Toronto, for example, periodically reported in the 1920s and 1930s that Dr Clara Benson, a senior member of the faculty of household science, provided laboratory space and equipment, making "possible the performing of some simple laboratory tests that were deemed necessary to complete the diagnosis in certain examinations."[87] Staff at Connaught Antitoxin Laboratories ran an immunization clinic for students attending the University of Toronto.[88] In the early 1920s, members of the faculty of dentistry at McGill University provided a dental examination to students undergoing the general medical examination.[89] In that decade, the Dalhousie Public Health Clinic became a de facto health services provider for students. The university paid one of the staff members of the clinic an honorarium to act as director of the service. All the staff carried out the annual physical exams, for which they received a regular fee of two dollars an examination.[90]

Administrators also drew on the resources of university, or local, hospitals. In some cases, university officials relied on reduced fees. In 1904, the examining physician at Victoria College discovered two students with curvature of the spine. She sent the students to a local orthopaedic hospital for treatment in its gymnasium. Normally this work cost twenty-five dollars a month but the attending specialist reduced the fee to ten.[91] In the mid-1930s, at the University of Alberta, administrators made arrangements with the university hospital so that, in order "to meet the average student's financial status," specialists charged minimum fees for examinations in non-emergency cases and operations.[92] In the years after the Second World War, Acadia University provided a significant donation for the erection of Eastern Kings Memorial Hospital on the condition that, if needed, four beds be reserved for students.[93]

Administrators also relied on the services of hospital personnel. Hospital staff helped with general examinations, provided urinalyses, and read chest X-rays.[94] In some cases, hospitals also provided work space. Dr F.C. Bell, general superintendent of the Vancouver General Hospital, allowed university medical officers to perform student examinations in the outpatient rooms at the hospital.[95] At times, disputes arose between hospital and university administrators over whether hospital staff provided such services gratis or whether that work was covered by general university contributions. Administrators of the university hospital at the University of Alberta argued that their staff provided numerous free hours to the care of university students. Hospital personnel complained that doctors, interns, and laboratory workers devoted considerable time to student medical examinations, without payment. By the early 1940s, for example, the hospital laboratory performed over 300 urinalyses a year without remuneration. University administrators, on the other hand, felt that since they already paid one large sum for clinical services, they did not need to pay any additional fees.[96]

In addition to relying on hospital services, from the 1930s through the 1960s, university authorities also drew on some outside funding sources. This was particularly true in the case of tuberculosis testing. In the early 1930s, McGill became one of the first institutions to X-ray large numbers of students, the result of funding provided by a private donor in combination with government contributions.[97] In the 1940s and 1950s, provincial departments of public health took over this work.

Students as Research Subjects

In obtaining funding for health services, physicians and university administrators also relied on the help of faculty whose research intersected with aspects of the student physical examinations. In the 1930s and 1940s, the medical officers at the University of Toronto reported a number of projects which had aided their work. In 1931–2, George Porter, director of the university health service, noted that Professor V. Harding and Dr L. Selby had, in conjunction with their research at the Banting Institute, initiated "special re-examinations of those students having positive sugar tests, thus making the diagnosis of diabetes more definite."[98] In the mid-1930s, Edith Gordon, medical adviser of women, noted that

she had been cooperating with Dr Melville Watson of the department
of gynaecology in his research on dysmenorrhoea.[99] In 1937–8, Gordon
noted that Dr B.L. Guyatt of the department of anatomy "arranged for
a high vitamin and chlorophyll product in sufficient quantities to give
to students whose haemoglobin was 70 per cent or lower, and who were
not, or did not wish to be under treatment elsewhere. More than fifty students were included in this group. Haemoglobin, red cell count, and dif-
ferential count were done monthly on those taking the product." That
year, Helen McMurrich, of the extension department, and Mr. Thomas
Cole, a representative of the Northern Electric Co., approached Gordon
about conducting hearing tests on a number of students. Wishing to promote their hard-of-hearing appliances and audiometers, they conducted
tests and lent their equipment for several years.[100] Some of this work continued into at least the late 1940s. The director of the university health
service, Charles Gossage, noted in 1947–8 that his office had cooperated
with dermatologists in the department of medicine to conduct "research
into the value of special sulphur lotion in the treatment of acne."[101]

Medical officers clearly saw this type of research activity as beneficial
to students. The medical adviser of women noted, for example, that Watson's research on dysmenorrhoea, allowed "a considerable number of
young women ... to avail themselves of certain treatment and supervision
offered by" that department.[102] She also reported that Guyatt's work on
haemoglobin had results that were "gratifying and in a few instances ...
almost spectacular."[103] The director of university health services commented that the work in dermatology was justified on the basis that
"apart from providing clinical research data, this made available to the
students valuable treatment for this troublesome condition."[104]

While administrators initially instituted health services in order to care
for students, physicians and scientists, and even the occasional entre-
preneur, quickly identified such programs as potential sources of cap-
tive research subjects. The provision of health services in the interests
of students thus blurred with the use of students as research subjects.
The introduction of audiometers may have helped the medical adviser
to identify students with hearing problems, but it was also clearly an attempt to sell this product to the university. Similarly, access to student
subjects helped further Watson and Guyatt's work. Indeed, at least some
faculty saw in the student body a means to develop their own faculties
and their individual research. In addition, some used university medical
exams as a means to provide training for their own students. In 1921–2,
the University Health Service at Toronto reported that the "Professor

of Pathological Chemistry had the urinalysis (a very important part of the examination) made for a large number by the medical students in his laboratory under his supervision, and he also did a large number of them himself."[105] In the early 1960s, the faculty of dentistry at the University of Manitoba had some of its students take on the task of student mouth examinations. In his annual report to the president, the chair of the faculty suggested that "this seemed a worthwhile venture for all concerned and should be continued."[106]

It was not a far step from combining research studies and student health to simply using student health results or student subjects for individual research disconnected from any benefits to the student. In 1936–7, the women's medical advisor at the University of Toronto noted that "Miss Kathleen McMurrich of the department of anatomy made anthropometric measurements on 100 women students in the medical office for a research problem in [sic] centre of gravity."[107] Similarly, in the late 1940s, the director of university health services at Toronto reported that "Dr T.G. Heaton, our physician in charge of tuberculosis, made a study of 'The Etiological Significance of Pulmonary Calcifications at the University of Toronto.'"[108] E.W. McHenry made use of student height and weight data for his broader surveys of Canadians' weight and nutrition.[109] In her reminiscences of graduate studies at Queen's University in the mid-1950s, Barbara Excell Hawgood notes that J.K.N. Jones, a carbohydrate chemist, drew on the available supply of graduate students as subjects for his "research project on the relationship of diet to blood fat levels." Hawgood relates, "I dutifully consumed a liquid diet (chocolate or strawberry flavoured) and at regular intervals presented myself for blood sampling, quite oblivious, in this double blind trial, as to whether I was in the corn oil group in which blood cholesterol was found to be quickly lowered or in the butter fat group in which blood cholesterol was observed to rise sharply."[110]

At least some faculty, then, saw the work of the university health services in the context of the larger research aims of the university, providing students as research subjects and facilitating student training. In the United States, Heather Munro Prescott has found that university researchers regularly recruited students for their own studies, both because they were an easily accessible pool of subjects and because of the belief that their ethnic, class, and educational backgrounds made them a good group from which to develop normative standards.[111] In the Canadian context, it is also clear that medical officers at university health services used faculty research interests to help fund their own departments.

Conclusion

Administrators drew on a variety of sources to help subsidize health programs for students: individual fees, the generosity of individual staff, university laboratories and hospital facilities, and faculty research. Not surprisingly, provisions for health services appeared in piecemeal fashion, according to institutional priorities, traditions, personalities, and finances. As a result, students' access to health facilities was often uneven, both within any given institution and across the country. Women's residences usually had the most extensive provisions, allowing students access to physicians, instructors in physical training, nurses, and dieticians. Male residents and male and female boarders often had less access to facilities. In general, larger urban universities had better overall provisions than smaller ones located in rural settings. Central Canadian and denominational universities were more likely to have developed compulsory physical training and medical examinations in tandem. By the 1940s, however, most universities provided some form of health service and many had compulsory physical training. Moreover, even in those universities which, for one reason or another, could not establish a health service, administrators advocated its need. That fact alone illuminates the way in which administrators and educators had come to perceive health as key to students' success and thus as an important service that should be provided by their institutions.

2
Ailments and Epidemics

University administrators supported the creation of health services at least in part to deal with the huge range of ailments that affected students on a yearly basis. A list of women's medical absences from class, kept by the warden at McGill's Royal Victoria College in the mid-1930s, is particularly illustrative of the variety and consistency of disease that appeared in residential institutions. Women most commonly absented themselves because of colds, influenza, and illness resulting from menstruation. Yet they also contracted diseases such as German measles, rheumatic fever, mumps, and chickenpox. They developed ear and eye trouble, infected teeth, blocked sinuses, indigestion, jaundice, and skin infections. And they suffered from various sprains, bone fractures, and breaks.[1] Administrators and medical staff at Royal Victoria College, as at other institutions, thus contended with both numerous common ailments and communicable diseases.

While ailments caused concern, communicable disease could threaten the functioning, if not existence, of the institution. The presence of such disease on campus was almost constant. At Victoria College, University of Toronto, for example, there was a case of typhoid fever in 1906, a diphtheria outbreak in 1911, a case of tuberculosis in 1912 and of diphtheria in 1915, influenza outbreaks from 1918 to 1920, a case of scarlet fever in 1918, tuberculosis in 1921, and scarlet fever again in 1923, a smallpox outbreak in 1927, a case of diphtheria in 1928, of typhoid fever in 1935–6, of diphtheria in 1937, and of scarlet fever in 1941. Students also periodically contracted measles and mumps.[2] Often one institution had to deal with a number of different communicable diseases in a given year. For example, in 1928–9 the nurse at the University of Alberta noted ten cases of scarlet fever, seven cases of German measles, and one case of mumps. And in 1947–8, the health service reported five cases of chickenpox, twenty-one of influenza, five of mononucleosis, two of mumps, two of rubella, and two of whooping cough.[3] Moreover, periodically these diseases also became epidemic. The 1911–12 diphtheria outbreak at Victoria College resulted in illness among sixteen students and staff. In the 1935–6 school year, German measles struck numerous students across the country: fourteen at Royal Victoria College, eighty-six at UBC, and ninety-one at the University of Alberta.[4] And of course significant numbers of students and staff at all institutions became ill as a result of the influenza epidemic of 1918–19 and the Asiatic flu in 1957.

Without vaccines, antibiotics, tetanus shots, and other medicines, even relatively common problems could become serious. Flu could turn into a fatal case of pneumonia. Sores could fester and infections spread unchecked. A toothache resulting from an abscess could lead to septicaemia and death. Acute appendicitis could result in a ruptured appendix leading to hospitalization or worse.[5] While the germ theory of disease became widespread in the late nineteenth century, the new field of bacteriology produced few immediate cures or treatments.[6] Diseases such as diphtheria, scarlet fever, and measles regularly swept through communities, resulting in high mortality rates, particularly among children and infants. A vaccine became available for both of the first two diseases in the mid-1920s but not until 1944 for the latter. A tetanus antitoxin was developed in 1904 for prophylactic use, but immunization against tetanus became widely available, at least in the United States, only after 1933. Tuberculosis remained a leading cause of death for young men and women until the discovery, in the late 1930s and early 1940s, of various chemotherapies such as sulfa compounds, penicillin, and antibiotics. Only then could physicians treat bacterial infections.[7]

Unfortunately, no run of records listing the diseases or ailments contracted by students over the course of numerous decades seems to exist at any one institution. Indeed, records tend to report only the most frequent illnesses in a given year or extraordinary cases. Thus it is difficult to track either persistence or change in disease at any one institution or commonalities across institutions. However, records do provide a sense of the variety of diseases found on campus and the kinds of personnel and facilities needed to address common student ailments. Information is also available on institutional reaction to contagious diseases, particularly in epidemic form. This is partly because of the paper trail left by university administrators attempting to contain epidemics and partly because it is easier to find public records, in student or local newspapers, of these events. This chapter will briefly examine the types of common ailments on campus. It then focuses on contagious diseases in order to illuminate their impact on residential institutions.

Ailments

From the records that do exist, it is clear that students suffered from a wide variety of illnesses. Within residences, administrators hired nurses and set up infirmaries in order to treat the most common problems: colds, flus, cramps, pains, and sprains. In 1936–7, for example, the physician at Victoria College noted, "the winter's work has been steady, with a constant stream of coughs, colds and influenza. Early in the year a mild head cold went through the residences. In December an intestinal upset affected about 15 girls and was troublesome but not serious ... In February, influenza of two types was prevalent."[8] In addition to colds and flu, college nurses treated minor ailments such as infected cuts, poison ivy, acute indigestion, sprained ankles, boils, and abscesses.[9]

Campus physicians and nurses also engaged in some preventative work. During medical examinations, physicians identified those students whom they believed might injure themselves by engaging in vigorous activity. In 1923, J.J.R. Macleod, head of physiology at the University of Toronto, impressed upon his president, Robert Falconer, the importance of the work of the medical examiner, George Porter. Macleod wrote,

> The examination which is given under his direction for the health of students is not a perfunctory examination but is one, as his statistics show, which is bound to reveal serious symptoms or abnormalities in all of the students examined. The fact that several of these each year include serious cardiac lesions, renal trouble, tuberculosis, hernia and high blood pressure show how important it is. It seems to me that without this that some students would suffer serious accidents, perhaps resulting in death, from being compelled to do physical exercise when they were not medically fit to do it.[10]

Physicians and directors of physical training also justified the implementation of medical examinations as a potential means of discovering an underlying, but previously undetected, disease, possibly saving a student's life. In 1926, R. Tait McKenzie spoke at the Congress of the Universities of the British Empire on the purpose of university medical examinations. One of the first physical training instructors at McGill University in the late nineteenth century and by the 1920s a leader in physical education in the United States, McKenzie noted that the aim of an examination was "to discover those handicaps or weaknesses or defects which are likely to interfere with the successful career of the student while at College and afterwards." Regarding the examination of students' lungs, McKenzie noted, "many a student comes to College with the incipient symptoms of tuberculosis or on the border-line of it, and, undertaking a very heavy course, he may do one of two things. He may take on too much work so as to run himself down, or he may engage in heavy athletic sports under the impression that it will do him good, and in this way will still further accelerate the progress of the disease."[11] Ten years later, H.J. Cody, president of the University of Toronto, addressed the same congress. In a session on "Physical Education in the Universities," Cody argued,

> It is possible for a student to come to a University and to be in the grip of some obscure disease of which he has no knowledge. Under this system of examination the existence of that disease is discovered in his first year, and his life is probably saved. Further, by calling in the aid of the psychiatric experts the medical director is able to make deductions as to the mental state of particular men; and very frequently these are raised from depression to good health in a way which could not be possible but for a compulsory medical examination.[12]

Medical examinations also allowed physicians to discover serious medical conditions at an early stage. The 1908–9 report of the physical director at the University of Toronto noted "two cases where the examination came at the most opportune times." Physicians discovered one student with "an abscess of the appendix" and another with a "hernia problem." Both students required operations.[13] Similarly, records at Victoria College indicate that over the years a number of students living in the women's residence suffered from appendicitis.[14]

The medical examination also allowed physicians to identify less serious issues that they felt could be rectified. Not surprisingly, given the amount of time students spent studying, many had previously undiagnosed eye "defects." If a physician detected a possible sight problem, he or she often recommended that the student have a second, more detailed eye exam or referred the student to a specialist. Physicians also noted such things as teeth that needed attention, nutritional deficiencies, and other ailments that could be readily treated.[15]

At places that linked medical examinations to physical training, physicians focused significant attention on students they believed to be in

need of remedial work. They regularly reported a number of "abnormalities." In 1934–5 the medical examiner at UBC noted an increase of
round shoulders in male students, an issue he attributed to the lack of
military training in schools.[16] The director of health services at the University of Toronto also complained about men's "round shoulders, flat
feet and spinal curvature."[17] Physicians made similar comments about female students. While in 1924 the medical adviser at the University of Toronto proclaimed co-eds at that institution to be "of Splendid type," she
also warned of the too numerous problems related to poor posture such
as "low shoulders, drooping heads, weak ankles."[18] In the 1920s, Edna
Guest, the medical examiner at Victoria College, lamented the number of students with uneven shoulders or hips or some spinal curvature
such as "functional Kyphosis."[19] Her successor, Marion Hilliard, noted in
1935, "all types of abnormality – scoliosis, kyphosis, protuberant abdo-
men, flat feet, etc."[20] Some of the concern about posture was quite serious. On occasion, physicians discovered cases of serious curvature of the
spine, requiring the referral of students to an orthopaedic hospital.[21] Yet
most of the diagnoses required less intervention, with students assigned
remedial exercises under the supervision of a gymnasium instructor.[22]

This type of general physical examination of students formed part of
the broader aims of the school health reform movement. By the 1920s,
many school districts had begun to institute physical examinations of
school children. The Committee on Students' Health in the faculty of
medicine at the University of Toronto recorded that routine physical
exams of 20,000 children in Toronto public schools in 1920 revealed
that 9,400 children were suffering from physical defects, 90 per cent of
which could be remedied when detected early and 3 per cent of which
required continued supervision.[23] Yet, the committee noted, this type of
work remained limited.[24] University health officers used the failure to
implement full medical inspection of schools and schoolchildren to justify the need for such programs at university. Many perceived university
screening programs as the last site in which to catch, and rectify, young
people's medical problems.

Contracting Communicable Diseases

Identifying physical "abnormalities," rooting out health dangers, and
tending to colds and minor ailments formed much of the annual and daily
work of campus physicians and nurses. This work alone kept health officials busy. The discovery of a student with symptoms of a communicable

disease complicated the work of the medical staff. The appearance of such diseases in epidemic form could seriously affect students and staff and on occasion bring the work of the university to a grinding halt.

Students contracted communicable diseases in a variety of ways. Some became infected at home and brought disease back to residence. For example, on Sunday, 18 October 1927, a first-year student returned to his residence room at Victoria College after having spent the weekend at home in a small town just north of Toronto. Although he had been sick at home, it was not until the day after he returned to residence that officials discovered he had contracted smallpox.[25] Similarly, in 1937–8, the dean of women at the University of Manitoba recorded that two cases – one of chickenpox and one of scarlet fever – had both been contracted at home.[26]

Students could also become infected while out at work. In March 1916, Marion Clark, the nurse at Victoria College, reported that "one of our Faculty [of Education] students went to supply [teach] in Belmont and found the school full of mumps. Out of a staff of four the principal [was] the only one on duty. I consulted a physician and he strongly advised her not being allowed to return to the hall for two weeks." The student moved in with a sister who lived in the city.[27]

Students were not the only ones responsible for the spread of diseases. In 1911–12, a waitress in the women's dining room at Victoria College contracted diphtheria, passing it on to three staff members, ten students, and three maids. Similarly, in 1937, administrators discovered one of the temporary maids to be a diphtheria carrier. She had not infected any students but was immediately sent to the isolation hospital.[28] Diphtheria was not the only disease brought in by staff. In February 1918, the dean of women recorded, "a mild case of scarlet fever had developed in the Hall, one of the maids having taken it. She had been removed immediately to the Isolation Hospital, and all precautions had been taken under the direction of the Health authorities. Over 2 weeks have elapsed and no other cases have developed."[29]

At times, diseases simply swept through whole communities. This is most evident in the case of influenza in 1918–19. Influenza first spread among troops and from there into the civilian population. It generally spread from east to west along communication lines and then from urban centres into more remote regions.[30] It occurred in three waves: a mild attack in the spring and summer of 1918; a virulent wave in the fall of 1918; and a less severe wave early in 1919. The influenza pandemic was unique at the time because it affected young adults the hardest. The global mortality rate is now estimated to have ranged between 50 and 100 million people, while that in Canada was about 50,000.[31] As in many other regions, it was the second wave, in October 1918, which severely hit Canadian universities. At Victoria College, for example, roughly 30 per cent of male residents and 45 per cent of women contracted influenza to some degree.[32] These rates of infection accord with similar patterns across Canada.[33]

But influenza was not the only disease that swept through Canadian communities and onto university campuses. In 1934–5, the Toronto University Health Service reported many cases of "measles which was so widely spread throughout the city."[34] In 1935–6, the University of Alberta experienced an outbreak of German measles, part of a larger, city-wide phenomenon.[35] In 1941–2, the director of the health service at UBC noted in his report to the president, his worry about "the increased incidence of Scarlet Fever in the Vancouver Metropolitan Area."[36] His fears proved unfounded, with only four students affected. UBC fared less well in 1957 when Asiatic influenza made inroads on campus, affecting 550 students.[37] Other institutions did little better. Asiatic influenza affected nearly 60 per cent of the student population at Acadia University, hundreds of students at the University of Toronto, 250 male students at Mount Allison University, and eighty students at McMaster University.[38]

Students who contracted a communicable disease risked passing it on to their room-mates and classmates. In the case of smallpox at Victoria College in 1927, the infected student passed the disease on to six of his housemates. Similarly, in November 1921 the dean of women at Victoria reported that one student was discovered "with an active tuberculosis of the lung which was just coming into the infective stage – and I feel we gave her, her only hope of cure, by its early discovery – and as she was not in a room by herself you may easily imagine what we saved her room-mate, and immediate friends – not to mention those who should have used dishes after her at table."[39] In 1929–30, a student at UBC contracted diphtheria and then unknowingly exposed numerous other students to it. Just over ten years later, UBC experienced a mumps epidemic, concentrated among second-year applied science students.[40]

Surveillance and Treatment of Communicable Diseases

The yearly appearance of communicable diseases led administrators to maintain a high degree of vigilance. Within school districts, teachers and school and public health nurses maintained a system of surveillance by identifying infected children, inspecting their playmates and siblings for contagion, and isolating the sick.[41] University administrators followed a similar routine. At Victoria College, for example, when the dean of women suspected anything unusual she immediately isolated the patient in the infirmary. If the case was mild – consisting, for example, of regular measles or mumps – the student usually remained in the infirmary to recover. Once a patient was released, the infirmary would be fumigated by the health department to ensure the safety of future patients.[42]

In more serious cases, administrators attempted to move the student to an isolation hospital.[43] On occasion, this proved impossible due to lack of space for infected students in local hospitals. In these cases, the patient generally remained in the infirmary. For example, in December 1915 a Victoria College student who had been moved to the infirmary developed measles. The nurse reported that "the physician strongly advised her being taken to Mrs. Macpherson's private hospital where only measles are taken but as there was not a vacant room at the time we have kept her in the infirmary which will be thoroughly fumigated as soon as it is vacated."[44] Nor were university health officials always happy with the solution of sending students to the isolation hospital, even when beds were available. In 1923, one Victoria College student who had contracted German measles was sent to the isolation hospital, where she then became infected with scarlet fever. Edna Guest, the college physician, reported to the residence management committee, "After this upsetting episode, we decided to try to isolate simple cases such as German measles and mumps in room 43A. This proved satisfactory for the cases that followed. Miss Stephenson, who is a graduate nurse, was very happy to look after the patients for three dollars a day and the girls were responsible for the fee."[45]

If administrators sometimes found it difficult to find individual students a place in an isolation hospital, doing so for a group of infected students often proved impossible. In these cases, they attempted to quarantine the sick within a wing of the residence. In 1904, administrators at the Macdonald Institute in Guelph faced two outbreaks of smallpox, resorting to quarantine in both cases.[46] During the 1911–12 diphtheria outbreak at Victoria College, which affected ten students, or nearly 10 per cent of residents, officials isolated those infected and hired three trained nurses to disinfect the rooms previously occupied by the patients. Dr Helen MacMurchy, the physician in charge, administered a diphtheria antitoxin.[47] University and health officials placed all residence students under quarantine for a few days, after which they sent all healthy students home. These efforts helped keep the outbreak in check until January, when there was a small recurrence. At that point, the maid who was originally infected fell ill again with diphtheria and was isolated, as was another student who was kept "in the hall infirmary for five weeks."[48] A similar situation occurred during an outbreak of German measles at the University of Alberta in 1935–6 which affected eighty-nine students. The director of medical services noted that "owing to the widespread contagion in the city the Infectious Disease hospital was wholly unable to take care of the epidemic."[49] As a result "the Medical Services were forced to treat their cases in the Infirmary and in a section of St. Joseph's College kindly rented to us for the occasion."[50]

Quarantine was an effective and common solution for known diseases such as diphtheria or smallpox. But administrators and doctors did not necessarily know how to cope with a new contagion. Like their counterparts outside the university, they were often slow to react to the spread of influenza in the fall of 1918. Officials of the University of Alberta initially simply warned students to avoid "places of congregation outside the Campus."[51] At Victoria College, the Women's Literary Society held an opening meeting in early October despite the presence of flu on campus and in the city.[52] During the same period, *The Varsity* noted that the medical examiner for men at the University of Toronto was in the process of performing the yearly medical examination, and "no doubt any incipient case of the 'flu' will be detected there."[53] Despite the editors' confidence in the examiners, the process itself involved a long line of half-naked men crammed together while waiting their turn and thus with ample opportunity to breathe all over each other, unwittingly infecting their classmates. Faced with the increasing spread of the disease among students, staff, and faculty, many university administrators resorted to the only known solution for containing the disease: they eliminated public meetings by cancelling classes.[54]

Impact of Epidemics on College Life

The periodic appearance of communicable diseases can tell us much about the impact of disease on the management of a residential institution and on institutions of higher education more generally. In severe cases, such as during the influenza epidemic, nursing care and convalescence time continued well beyond the epidemic itself. By mid-November 1918, for example, the influenza crisis had eased at Victoria College but the effects continued to be felt. The dean of women wrote, "As the students recovered, but were not able to come downstairs, a small dining-room was set up in one of the rooms and the students set their own table and washed their own dishes as they were able. It gave them occupation. Even after they were able to be downstairs, they had still to take tonics, and were long in recovering strength. Some of them still are easily fatigued, and will not feel really well for some time to come."[55] Thus the strain on staff, and on the institution and its resources, had both immediate and long-term effects.

The impact of these diseases was, of course, felt most significantly by the students affected. Most recovered from their illnesses but lost some portion of their school year. During the 1911–12 diphtheria outbreak at Victoria College, sixty-seven female residents could not write their December examinations due to the quarantine.[56] Similarly, in the spring of 1919, influenza continued to take its toll. Eleven students wrote their examination papers while still in bed.[57] Some students lost half a year or a year of schooling. In April 1916, the nurse wrote, "our student who had measles came back from the hospital on March 29th and has been ill in all 8 weeks since entering, 3 weeks of which she spent at home, 3 weeks in the infirmary, and two in hospital. She hopes to write on most of her examinations and those she fails in will try in fall so she will not lose her year."[58] Other students found they could not continue their education. Students who developed diseases such as tuberculosis and rheumatic fever often left university permanently.[59] And, of course, some students died.[60]

Not only students but staff too contracted communicable diseases. In her study of nursing in twentieth-century Canada, Kathryn McPherson notes the risks nurses in hospitals and sanatoriums faced to their own health.[61] Though such risks were much smaller in a university residential institution, they still existed. During the influenza outbreak, for example, Miss Gregory, the nurse at Victoria College, became ill.[62] Other staff equally fell prey to communicable diseases. In 1907, the instructor in physical culture, Miss Armington, was diagnosed with tuberculosis.[63] An outbreak of influenza in February 1920 left "the janitor, cook, both parlor-maids, two heads of houses, as well as 12 students" ill.[64] Similarly, in 1928 Margaret Addison, the dean of women, contracted diphtheria and spent the spring in an isolation hospital.[65] Staff also suffered from less deadly contagion passed around a residential institution. The dean of women at the University of Manitoba noted in 1936–7 that there were a number of colds and cases of flu. She herself was sick in the fall and had to hire a private nurse.[66]

The appearance of epidemics also took an emotional toll on residence staff. During the 1911–12 diphtheria outbreak at Victoria College, Margaret Addison and the directress of physical education, Emma Scott Raff, neither of whom, incidentally, had any nursing training, had the main responsibility for tending the sick.[67] The reliance on university staff was also a feature of the influenza epidemic. Acquiring trained nurses during the outbreak was a common difficulty across Canada, as indeed elsewhere in the world. The war had depleted the ranks of trained nurses and those remaining were needed in public and military hospitals.[68] At the University of Alberta, authorities turned the basement of Athabasca Hall into an infirmary for thirty, with the "south end for women and the north end for men." The president of the university noted that "the impossibility of securing competent nurses during very much of the time was a matter of intense concern and laid an extremely heavy burden upon Miss Russell, the House Superintendent and her staff."[69] At Annesley Hall, Margaret Addison could initially secure only two partially trained nurses for twenty students. This increased to one trained nurse and three assistants for twenty-five patients. But the residence had lost its cook, so Miss Elliot, the house director, with the help of one of the dons, prepared all the meals.[70] At UBC, the lack of facilities required that university authorities convert the auditorium and adjacent classrooms into temporary hospital wards. Both staff and students assisted with "orderly and nursing duties."[71] Similarly in 1957–8, with the outbreak of Asiatic flu at the University of Toronto, care took place in the residences, with the assistance of residence officials.[72]

Deans of women and other university staff thus often took on the responsibility of caring for the sick, becoming temporary nurses, sickbed companions, and cooks. Women have long been relied upon as caregivers, a role imposed upon them, and seen as intrinsic to their nature, but one which at times they have also taken upon themselves as part of their civic duty.[73] The added burden of such work must not be overlooked. The comments of the dean of women at the University of Manitoba are illustrative. In 1939–40, the university hired a graduate nurse for much of the second term during a flu epidemic. Expressing her gratitude for the provision of the nurse, the dean wrote, "She set me free from the cramping anxiety connected with illness with which I am not especially trained to deal, and also from the physical tie of daily sickroom routine (taking of temperature, signing orders for trays, attending the doctor on his rounds, supplying prescribed medicine, and so on) which in the past had often for long periods prevented my attending to anything outside the Residence."[74]

Despite the negative effects of illness and epidemics, in some cases
students and staff perceived a positive side to the spread of disease. Students, in particular, often embraced school closure. In 1918, at the University of Alberta, administrators decided that the university should be
closed and since there was talk of quarantining, the city students wishing to go home should do so. The provost complained, "I immediately
sent word through the corridors quite expecting that the news would
be received with deep concern by the students for it looked as if our
whole year's work might be brought to an end almost before it had got
properly under way. But if I expected the students to reflect my own
serious concern in this matter I was certainly to be disappointed. With
a display of the utmost gaiety they hurried their belongings into their
hand bags ..."[75] Students at Mount Allison Ladies' College equally en-
joyed the break, at least prior to the onset of the epidemic. With news of
the spread of influenza, university administrators quickly quarantined
students to the college. In the initial days, students held recitals, prom-
enades, and had hikes in the country "to keep strong." Recalling the
nursing aid of instructors, one student wrote that "none of us will ever
forget our kind nurses and the good times we had with them in the hospital."[76] Similarly, in 1927 Mary Dulhanty contracted measles while she
attended Saint Vincent Academy. She was isolated for over two weeks
along with nine other students and recorded in her diary that they "had
a marvelous time." For Dulhanty and her fellow students, convalescence
offered a period of leniency from school restrictions, with students having fun washing their own dishes, putting on plays, and in Dulhanty's
words, making "as much racket as we could."[77]

Impact of Epidemics on Health Provisions

Aside from providing students with a temporary break from school, the
occurrence of outbreaks had some positive long-term effects. Government officials and private agencies often reacted to outbreaks of disease
by expanding and reorganizing their health facilities.[78] On occasion,
university administrators did the same thing. Historian Heather Munro
Prescott notes that after a typhoid epidemic at Cornell University in
1903, in which infirmary services proved insufficient, officials increased
the size of the infirmary, hired more nurses and doctors, and built a diagnostic laboratory, resulting, by World War One, in one of the best health
services in the country.[79] It was owing at least in part to the influenza epidemic that the University of Toronto developed a basic university health

services infrastructure in the 1920s. Other institutions did likewise. In 1925–6, for example, Acadia added to its existing health facilities by purchasing a house to be used for contagious diseases.[80]

Some administrators took lessons from the immediate past, becoming much more alert to the serious consequences of influenza. In 1920, there was a significant amount of flu on the University of Toronto campus. Fearing a recurrence of the epidemic of the previous year, Principal Hutton of University College cancelled all social functions indefinitely.[81] In 1928–9, as a result of the prevalence of influenza among residence students at the University of Alberta, administrators cancelled classes a week before the Christmas vacation.[82] At Victoria College, administrators drew on the lessons of their previous experiences with influenza and diphtheria in order to contend with the 1927 smallpox outbreak. They immediately quarantined students who had been exposed to those infected and cancelled all social activities for the week. The student journal triumphantly declared that, "thanks to these prompt measures, the epidemic was much less severe than the earlier dreadful outbreaks of diphtheria and influenza."[83]

Compulsory vaccination also became a means of controlling the spread of disease. In the early twentieth century, this was still a new procedure that raised significant controversy. Indeed, in 1905 one student, faced with the requirement of revaccination, turned down her acceptance to the Macdonald Institute in Guelph. She noted, "… it is some years since I was vaccinated, and I am *very much* against it. The cases in Galt a short time since resulted in illness worse than small-pox itself."[84] Yet outbreaks forced administrators to act. During the smallpox epidemic of 1885 at McGill, the principal and the heads of various faculties ensured the vaccination of all students.[85] By the time of the Victoria College outbreak in 1927, Ontario had, for some time, made vaccination mandatory in the case of an outbreak. While the city health officer required all Victoria students to obtain vaccinations before returning to lectures, in this case almost 500 University of Toronto students also clamoured at the opportunity to receive a free vaccination. Moreover, as a result of the outbreak, the board of governors decided that all future first-year students would require vaccination prior to registration, a decision which also affected Victoria's incoming students.[86] Administrators praised such programs in the belief that they reduced incidents of contagion. For example, when Vancouver experienced a small outbreak of smallpox in October 1928, the medical examiner attributed the universities' avoidance of the disease to the large number of vaccinated students.[87]

As vaccination became more common for other diseases, administrators and medical officers expanded susceptibility tests and immunization requirements as well as providing free inoculations. For example, in the 1920s, students at the University of Toronto and McGill University needed to be vaccinated against smallpox prior to registration, a requirement extended to students at most universities through the 1930s and 1940s. Beyond that, regulations differed by institution. For example, by 1941 the University of Alberta expected students to be immunized against typhoid, scarlet fever, diphtheria, and, with the creation of the new BCG vaccine, against tuberculosis. In addition, Alberta's medical officers performed a Schick test to determine susceptibility to diphtheria, and a Wassermann test to detect the presence of syphilis. At Dalhousie, medical staff performed a Dick test to determine susceptibility to scarlet fever, as well as Schick and Wassermann tests. Queen's provided immunization for typhoid and performed Schick and Dick tests. Toronto performed these tests only if they believed them to be necessary. Staff at McGill provided the Wassermann test on demand. By 1945 the medical exam at the University of Montreal included a Wassermann test.[88] Health services also began to pay attention to new threats. As a result of the prevalence of acute poliomyelitis and an epidemic of encephalitis in the prairie provinces and parts of British Columbia in the summer of 1941, students arriving at UBC in the fall of that year had to report to the health office.[89] In addition, by the end of the Second World War, many institutions had begun to regularly test new students for tuberculosis.

The silver lining of the outbreaks, then, was that administrators often paid greater attention to student health. Many students gained at least some access to nurses, physicians, basic medical treatment, vaccinations, and early screening programs. Students' ill health, and particularly epidemics, drew administrators' attention to the need to address not only students' intellectual, but also their physical, development.

Class Understandings of Disease

As administrators articulated their concerns about student health, however, they also revealed, both directly and indirectly, beliefs common to their own class and ethnic position about sites of contagion and carriers of disease. The vision of the university as healthy was at times juxtaposed against depictions of local communities as diseased. This was particularly true in urban centres. The instance in 1916 of the student at Victoria College who came into contact with mumps while substitute teaching in Belmont is a case in point. In her report on the incident, the nurse stated that she hoped in future there would be no need to take in education students in order to fill residence spaces, as many cases of illness, "have been traced directly to infection contracted while teaching in the public schools, especially is this true in the schools situated in the Ward, as that is where many of our contagious diseases are started which become epidemic."[90] The Ward, situated just southeast of the university, was Toronto's slum district, home to many new immigrants. While the nurse's comments pinpointed the infectious nature of all schools, they also highlighted her concerns about the working class in general and the growing immigrant population in the city in particular.

While the nurse's report highlighted fears about students becoming contaminated through contact with groups beyond campus bounds, administrators also worried about the maids, cooks, and janitors employed to maintain and service the institution. Historians have found that despite the bacteriological revolution, public health officials and programs continued to reinforce beliefs about marginal groups such as women, immigrants, or the poor as carriers of disease. Class, gender, and race became intertwining factors which exacerbated fears about the spread of contagion. In particular, medical experts perceived domestics and cooks, usually women and often poor immigrants, as carriers because of the nature of their jobs, which brought them into contact with food and water. Their poverty, which led them to live in neighbourhoods known to be overcrowded and often unsanitary, made them more suspect.[91]

An incident at Mount Allison is illustrative. In the 1930s, the nurse reported an elevated number of sore throats among students. Concerned about this development, she requested that Dr C.L. Glass, the university's medical advisor, A.J. Colpitts, the manager of the institution's farms, and Professor Roy Fraser, head of the department of biology, investigate the situation. According to the report of the president, they "found that the germs of the disease were present in the mouth of the man who was pasteurizing the milk and of many of the maids." The president noted that "this, of course, was to be expected." He recommended, however, "that greater care should be taken in the pasteurization of the milk, especially in the washing of the milk utensils, and recommended that an electric dishwasher be secured for the Residence, and if found satisfactory that such be installed also in the other residences." The president also supported the recommendation "that more general use be made of the steam now in all of the buildings and that instruction in how to avoid contamination and infection be given to those in charge of pasteurization, those who carry the milk and to the maids and others who handle the milk, the food in general, and the dishes."[92]

Administrators' concerns about sanitary conditions in the kitchen focused the blame less on the university's lack of sanitary facilities and more on its staff. At some institutions, concern about the threat posed by staff to students resulted in increased medical surveillance. At Victoria College, for example, administrators attempted to ensure the health of staff members early on through an interview process and, by the 1930s, with medical examinations.[93] Directed primarily towards the surveillance of maids, as the physician noted,

> We examine this group primarily for the safety of the students, and secondly that we may check any condition which may interfere with their work – and finally, for the sake of the woman herself. At the present time we can only be sure that they are not carrying any disease or harmful condition. In the near future we may consider how we may help them to enjoy life more because their flat feet are not so flat and their diet is intelligently chosen.[94]

Similarly, by the 1940s, the university physician at Acadia undertook examinations of custodial and dining-hall staff and, as he reported to the president, "any found physically unfit were dismissed."[95]

Administrators' actions speak volumes to their beliefs about disease as primarily a threat arising from outside the student population. Sometimes, of course, that threat was real. Yet it was also imagined. For example, while the dean of women at Victoria College cited students' practice teaching in the Ward as a danger, there is no evidence that students in fact brought disease into residence as a result of contact with children from that area. Moreover, if staff occasionally posed a threat to students, students were more likely to spread, and contract, disease among those they knew: classmates, roommates, friends, and family members. And, although this was not acknowledged, students equally posed a threat to the well-being of staff.

Conclusion

Concern about disease was a serious issue, and, without doubt, disease was a common and perennial problem. Regular and communicable disease could have a devastating effect on both students and institutions of higher education. It threatened the health of students and staff and devoured university resources. Some students and staff died or were found to have serious health problems. The lack of medical resources meant some fell through the cracks. Deans of women and men, those first accountable for student health, found much of their time devoted to caring for the sick. In cases of epidemics, institutions felt the financial strain resulting from the care of numerous students.

Administrators' need to maintain a functioning institution, their fear of loss of income, their sense of responsibility as *in loco parentis*, all led them to search out means of providing medical services. Though the reasons remain unclear, some diseases such as smallpox, measles, and scarlet fever, were already becoming less prevalent in the nineteenth century. Vaccination would gradually aid in diminishing the presence of contagion. By the 1930s, for example, diphtheria had become relatively uncommon.[96] The invention of penicillin, sulfa drugs, and antibiotics would fundamentally change societal experience and understanding of illness. Yet in the first half of the twentieth century, children and adults had more in common with their forebears than their late-twentieth-century relatives in terms of their susceptibility to, and fear of, disease.

3

Physical Culture and Character Formation

Despite the very real threat posed by disease, evidence suggests that at least in some institutions students seem to have been in remarkably good health. At the University of Toronto, where continuous statistical reports on the overall health of male and female students exist for most of the period from the 1920s to the 1950s, along with more sporadic reports thereafter, medical examiners generally found over 90 per cent of male students and 80 per cent of female students to be in sound physical shape (see Appendix).[1] The few statistics available at other universities suggest a similar trend. Why, then, the concern of administrators and students with creating a variety of medical services and health programs? In the early decades of the twentieth century, the actual presence of disease was but one reason for the establishment of some form of infirmary or health service. Other priorities and concerns also animated the actions of administrators and health experts. This chapter and the next analyse educators' specific health concerns, to try to make sense of university officials' understanding of what constituted "health" and to examine the broad influences shaping their desire to minister to all aspects of the student body.

International Systems of Physical Culture

By the turn of the century physical training had become a key component of administrators' and medical experts' vision of the healthy student body. The physical educators employed in universities drew on a number of systems of physical education that had become prominent by the late nineteenth century. The German system of gymnastics developed by J.C.F. Guts Muths and Ludwig Jahn, and the Swedish version developed by Per Henrik Ling, played foundational roles in the growth and spread of physical training. By the 1890s, these systems had gained hold in England and were taught in female schools of physical training and in private girls' schools. The German system "emphasized strength, and included marching, singing, free exercises to music with wands, dumb bells and clubs and apparatus work on the vaulting horse, ropes, rings, ladders and bars."[2] In the Swedish system, educators discarded handheld weights but employed some light floor equipment such as ladders, bars, and boxes.[3] They focused on "a series of free-standing exercises performed in unison, [which] systematically flexed and extended every muscle group in the body."[4] The Swedish system gained adherents as a method of physical training for young and more delicate bodies such as those of children and women. Ling emphasized the importance of building strength and skill gradually without putting undue strain on the body or creating unwanted physical changes.[5] At the same time, he emphasized the importance of physical exercise as a form of therapeutics – developing a variety of corrective exercises.[6]

At the turn of the century, the Swedish method began to eclipse the German system. In the early years of the twentieth century, Swedish gymnastics became incorporated into the British educational system.[7] Combined with traditional military drill, it formed the core of the courses of the Strathcona Trust Fund that spread throughout Canada in the early decades of the century.[8] In the United States, Ling's system also gained prominence through the work of physician and physical educator Dudley Sargent who drew on it, along with other systems current on the Continent and in the United States, in order to create his own unique method.[9] Sargent employed both light and heavy apparatus such as weights, Indian clubs, dumb-bells, horizontal bars and rings, inclined planes and rowing machines, and he focused on both individual and group work.[10]

Sargent also incorporated the methods of France's François Delsarte into his training program.[11] A vocal and dramatics teacher, Delsarte aimed to improve students' projection and theatrics through the use of specific poses and gestures. Delsarte's methods, along with those of Émile Dalcroze and Rudolf Laban, would reshape ideas about movement in the fields of physical education, modern dance, and theatre. Delsartism became popular in the northeastern United States and the Maritimes, especially among middle-class women and those connected to the Chautauqua adult-education movement.[12]

The northeastern United States, particularly the area in and around Boston, became a particular focal point in the development and teaching of physical culture. In 1879, Sargent was appointed director of Harvard's Hemenway Gymnasium and assistant professor of physical training at Harvard. In 1881, he established the Sargent Normal School of Physical Education in Cambridge, Massachusetts, for women studying at Harvard's women's college, Harvard Annex (later Radcliffe College). He later created a summer school program at Harvard's Hemenway Gymnasium, open to both men and women. In 1889, Mary Hemenway, a Boston philanthropist, founded the Boston Normal School of Gymnastics, headed by Baron Nils Posse, a graduate of the Royal Central Gymnastics Institute in Stockholm, a gymnasium established to promote Ling's methods. The following year, Posse established the Posse Normal School of Physical Education in Boston. Meanwhile, in 1887, the YMCA founded the Physical Department of the International Young Men's Christian Association Training School (later Springfield College) in Springfield, Massachusetts. Headed by Luther Gulick, the school drew on a variety of regimes.[13]

While these schools, and the training methods they focused on, remained influential into the twentieth century, new approaches and sites of practice also gained influence. In the 1920s, the natural method developed at Columbia University gained some adherents. In the 1930s, physical educators became enthusiastic about a system of Danish gymnastics developed by Niels Bukh. Bukh toured Britain, the United States, and Canada in the 1920s, promoting his own version of gymnastics – a system which would gradually become incorporated into the British, and later Canadian, school system.[14]

These international schools and systems of physical culture would have a significant impact on developments in Canada. By the turn of the century, physical educators trained in the German and Swedish methods, as well as those developed by Delsarte, began to find positions in Canadian universities. Some had received their training overseas. For example, Ethel Cartwright, physical director for women at Royal Victoria College, McGill University, from 1906 until 1927, and later head of the department of physical education (women) at the University of Saskatchewan from 1929 to 1943, trained at Chelsea College of Physical Education in England, one of the first institutions in London to offer a specialist course in physical education.[15] That institution focused on German gymnastics, though it included training in Swedish exercises and English military drill.[16] Emma Scott Raff, director of physical culture at Victoria

College from 1902 to 1913 as well as at The School of Expression, later the Margaret Eaton School, from 1900 to 1924, was influenced by the Delsarte method through her training at the Curry School of Expression in Boston and the Gower St. Academy in London, England. She was also familiar with Swedish principles, a central pillar of the program at the Margaret Eaton School.[17] Many of the first instructors in physical education, however, received their training in the United States, at schools in and around Boston, such as the Posse Gymnasium, the Harvard Summer School Program, and especially the Sargent School.[18] In the interwar years, the Margaret Eaton School became a source of qualified instructors, as did universities such as Columbia in the United States and McGill in Canada.[19]

Just as many of the first female physical educators seem to have trained under Sargent, so too did some of the first male physical educators. For example, R. Tait McKenzie, an instructor in gymnastics at McGill in the 1890s and its first medical director from 1901 to 1904, attended the Harvard Summer School program.[20] However, many more received their training at Springfield College in Springfield, Massachusetts. A.S. Lamb, who graduated from the College in 1912, held the position of physical director at McGill University from 1912 until 1921, when he became director of the department of physical education and athletics, a position he held until 1949. William Terry Osborne, physical director at Acadia University from the 1920s until 1946, received his bachelor of physical education from Springfield as did Fred Kelly, who joined the staff in 1927 and later headed the department until 1967. John Howard Crocker, director of physical education at the University of Western Ontario from 1930 to 1949 had extensive practical experience with the YMCA as well as an MA from Springfield.[21] In addition, by the 1930s, Danish gymnastics had begun to filter into university programs. Some instructors received their training in these new methods directly from the source. In 1932–3, for example, W.H. Martin, a member of the gymnasium staff at the University of Toronto voluntarily travelled to Ollerup, Denmark, and took a special course in Danish fundamental gymnastics under Niels Bukh. On his return, he introduced some of this work into the regular gymnastics classes.[22]

The Programs

Given the training of many Canadian educators it is not surprising that they established programs based on European and American systems of physical education. Physical educators at Toronto and McGill's women's residences, who instituted some of the first compulsory programs, drew in particular on these systems. They tended to include a number of common elements: some form of gymnasium work, corrective exercises where necessary, introduction to a variety of games and sports, as well as work in aesthetics and deportment. Gymnastics usually formed the core of the program, though it differed according to the training of the instructors. For example, beginning in 1902, University College engaged for several years a Miss White, who taught "'exercise with dumbbells, wands and Indian clubs.'"[23] At Royal Victoria College at McGill, Ethel Cartwright introduced her students to a form of gymnastics clearly influenced by German methods which used a variety of apparatus and free gymnastics work such as barbell and wand exercises, Indian club swinging, balance beam exercises, horse exercises, and vaulting, as well as squad drill and tactical marching, skipping, running and jumping, and games such as captain ball.[24]

At Victoria College, Emma Scott Raff drew on both the Swedish system and Delsarte's methods. Swedish gymnastics worked well with the limited space of Victoria's basement gymnasium. Students could use light floor apparatus such as boxes and then clear these away for free-standing exercises.[25] Scott Raff drew on Delsarte's system by emphasizing aesthetic movements along with scientific breathing and fundamental principles which included deep breathing, relaxation, extension of muscles, and expansion.[26] She was interested in expression, poise, and movement of the body. As she stated in 1905, "In the work this year, we have laid more stress on freedom of the body than development of muscle. Development has been worked for by expansion and free standing exercises with less use of apparatus, relaxation, and poise of body and individual corrective work."[27]

Whatever form of gymnastics work they used, female physical educators at the University of Toronto and McGill University combined an emphasis on that activity with both dance and sports. For example, students learned a variety of German or Swedish folk dances in order to develop grace and poise.[28] Instructors also introduced them to both individual and team sports. Physical educators in England and the United States commonly combined gymnastics with sports considered appropriately feminine – such as netball, lacrosse, and field hockey – in which they could teach skills and avoid physical contact or aggressive plays.[29] At Victoria College and McGill University, physical instructors exposed students to indoor games such as captain ball, centre ball, basketball, fencing, tennis, and hockey.[30]

Physical educators also focused on improving student posture and carriage. At both Victoria College and McGill University, deans of women and physical instructors emphasized the importance of classes on deportment and proper habits of sitting, standing, walking, studying, and methods of breathing.[31] In 1905, Lelia Davis, medical examiner at Victoria College, noted,

> Some girls, who have had but little previous exercise, or who possess by nature rather weak physical frames, come in with a lax, undeveloped muscular system and a more or less fixed habit of falling into a wrong position of standing or sitting. This, if left uncorrected, is liable to develop into a permanent faulty position. The aim is to strengthen the body generally and develop the muscular system, and to correct the wrong habits which are largely the result of carelessness and physical weakness, by means of suitable exercises and the development of a proper mental conception of normal form and position.[32]

Wartime conditions did not significantly change the emphasis of physical training for women. While universities instituted military drill for men, no equivalent requirement existed for women.[33] After the war, however, more universities began to institute compulsory programs. In general, these new programs mirrored those established in Canada and the United States prior to the war, with gymnastics, folk dancing, and the promotion of posture often taking centre stage. In the 1920s, for example, the University of Western Ontario (UWO) and the University of Saskatchewan offered these elements of physical culture. Similarly, students at Mount St. Bernard College, the female college at St. Francis Xavier University, engaged in "March Tactics, Setting Up Exercises, Folk Dancing, and Formal Gymnastics."[34]

Programs did not, however, remain static. In the 1930s, some places switched from Swedish gymnastics to Danish.[35] Others added to their dance options. In addition to folk dancing, for example, McGill offered interpretive dance, while UWO offered "simple fold and artistic dancing."[36] Physical educators also attempted to expose students to the breadth and variety of activities that had developed since the nineteenth century. At Acadia University, compulsory fall term activities included field hockey, softball, hiking, basketball, and swimming. In the winter, they consisted, for first-year students, of basketball, volleyball, badminton, skiing, dancing (modern, interpretative, square, Virginia reel, waltz variations), and light and Danish gymnastics. Sophomores focused on skiing, badminton, volleyball, dancing (modern and advanced

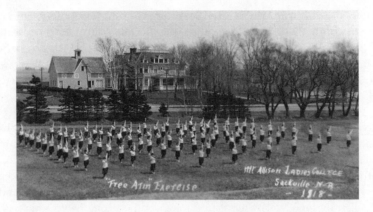

3.1 Mount Allison Ladies' College, "free arm" exercise lawn drill, 1918.
Mt. Allison University Archives, Ref. 8038/2.

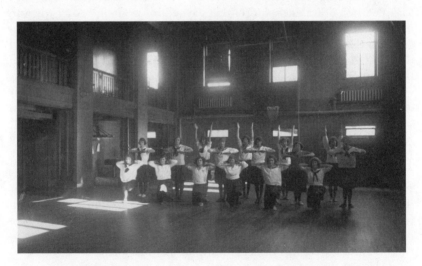

3.2 Girls in gymnasium, Household Science Building, University of Toronto,
1922. University of Toronto Archives, Digital Image 2009–55–8.

techniques), light and some heavy gymnastics, basketball, team game coaching, and safety education.[37]

By the beginning of the First World War, then, at least some institutions had fairly developed women's physical culture programs. The situation for male students was considerably different. Although physical training was not compulsory for most male students prior to the First World War, some institutions did hire physical instructors and provide gymnasium facilities. In this period, the men's voluntary programs tended to parallel those for women, offering gymnasium work, a variety of games and sports, as well as corrective exercises. In the 1880s, men at Dalhousie could take lessons in "club swinging, vaulting, wrestling, fencing and the use of rings and dumbbells."[38] At Mount Allison, instructors trained students in club and dumb-bell drill; work on high, low, and parallel bars; tumbling; and ring work.[39] At McGill, the program consisted of "free exercises, bar-bells and clubs, folk dancing and gymnastic games, with a limited amount of apparatus work"[40] as well as basketball, boxing, fencing, wrestling, and handball.[41] As in the case of female students, instructors provided male students found to be "defective" with exercises for "improvement in carriage and physique."[42]

With the onset of the First World War, some universities instituted compulsory exercises for men in the form of military drill, instruction which, at some institutions, followed the Swedish methods-based course of the Strathcona Trust.[43] Men's compulsory programs became more common in the interwar years. As with those for women, no single program dominated Canadian universities. Indeed, they differed according to developing priorities and, in particular, to the facilities available. Yet there were some commonalities. At most places, men on a university sports team or in the Canadian Officers' Training Corps (COTC) were exempt from physical training while engaged in those activities. Those not exempt from physical training participated in gymnasium work, sports, or games. For example, immediately after the war, UWO established a program focusing on drill, exercises, and outdoor and indoor games.[44] At Toronto, gymnasium work consisted of activities such as Swedish drills, setting-up exercises, boxing, and wrestling. Sports and games included fencing, indoor track, interfaculty rugby, association football, hockey, basketball, indoor baseball, and water polo.[45] At Acadia, men played soccer during the better weather in the fall. In the winter, activities moved indoors with freshmen engaged in "fundamental gymnastics, light gymnastics, heavy gymnastics, individual skills, team games ... and corrective gymnastics where needed" and sophomores in "advanced gymnastics, team games, theory of team games, safety education."[46]

With the outbreak of the Second World War, administrators approved the reformation of COTC units, most of which had become dormant after the First World War, and instituted compulsory military training for physically fit male students either in the COTC or in an auxiliary corp. The National Resources Mobilization Act of 1940 permitted the conscription of young men for home defence. Initially, students who complied with these regulations and continued in good academic standing could remain in their programs until graduation. By 1944, however, the National Selective Service had decided that arts students who placed in the lower half of their class could face conscription for war-related work.[47] Several universities also instituted compulsory training for women.[48] As during the previous war, during the Second World War educators came to worry about the fitness of their students, a concern that continued in the post-war period, particularly with the onset of the Cold War. This was articulated powerfully in the American context, where politicians raised anxieties about the soft bodies of young men unable to combat the communist threat.[49] As a result, universities continued to support compulsory physical education programs. As we saw in chapter 1, several universities that had not previously had such programs instituted them. Others continued on with their programs, often stressing pre-war elements such as folk dancing and the promotion of good posture for women, and gymnastics as well as individual and team sports for both sexes.[50]

The Promotion of Values

During the first half of the twentieth century, then, administrators at most English-Canadian universities not only instituted physical training, but also hired instructors who focused that training around a core set of requirements, including floor exercises, games and sports, and corrective exercises. What were the aims of such programs? The systems employed by physical educators were not simply about physical development. Rather, they promoted specific ideas about morality, spiritual development, and intellectual growth which had particular implications for character formation and gender ideals.

Physical educators drew on training systems that both reflected and reinforced aspects of manhood and womanhood that they hoped to instil in students. They used their beliefs about character formation to argue for, and justify, the creation and expansion of university programs in physical culture in the first four decades of the twentieth century. The physical director of the University of Toronto stated in 1912–13 that gymnasium work "can build a man up physically, and that means morally to a great extent."[51] In 1914–15, administrators at McGill supported physical culture with the aim of creating an "able-bodied manhood" or a "robust and manly type."[52] Similar sentiments held in the decades after the war. In the 1930s, Warren Stevens, athletic director at the University of Toronto, stated in a report to the senate recommending the creation of a school of health and physical education, that athletics provided the means by which to teach "bodily health and fine ideals of conduct."[53] Later in that decade, S.A. Korning, associate professor of physical education at Dalhousie, phrased his aims as "the development of valuable qualities of will and character,"[54] while the director of physical education at Acadia University stated that "besides the physical development, one of the important functions of a department such as this, is to grasp the opportunity of teachable moments in character education at their flood rather than attempting to drive dry theoretical fodder down unwelcome throats."[55]

What did educators mean by *manhood* and *womanhood?* They rarely laid this out explicitly, likely in the assumption that their audience would understand the key characteristics implied. When they did do so, however, they tended to emphasize the values and ideals that had developed around nineteenth-century middle-class amateur sport. Historians have now illuminated those ideals fairly extensively. For men, they included values such as "fair play, physical hardiness, physical and mental well-being, courage, endurance, teamwork, efficiency, self-restraint, innovation, competitiveness, and respect for others."[56] Proponents of amateur sport emphasized individual responsibility and personal development through sublimation of the self in the service of others, and ultimately, of the nation. And service itself became the tangible evidence of one's character, illustrative of such values as charity or honesty.[57] While the ideal of amateur sport was, in its origins, a masculine one, educators came to see games and sports as providing women with qualities such as organization, discipline, respect for authority, determination, self-reliance, self-control, selflessness, teamwork, and service to others.[58]

Physical educators and medical officers in Canadian universities continued to advocate the development of such ideals in the twentieth century. In 1912–13, the physical director at the University of Toronto

‸‸‸‸d that sport taught young men "self-reliance, self-control, un-selfishness, persistence, and a spirit of fair play that makes him his best self."[59] During World War One, the rhetoric on campus often reinforced values such as duty, courage, and sacrifice, twinning these with physical strength and virility.[60] In an article published in 1923 in the Ontario Educational Association's *Yearbook and Proceedings*, A.S. Lamb noted the importance of physical education in developing such qualities as "initiative, leadership, honesty, loyalty, courage, self-control, modesty in victory, fortitude in defeat."[61] In a companion piece, Ethel Cartwright, physical director for women at McGill University, argued that physical education was important for girls and women, as it created "self discipline, self control, self reliance, unselfishness, honesty, loyalty, habits of ready obedience, co-operation, a spirit of service overshadowing a spirit of gain."[62] Similarly, Edith Gordon, medical adviser for women at the University of Toronto, noted that it was important for girls "to learn the rules of the game; to play fair; to co-operate with team mates; to meet defeat or victory with dignity; to have a sense of responsibility; to be unselfish; to maintain self-control under every circumstance."[63]

While physical educators wanted to develop moral character, they also aimed for mental prowess. Much of the rhetoric around physical culture emphasized the interconnection of mind and body. In the first decade of the century, Emma Scott Raff argued that for "this work to be of value [it] must be joyous, a co-ordination of mind and body, without which no real strength or beauty can be evolved."[64] Similarly, F.H. Harvey, the medical director at McGill, believed that the aim was "to secure harmonious development and physical efficiency."[65] This emphasis remained prominent at Toronto and McGill in later years.[66]

The belief in the connection between mind and body evolved from a variety of sources. It was central to the ideas of Ling and Delsarte, who sought to reunite mind and body.[67] Developing his methods in the early nineteenth century, Ling was reacting to what he considered to be an unhealthy emphasis by German physical educators on the isolation and development of individual body parts. Rather, he focused on the flow of the whole body and the creation of coordinated movement.[68] Delsarte, too, believed in balancing mind and body. Decrying the mechanization of the Industrial Revolution, which had led to "'artificiality' in movement patterns of work and leisure," Delsarte instead took up the ideals of romanticism, emphasizing a natural flow in body movement.[69] YMCA leaders equally focused on the mind-body-spirit triad.

In justifying the need for greater expression of the body and freedom of movement, some educators drew on the Victorian enthusiasm for the heritage of Greece. Blaming the public school system for "defects in the youth of our nation," Edith Gordon contrasted the medieval influence on "modern education in its attitude towards the body"– which emphasized a "policy of repression" – with the more favourable Greek model – which accented the individual as possessed of a complex nature, in which each part "required developing and training," and emphasized bodily expression.[70] Similarly, George Porter, the director of the men's health services at the University of Toronto from 1922 to 1941, argued that "physical education should follow the Greek ideal and aim at 'the harmonious development of all the individual faculties' and in the process of body building not only should the muscles be considered but the nerves, the eye, the brain and the heart."[71]

The ideals of manhood and womanhood, however, required more than perfecting mind and body. Many educators believed they could be achieved only through spiritual development, something that itself would be furthered through good health. Rev. D. Bruce Macdonald, a past chairman of the board of governors of the University of Toronto, laid out this position in a 1924 article on the importance of play in the education of children. He explained, "Man is created in the image of God. The body is the temple of the soul, and is consequently worthy of all reverence." Macdonald continued, "There is much truth in the statement that it is easier to be a good Christian when possessed of a good liver. Intellectual processes are keener and more effective when the waste products of the body are being properly eliminated. This acceptable condition of well-being is largely obtained through proper exercise, play, athletic activity ..."[72]

The ideas propagated by physical educators, health experts, and educators concerned about students' physical development built on, and drew from, a rhetoric common among administrators. In the late-nineteenth and early-twentieth centuries, Canadian universities were shaped by the ideal of the university as a moral community. This notion was already being challenged by the gradual growth in emphasis on research, on social scientific methods, and on a culture of utility as evident in the development of professional education. Yet for the moment, the idea of the moral community continued to hold sway. The form and nature of Christianity was, however, undergoing significant change. Reacting to the effects of industrialization, in the late nineteenth century some

Christians began to emphasize the importance of a social Christianity, which supported the need for significant economic reform such as the introduction of fair wages, the right of labour to organize, and the amelioration of living conditions. Only the improvement of individual and social welfare, rather than just the eradication of individual sin, would elevate the human spirit.[73]

The belief in the university as a moral community tended to be stronger in denominational institutions, or those with denominational roots, than in non-denominational institutions and also stronger in universities in central and eastern Canada than in those west of Ontario. Yet, not surprisingly in a still largely Anglo-Saxon country, the ideals and aims of Christianity permeated all these institutions. Within many universities, this translated into an aim to develop intellectually, morally, physically, and spiritually sound citizens.[74]

The Practical Aims of Physical Training

The views of physical educators and medical officers were never systematic. They drew on the language common at the time in progressive circles and among educational theorists, picking from this or that theory to make their case for the role of physical education and medical examinations as necessary for human elevation. Yet they also translated their high ideals – of character formation, unity of mind and body, Christian idealism – into very practical aims of addressing their perceived concerns about the student body.

While physical educators echoed the aims and values of proponents of middle-class amateur sport, they also believed physical training had aims separate from, and superior to, athletics, which made it a crucial component for all levels of schooling. Indeed, they felt that they could reach a far greater number of students through physical training than through athletics. Through such training, physical educators aimed to impart the ideals of manhood and womanhood not to what they considered the few exceptional athletes, but rather to all students.[75] This was a refrain constantly repeated by North American physical educators. No doubt it provided a central justification for the expansion of programs in physical training and the need for more resources. But their belief in the need to reach all students also corresponded to more general views of education as a means of mental, moral, spiritual, and physical development and improvement.

Educators asserted that physical training would increase students' mental prowess by countering the negative effects of a sedentary lifestyle and the stress caused by too much studying. In 1908–9, the physical director of men at the University of Toronto argued the importance of introducing compulsory physical examinations and training in order to reach students who did little else but study and, as a result, left the university in poorer physical condition than when they entered.[76] In 1913–14, the Principal of McGill University warned that many men "are commencing an arduous and exacting course of study under conditions of physical immaturity."[77] A year later, he justified the need for compulsory military drill or physical training on the basis that while the college years were a time for physical improvement, "they are often just the years, especially under the normal conditions of city life, in which the building of the body is neglected by a considerable portion of college students."[78] Female students came under equal scrutiny. In 1906–7 Ethel Cartwright argued for "organised physical work for every body to counteract the harmful effects of too close an application to study, and to build up healthy vigorous bodies and constitutions, to increase by natural methods students' mental capabilities, and so help them to become when leaving, the healthy, vigorous, enthusiastic people Students just through College should be."[79] In a session on "Physical Education in the Universities," at the fifth Quinquennial Congress of the Universities of the British Empire, Professor John Hughes of McGill spoke in particular of the need for medical supervision of female students. Reiterating a belief common at the turn of the century, Hughes argued, "Women students on the whole are more inclined than men students to strain themselves by overwork. (That is my experience, and I have found in conversation with colleagues that they share that view.)"[80]

While administrators scrutinized students' study habits, women came under extra scrutiny for their propensity to oversocialize. In 1903, Margaret Addison, the dean of residence at Victoria College reported to the committee of management that the students were "physical wrecks" in part due to their excessive socializing.[81] Twenty years later, the medical examiner at the University of Toronto, Edith Gordon, argued for the necessity of compulsory examinations and physical training to "protect both the over-zealous student and the social butterfly from the results of their own indiscretion – the girls who come to college exclusively for purposes of education and the girls who come exclusively for purposes of co-education."[82]

If educators aimed to use physical education to shape students' character and counter the ill effects of university life, their ultimate aim was to train students for their role as productive citizens. In the 1920s A. S. Lamb argued that McGill needed to produce "graduates who are physically as well as mentally fitted for their life-work."[83] John Howard Crocker, director of physical education for men at the University of Western Ontario from 1930 to 1947, believed physical education to be central to the progress of the individual and the aims of the university in creating citizens. In the 1931 student yearbook he wrote,

> The University seeks through the education of the mind and body to prepare its students to take their responsibilities as Canadian citizens. A solid foundation of a healthy body and a sound mind must be the corner stones upon which their careers are built and education will only be complete when students have a full conception of their individual responsibilities.[84]

Drawing on the rhetoric of the past thirty years, Warren Stevens, an athletic coach at the University of Toronto, wrote in the magazine *Health* in 1935,

> The late President Theodore Roosevelt summed the matter up correctly when he said in speaking of education for a growing body, "What we have a right to expect from an American boy is that he shall turn out to be a good American man." What part has athletics in this educational process, the aim of which is to develop good citizens? Few people get to know their friends as a football coach knows his players, and one thing he invariably wants to know about a player is, "What happens when he gets bumped?" This is the test of life as well as of the athletic field. Modern athletic contests such as football provide hard bumps, educating knocks, bumps that bring out the best in boys, and show up the worst.[85]

Educators in the early 1940s reiterated this link between athletics, character, and good citizenship. One historian has argued that, concerned about the deterioration of the male body, proponents of physical culture in interwar Britain emphasized "the cultivation of a fit male body as an obligation of citizenship and a patriotic response to the needs of the British Empire."[86] A 1940 memorandum on physical education at McGill stated, "Youth is the period in which habits are formed that will materially affect the health status of our future citizens."[87] Indeed, administrators at that institution pressed upon students the need to engage in physical training as a responsibility to themselves and their country, reminding them that they had "a definite obligation to themselves and to their country to do everything possible for greater physical efficiency."[88] For men, the qualities of manhood would stand them in good stead for the work world ahead of them and for service to the nation, most pressingly, in this period, in the form of military service.

Women's roles, however, were in flux. While higher education was often seen as a means to better train women for their roles as mothers, increasingly voices could be heard emphasizing the importance of education to train women for participation in the workforce and public life – an issue we'll return to in chapter 5. Still, in the early decades of the twentieth century, women continued to marry and most expected to do so. Indeed, a 1938 survey of university students in Canada found that women not only assumed that they would marry but preferred the option of marriage to career.[89] Generally of practical mind, physical educators worked within that reality. Yet, like the physicians of the day, they also conflated women's social position and their biology, believing women's lives and nature to be different from that of men, and thus that men and women required different forms of physical training. Some historians of sport have emphasized the conservative view that medical experts and physical educators held of women's bodies and the limiting impact this had on the development of women's sport.[90] In Canada, conservative voices included prominent physical educators such as A.S. Lamb, Ethel Cartwright, and her successor, Jessie Herriott, all at McGill; Florence Somers, a faculty member at the Margaret Eaton School and later at the School of Physical Education, University of Toronto; and Helen Bryans, at the Ontario College of Education. These educators embraced the "girls' rules" and "play days" movements that developed in the United States. The former arose in the late nineteenth century and spread in the early decades of the twentieth century as a means to limit physical contact and the intensity of competition in women's sport and to keep women's sport under the control of female educators. The latter developed in the 1920s and 1930s as a means of extending female sport to all women, not just the athletically inclined.[91]

The ideas of conservative educators are exemplified in a 1923 article by Ethel Cartwright that appeared in the Ontario Educational Association *Yearbook*. Cartwright wrote, "Girls should be impressed with the fact that Physical Education does not strive to make them men's physical equal, but it aims at perfecting their womanhood."[92] In view of this, she argued, they should engage in moderate exercise that limited jumping and avoid sports and games that could cause strain. She did not oppose competition but discouraged overly strenuous forms, such as running hard for more than a hundred yards. She urged caution in regard to girls' and women's involvement in sports leagues involving strain and travel.[93] Adhering to late-nineteenth-century views of menstrual disability, Cartwright also argued that "during the menstrual period they should not be allowed to compete. It is criminal to run the risk of sacrificing the health of an individual for the sake of a game ..."[94] Such views clearly linked women's abilities to their biology. In addition, Cartwright, like her American colleagues, used the idea of female difference as a means of keeping female physical educators in control of women's sport. Trained women teachers, she argued, should be in charge as "they are in intimate touch with the girls' health and have a wonderful opportunity to teach hygiene and healthful habits ..."[95]

This opposition to intense competition was not held by all. A Toronto group, led by Alexandrine Gibb, a sportswoman and journalist, and that included A.E.M. Parkes, secretary-treasurer of the University of Toronto Women's Athletic Association, supported women's competition.[96] Yet, while real division existed within the women's athletic community, particularly regarding the issue of competition, progressive educators often echoed their more conservative compatriots. Mossie May Waddington Kirkwood, dean of women at University College in the 1920s, and later of St. Hilda's College, was a strong advocate of women engaging in not only sports but also professional careers. Yet in 1923 she argued that to avoid students' becoming overtaxed they should only be allowed to play on either the hockey or basketball team, and that the sport be chosen in consultation with the medical adviser and managers of the teams.[97] Similarly, in the late 1920s, as the debate over competition was heating up, Edith Gordon spoke on the topic of "Physical Examinations and Medical Inspection" at the Women's Building at the Canadian National Exhibition. Gordon was not opposed to women's competition. Indeed, she argued that competition helped develop such qualities as fair play, teamwork, responsibility, and self-control – qualities, she argued, which were "valuable to the individual and the community." Yet she too noted that the "dangers to be avoided were the desire to win at any price, the physical and nervous strain in the formative years, participating in strenuous games without physical examination and sometimes without previous training."[98] Moreover, Gibb, Parkes, and Gordon worked alongside Cartwright to found the Women's Amateur Athletic Federation of Canada in 1926. In keeping with the beliefs and expectations that had developed within women's athletic programs since the nineteenth century, and as a means to assuage fears about women's participation in sport, that body required female athletes, unlike the men involved in the Amateur Athletic Union, to have annual medical examinations.[99]

As Bruce Kidd argues, in many respects both conservative and more progressive physical educators advanced the cause of women's sport simply by promoting women's physical activity. Despite women's newfound freedoms after the First World War, prominent voices continued to oppose aspects of women's athletics. As late as 1929, for example, Dr J.W.S. McCullough, the Ontario provincial government inspector of health, publicly stated, "I don't think it is a good thing for girls to go in for sports generally ... It is all right, perhaps for girls to play tennis, golf and the like but they should not compete in the general sports of men, such as running, jumping, basketball and hockey. It's not the proper thing for girls at all."[100] Similarly, A.S. Lamb continuously worked against the inclusion of women in international competition. Moreover, female athletes often had less access to athletic facilities and financial support and were often denied equal opportunities to compete for athletic awards.[101]

The concern about maintaining young women's femininity became prominent during the Second World War. While several institutions introduced physical training, administrators at others voiced concerns about women engaging in military drill. Historians Nancy Kiefer and Ruth Roach Pierson argue that at the University of Toronto authorities rejected the idea of the creation of a female Canadian Officers' Training Corps, fearing "the implications that military drill and discipline and the donning of a uniform would have for the 'femininity' of the coeds."[102] Such attitudes existed elsewhere. While men at Acadia University engaged in military training, the university provided a course to "Freshmen Girls" that stressed "good posture and mobility" as well as personal hygiene.[103]

Proponents of women's physical culture and athletics, then, had much to overcome. While real differences existed between female physical educators, they also held many beliefs and attitudes in common. To varying degrees, both conservative and progressive proponents of women's sport adhered to a notion of women's difference. Yet they also encouraged women to express themselves physically, to explore the movement of their body, and to attempt new activities. Examining the impact of female physical educators on women's sport in the United States, Martha Verbrugge argues that, generally, they were neither accommodationist nor radical.[104] They emphasized sex difference not only because they believed in the biological difference between men and women, but also because it provided a useful means to argue for equal facilities and for their own positions as educators. Verbrugge writes, "They regarded the female body as disadvantaged, but still trainable; women's skills as limited, yet important; women's sports as tame compared to men's, but challenging in their own right. To female physical educators, sex differences were both enabling and disabling factors in women's lives."[105]

The impact on female students was mixed. On the one hand, women's opportunities to engage in physical culture and in different forms of exercise increased in the first half of the twentieth century. On the other hand, this occurred within bounds considered respectable at the time. Examining the English context, Kathleen McCrone argues that "the very act of 'playing the game' transgressed traditional gender roles and within socially accepted limits, opened up new possibilities for women."[106] Similarly, Anna Lathrop argues that, in promoting physical culture, the educators at the Margaret Eaton School often exposed women to new types of activities and new ways of movement. Yet at the same time, Lathrop notes, many of the exercises did not have the physical component necessary "to build [the] physical strength and cardiovascular endurance" that would have improved students physically.[107] Indeed, in the early years that was often not the intention of physical culture at all. The statement of justification for the physical training program for women at McGill noted that the training was based "on Anatomical and Physiological laws" to produce greatest health and efficiency. It continued, "To this end all undue exertion is avoided, and the work is made as recreational as possible. The exercises are largely of a corrective nature to counteract bad and harmful positions so often assumed during study hours."[108] At McGill, as elsewhere, posture, stature, and comeliness seem to have been valued to a greater extent than physical exertion or endurance.

Both men's and women's activities, then, reflected and reinforced the social and cultural ideas of health experts. Physical educators focused on systems of gymnastics aimed at balancing the body, exercises that developed strength gradually without injury, team sports that reinforced notions of fair play, corrective exercises for poor posture or uneven development, and the encouragement of lifelong participation in exercise and sport. Most importantly, educators believed that both male and female students needed guidance in training their bodies. Their ultimate aim was to create better citizens. Yet the forms of citizenship envisioned for male and female students were significantly gendered. The nineteenth-century notion of women's important role as guardians of the race remained prominent in university administrators' rhetoric into the early decades of the twentieth century. The ultimate sacrifice for male students came through military service. This gendered division of national service was reflected in the types of exercises assigned. Women's activities tended to be much lighter and less demanding than those of men and emphasized little or no physical contact. Men engaged in more strenuous activity, learning skills to strengthen the body and encourage endurance and toughness. Exercises thus reinforced beliefs in natural difference. The physical culture programs also aided the institutional- ization of difference – both in the types of exercise and sport offered to men and women and in the sex segregation of classes. While the latter remained a feature of some academic courses at some institutions into the early twentieth century, physical education programs reinforced that trend well into the post–Second World War period.[109]

Students' Perception of Physical Training

While physical educators' and physicians' beliefs about the positive ben- efits of compulsory physical training abound, students' reactions remain largely hidden from the historical record. The responses that do appear are, not surprisingly, mixed. Some found that they benefitted signifi- cantly from their time in the gymnasium. In 1903, physical educators at Victoria College asked senior students to write down their experiences. One noted, "I did better work when faithful to the gymnasium than at any other time." Another stated that "the Gymnasium work here has taught me the value of systematic exercise to a woman." Edith A. Weekes wrote that "the practice and training I have had in physical culture this winter, has not only benefitted me physically, but the exercises and the precept and example of our teachers have given me a new appreciation of and reverence for the mechanism of my body."[110] Several years later, another student told Scott Raff, "the work in this gymnasium this year has meant for me an increase of physical strength, freedom from severe colds and a greater capacity for work and study than I would have had otherwise."[111] Clearly, these responses, provided to Scott Raff and other residence of- ficials, must be taken with caution. But they indicate that some students found their exposure to physical education useful. Instructors at Victoria often reported enthusiastic responses to the work in the gymnasium and in some cases to the classes on deportment.[112]

However, on occasion, students recorded outright dislike for physical training. In 1921, in a letter to the editor of the University of Toronto student newspaper, *The Varsity*, a male student complained that physical training decreased interest in physical activity. He wrote,

> This morning when we arrived at Hart House we were informed that if we wanted our attendance taken we had to go into the tank. Personally I detest swimming, even though I can swim, therefore, along with a number of others I did not attempt to have my attendance taken ... surely university students are old enough to know what they like and what they don't like and should be allowed to have some say in what they have to do and not be treated like school children.[113]

Phyllis Peterson's experience at McGill in the 1920s was not much better: "My exposure at that time to fencing, gymnasium and aesthetic dancing soured me on anything more strenuous than opening and shutting windows for the rest of my life."[114] Thirty years later, the university physician at the University of Western Ontario complained about the steady stream of students seeking medical certificates to excuse them from physical training for either the whole course, due to disability, or some portion of the course, due to "temporary illness, imaginary or real." The physician went on to state, "The fact that there is this constant demand for medical certificates makes me feel that there is some lack of rapport between the instructors and their classes."[115] Indeed, some students found ingenious ways to avoid exercise. As a student at the University of Toronto in the early 1960s, Archie Campbell, who disliked sport, was able to secure a spot for himself and a friend in a kinesiology research study that allowed them to avoid physical education classes for much of the year.[116]

Such visceral reactions to physical training are rare. Yet it is clear that larger numbers resisted the imposition of physical exercise. Editorials in student newspapers occasionally berated students for failing to use the gymnastics facilities—evidence of a belief on the part of some students in the importance of physical exercise and, equally, of the reluctance on the part of others to use the facilities available. Similarly, in some years, students at Victoria College readily attended physical training classes, while in other years instructors deplored their indifference to the work.[117] This was also frequently a refrain within the voluntary men's program at the University of Toronto prior to the First World War.[118] One way students made their dislike of, or simply disinterest in, these programs known was through absenteeism. Instructors had little sway in the case of voluntary programs.[119] Yet making the programs compulsory did not completely eliminate the problem either. To combat absentee-ism, physical educators could exert moral suasion. In 1906–7 Emma Scott Raff posted the names of residents in her office, and each day students had to register the physical activity they had done.[120] Physical instructors could also report students to a higher authority. At some institutions with compulsory attendance, they sent a list of absent students to the head of those students' respective faculties. This occurred well into the period after the Second World War.[121] Other institutions instituted fines for non-compliance.[122] Yet as the physical director for women at Dalhou-sie University noted several times in the late 1940s and early 1950s, some students simply did not attend as "they know that nothing will happen to them if they do not come."[123]

While some students simply refused to attend classes, other students protested certain aspects of the program. At Victoria College, in 1910, first- and second-year students grumbled about the inequities of the program. Scott Raff noted,

> The work in deportment has not been satisfactory. In the beginning of the season, I started after-dinner lectures on deportment to have such reports as "The Seniors do so-and-so." The Seniors were consulted and asked to cooperate in this work and an outline given of things that we must be care-ful not to do, and of others that we must very carefully observe, as they do in other well-regulated families. With one or two exceptions we have had no help from the Seniors. They are constantly breaking these unwritten rules.[124]

A much different case occurred in the 1930s at Dalhousie University, where students pressured the administration to fire a physical instruc-tor from Sweden who focused on teaching European activities such as handball instead of North American games such as football, basketball, or softball.[125]

Attitudes towards physical training also differed according to access to gym facilities. In the early 1920s, some female students at the University of Toronto advocated the creation of compulsory physical training as a means of gaining access to better athletic facilities. As early as 1913, female supporters of women's athletics had been told that their own op-portunities would increase only after they had done so for men. In 1913, for example Helen MacMurchy, Ivy Coventry, and two undergraduate students met with James Barton, the director of physical education, to

UNIVERSITY OF TORONTO
PHYSICAL EDUCATION FOR WOMEN
ATTENDANCE RECORD 1950-51

Name .... No. ....

Week Ending	October	November	December	January
	13 : 20 : 27	3 : 10 : 17 : 24	1 : 8 : 15	5 : 12
Gymnastics	: :	: : :	: :	:
Elective	: :	: : :	: :	:

Second Term	January	February	March	April
	19 : 26	2 : 9 : 16 : 23	2 : 9 : 16 : 23 : 30	6
Gymnastics	:	: : :	: : : :	
Elective	:	: : :	: : : :	

THIS CARD IS FOR YOUR CONVENIENCE ONLY

REGULATIONS

1. First Term: October 10th to January 12th .... 12 weeks
   Second Term: January 15th to April 6th .... 12 weeks
2. Requirement: 2 classes a week, with at least 9 periods attended in each class, each term.
3. Medical Exemption: Exemption for sickness will be granted only if student is absent from college *for a week or more* and on return to college reports to the Health Service with a doctor's certificate.
4. Students who do not have the required number of classes will be considered as having failed in Physical Education and
   (i) Will be required to take Physical Education in second year and pay the supplemental fee of $10.00.
   (ii) Will not be eligible for University prizes and scholarships of the first year.

3.3 Attendance Record, 1950–1, Physical Education for Women, University of Toronto. University of Toronto Archives, A83–0046/001.

discuss plans for the formation of an athletic association for women. During this meeting, the women expressed the desire that all women have a physical examination and that exercise be compulsory. Barton figured that "there would certainly be some difficulty in enforcing this until the same was required of the men."[126] In this case, women's demands for compulsory training would gain force once university authorities instituted compulsory military drill for men during the war.

Access to facilities, equipment, and instructors equally led some students at UBC to push for the implementation of physical training. At the end of the Second World War, students called for the termination of compulsory military drill for men but argued in favour of gymnastics instruction for all students. In the 1930s, the Alma Mater Society had requested access to voluntary physical training, and in 1936 the University finally hired both a male and female instructor. In 1939, in an attempt to pressure the university to increase athletic facilities, the student council requested that physical education be made compulsory. While military drill became mandatory for men, the Women's Undergraduate Society had to continue to exert pressure on the administration, finally succeeding in 1942–3 in having compulsory war work introduced for female students. The university instituted two hours a week, of which one hour was spent in "keep-fit classes." While compulsory training ended after the war, the gymnasium instructors hired in the 1930s due to student pressure laid the groundwork for the creation of a degree program in physical education.[127]

Conclusion

If some students protested compulsory physical training, either directly or through more passive means, most seem to have accepted it as part of university life. For doctors, physical educators, and administrators, physical culture became one means of ensuring the health of the student body. Yet health was not just an end unto itself. Historians have illustrated the way in which educators envisioned the university and all its component parts – the liberal arts curriculum, residence life, the dining hall, and various extracurricular activities – as aimed at creating and shaping upright citizens of moral character. By the early twentieth century, physical culture had become one more means of instilling the values and ideals of middle-class society. Physical educators believed that the assigned exercises, forms of dance, and sports, could help inculcate particular values that would stand students in good stead for their future endeavours and enable them to contribute in myriad ways to the nation. Through exercise, the abstract ideals of health, morality, spiritual development, and intellectual growth could become reality. In other words, character would become writ on the body. Yet physical training was never sufficient in and of itself to create character. Rather, it formed one part of a broader attempt to ensure the conditions in which a healthy body could thrive and thus from which character could emerge. It is to this larger vision of health that we now turn.

4
Health in Home and Body

The nineteenth century was a period of great enthusiasm for science. First applied to industrial development, the scientific method was soon used to attempt to understand various social issues and problems. Physicians, scientists, and intellectuals, for example, turned their attention towards gaining insight into creating the conditions for improved individual and national development. They did so in myriad ways: the creation of a public health movement; the application of statistical analysis as an approach to understanding the human body; the adaption of evolutionary theory to social and cultural development; and investigations into the nature and forms of human sexuality, among others. With the growing emphasis on research, universities often became centres for the development and implementation of new ideas. In the twentieth century, an emerging cadre of university-based experts would come to dominate such divergent fields as bacteriology, public health, social work, and child psychology.

Not surprisingly, given the number of experts on campus and their growing societal influence, university administrators and faculty not only kept abreast of current developments but attempted to apply some of these to campus practices. Yet in doing so, they neither jettisoned the old nor fully embraced the new. Rather, they adapted what they found to be useful and practical. They readily accepted principles of vaccination, isolation of the sick, physical examination, and other elements of preventative medicine. Yet these continued to be intermixed with the existing practice of sanitary science and adherence to Christian moral precepts. Moreover, even as educators came to place great weight on the objectivity of the scientific method, their endeavours remained imbued with social and cultural bias. This chapter examines the way in which new ideas in medicine and the social sciences became applied to the student body as well as how those ideas were refracted through existing belief and value systems. It does so by focusing on three issues that emerged as concerns in the written record: endeavouring to create a pure living environment; ensuring the means for bodily growth; and providing instruction in health rules and knowledge for good personal hygiene and healthy living.

The Living Environment

Historians have fully documented the way in which university administrators and alumnae understood residence life as a means of developing and maintaining student morality.[1] Less well documented is the way in which they perceived the healthy nature of the students' living environment as facilitating the preconditions for a moral life.[2] Records at Victoria and University Colleges in particular reveal that doctors, nurses, and deans of women spent as much time attempting to create a healthy residential environment as they did rooting out students' pre-existing physical defects. At Victoria College, for example, medical staff did not simply perform examinations and attend the sick, but also regularly inspected the residences, assessing living and dining conditions, study facilities, and recreational possibilities.[3] No such records exist for University College, but there, the alumnae association submitted a report to college officials in the late 1920s that condemned the lack of formal residential facilities for women and provided a detailed indictment of the existing living arrangements and housing conditions available to students.[4] Together, these records provide insight into some of the health concerns of administrators and health experts.

In expressing their anxieties regarding student health at these institutions, as at others, university officials and physicians drew on late-nineteenth- and early-twentieth-century sanitary science. Prior to germ theory, which identifies microorganisms as the culprit of disease, explanations for illness often rested on "miasma" theory. The latter attributed disease to poisons released into the atmosphere from a variety of sources: human, animal, and organic waste and decay; the breath, skin, and clothing of the sick; or even the exhalation of the healthy. Sanitarians, those who practiced sanitary science, focused on cleanliness – of the streets, the household, and the individual. Nancy Tomes argues that even as Americans began to accept germ theory – covering their mouths to cough and noses to sneeze, or eliminating the shared drinking cup – they continued to understand disease as residing in dust or transferred by flies.[5] In the early decades of the twentieth century, health experts wedded germ theory and sanitary science, building their efforts to prevent the spread of germs onto practices of "ventilation, disinfection, isolation of the ill, and general cleanliness."[6]

Sanitary science, however, was much more than a method of attacking the presence and spread of disease. Sanitarians believed that by implementing its practices they could both bring some order to their world and help improve it. Suellen Hoy notes that American sanitarians drew on contemporary beliefs about national progress to reinforce the idea that "filth bred chaos and barbarism, while cleanliness ensured order and advancement." During a period of significant industrialization, sanitarians encouraged the belief among many "middle-class Americans that cleaning the environment of its most offensive nuisances would alleviate the major sources of urban decay."[7] Such beliefs held in Canada too. For example, in 1905 the Toronto medical health officer, Dr Charles Hastings, noted "mental, moral and physical degeneration go hand in hand. This is well attested by observations made in children's courts in the various cities. Insufficient and improper feeding, badly ventilated homes, environments of filth and dirt constitute the very hot-beds in which criminals are bred."[8]

Such theories informed health practices within university residences as well as ideas about suitable conditions in boarding houses. Air quality, ventilation, and overcrowding became key issues. In the early 1920s, the medical adviser for female students at the University of Toronto suggested that students should have access to "single rooms, large windows, and adequate ventilation."[9] She criticized the university's residence facilities, particularly those that consisted of "old houses with large rooms that necessitate the placing of two or three students in one room with a single window and no provision for cross ventilation."[10]

At Victoria College in the 1930s, nurses and physicians attributed colds – the most common student complaint – to the quality of the air. This had been a common worry earlier in the century, with family members and nurses blaming uneven or insufficient heating as the culprit for students' colds.[11] Health experts raised similar concerns in the 1930s, after inspections revealed broken and draughty windows.[12] In the fall of 1932, Edna Guest noted the significant number of "mildly congested sore throats." She linked the increase to the atmosphere, a regular problem in the city when the population began to light furnaces and stay indoors, and recommended that an expert opinion be sought on the heating system in the residence.[13]

Physicians also argued that poor air quality resulted from overcrowding. Despite the routine placement of two to four students in each room, medical officers and educational authorities had begun to question the wisdom of that practice. In the 1920s the University College alumnae association stressed the necessity of one, and no more than two, students per room.[14] In 1927, Victoria's physician noted a serious problem of overcrowding in residences. She wrote of one residence, "almost no floor space when the necessary study-tables and other furniture are in place ... with two girls, and sometimes three, where one ought to be; and it takes little imagination to realize how poisonous the air in these rooms must get after even one hour with two, three or four girls studying in them ..."[15]

While physicians attributed sickness to drafts and closed-in conditions, they believed fresh cold air and proper ventilation to be key for good health. In 1905, the dean at Victoria noted, "the healthy exercise out of doors on the open air rink, and the airiness of our building have been strong factors in keeping our young ladies well."[16] Similarly, in March 1916, the nurse at Victoria reported an improvement in student health, stating that the "cold weather and outdoor sports have helped greatly."[17]

Residences may have had their problems, but administrators and university health officials generally deemed them healthier than boarding houses. From at least the late nineteenth century, students and university staff recognized the problem of finding good boarding. At universities such as Toronto and McGill, members of the campus branch of the YM/YWCA, and after 1921 of the Student Christian Movement, met new students arriving alone by train and guided them to campus or boarding houses. These student groups initiated such activities in recognition that many students from rural areas and small towns would feel overwhelmed arriving in a larger urban centre and would find it difficult to locate good boarding houses on their own. In some cases, such as at McGill, the Student Christian Association and the University Health Services co-operated to inspect boarding houses and provide new students with a list of approved housing.[18]

Despite these efforts, reports by medical officers, as well as the occasional survey of student housing, suggest that at least some students had difficulty finding proper lodgings. A 1910 report by the dean of women at Victoria is illustrative. She noted that a young woman "came to Toronto, a stranger, and entered an ordinary boarding house. Through neglect and unwholesome surroundings she became a physical wreck and went home to die."[19] In the 1920s, the alumnae association of University College complained about the uncleanliness of lodgings, stating that "clean linen is very difficult to get and two different groups of students have had to leave houses on account of vermin."[20] In the early 1930s, the acting dean of women at Victoria reported similar problems. "Boarding houses in this district," she noted, "may be over-run with bedbugs, and one student, who thought she had developed hives, was seriously poisoned by the bites of these parasites. Another student, trying to live on three dollars a week, for both board and room, and needless to say living under very poor conditions, contracted two skin diseases, which were early diagnosed by the physician. A Victoria Women's Bursary came to the rescue in each case."[21]

The University College Alumnae Association attributed one of the causes for both the scarcity and poor quality of housing to the increasing number of immigrants boarding near the university – an area "formerly of a very high character." "The inroad of the foreign population," the association report stressed, had resulted in "great overcrowding and lack of cleanliness [sic] ... and a general lowering of the tone of the district ... Five times in two months examples of indecent behaviour and attempted assault have been reported to the police."[22] Administrators thus attributed lack of cleanliness not to the slum conditions and urban poverty that had developed in areas around the university but rather to the immigrants living there. Suellen Hoy notes of the American context, "Cleanliness became something more than a way to prevent epidemics and make cities liveable – it became a route to citizenship, to becoming American."[23] In the shift from public to private health, cleanliness was elevated to a sign of personal virtue and a badge of patriotism.[24]

The University College Alumnae Association worried not only about the unwholesome locations of boarding houses, but also about their quality and nature. A prime concern regarded the mixing of the sexes. In one case where a student was too sick to go out for food, "the Head of the Women's Union went to see her [and] she found the girl lying in bed and a male undergraduate making up her fire, he having been commissioned to do so by the landlady."[25] In other instances, investigators were alarmed to find men and women boarding in the same houses. As with college residences, they believed students should live in single-sex accommodation that had sitting rooms to receive visitors of the opposite sex.[26]

Members of the alumnae association also raised concerns about single-sex cohabitation and sleeping arrangements, particularly the

sharing of double beds.[27] Neil Sutherland argues that in the first half of
the twentieth century, significant numbers of siblings shared not only
rooms, but also beds.[28] Many university students would have grown up
well accustomed to such practices and thus thought little about doing so
with their room-mates.[29] By the 1920s, however, health experts frowned
on this practice. The emphasis on single beds was due in part to new
ideas of preventative health. It may also have been the result of changing ideas about sexuality. Michael Bliss points out that the sex manual,
What a Young Wife Ought to Know, one of a bestselling series in Canada in
the early decades of the twentieth century, advised that in order to avoid
sexual experimentation, mothers ought not to allow young children to
sleep together.[30]

Many boarding houses also lacked proper cooking facilities or provision of meals. In some boarding houses, the owner provided daily sit-
down meals for lodgers. Others, however, simply placed a hotplate in
the room for heating food, or worse still, had no cooking facilities at
all, so that students had to seek out meals at local lunch counters. In
their report, the alumnae association of University College stressed the
importance of room and board being provided in the same house or
within proximity to each other.[31] Educators at many universities believed
the dining room to be a site of healthy and moral living. Students gained
a sit-down dinner that not only included nutritious meals, but also provided them with an opportunity to learn dining etiquette, the art of po-
lite conversation, and general comportment for public life. As such, the
dining room acted as an extension of the residence hall – a place where
students could gain the refinement and cultivation deemed necessary
for their future endeavours and in order for them to take their place
as the future leaders of the nation.[32] In addition, in many residences,
where students lined up to enter the dining hall, it provided nurses and
administrators with an easy means to assess weight and pallor. Thus the
dining room could also act as a site of surveillance of student behaviour,
morality, and health.

For many officials and graduates of the university, living environment
played a key role in ensuring students' health and morality. The physical
conditions of the building aided the emergence, or prohibited the development, of a student's well-being. University officials and concerned
citizens envisioned residence not simply as a place where they could
oversee student comportment, but also as an edifice that structured
and shaped student conduct and morality. The atmosphere, ventilation,
lighting, dining facilities, number of roommates, location, and cleanliness all played a determining role in evaluations about the health and

moral standards of students' living conditions. A clean, wholesome, and moral living environment was a first step to ensuring the development of character.

Bodily Growth

By the turn of the century, educators had also begun to equate the formation of character with physical growth. Beginning in the 1860s, several American campus physicians and physical directors began to collect the anthropometric measurements of male students, an undertaking that by the 1890s had spread to significant numbers of male, female, and co-educational institutions.[33] Anthropometry, or the measurement of human bodies, developed in the eighteenth and nineteenth centuries as part of the broader rise of statistical analysis and the desire to measure and compare human variability.[34] Proponents of anthropometry recorded a variety of information, such as height, weight, arm span, forearm girth, size of legs, and circumference of the chest, in order to create a body of growth data. Such data were collected for a variety of reasons. In the eighteenth century, these measurements were used in Europe, and by the nineteenth century, in the United States, to determine the physical fitness of men for war. Through the nineteenth century, British reformers developed growth studies to help reform the working and living conditions of poor children and identify those in ill health. In Britain and the United States, school surveys and infant welfare clinics developed out of that work. The rise of anthropometry also led to a variety of surveys of those housed in prisons and reformatories, which came to link various physical traits to criminality.[35] Some physical anthropologists drew on anthropometric measurements in order to identify different racial or ethnic groups and to seek out differences between the sexes. As eugenics became popular, these types of measurements often became a means of identifying individuals and groups with supposedly deficient or superior racial, gender, and moral characteristics.[36]

With various origins and different intents, the aim in collecting all of this early statistical data was to harness the methods of the natural sciences to the study of human society by uncovering "general truths about mass phenomenon."[37] The aim was to compile statistics on individual variability in order to understand, and develop, general laws about societal behaviour. By the turn of the century, many moral and social reformers would draw on the methods and analysis provided by experts in the newly emerging fields of social sciences as a means of working towards the betterment of human society.

Within American universities, physicians and physical educators interested in athletic development implemented the collection of anthropometric measurements in order to assess physical development and help students to avoid the asymmetry that they believed resulted from focusing on a single sport.[38] Some health experts also focused on creating an average or standard by which individual students could be measured. In the United States, Dudley Sargent provided some of the most extensive early co-sexual studies to determine the measurement of the average male and female bodies. Using this data, Sargent employed R. Tait McKenzie to create a series of statues depicting the average American college student and had these displayed at the 1893 Chicago World's Columbian Exposition.[39] Jacqueline Urla and Alan C. Swedlund have argued that Sargent's work was part of a larger trend by the early twentieth century to identify the average American of each sex. Sargent derived the measurements for his average male and female bodies largely from statistical composites of young, white, elite college students. As Urla and Swedlund note, "although anthropometric studies … were ostensibly descriptive rather than prescriptive, the normal or average and the ideal were routinely conflated."[40] Indeed, Wendy Kline notes that the enthusiasm for statistics and measurement "led to an increasing emphasis on 'normality' as a central organizing principal of modern civilization."[41] In the case of physical education, the physical dimensions of the average American thus equated normality with the white middle-class Anglo-Saxon body at the expense of other American bodies. Indeed, as with most of these statistical composites of body types, few men and women, including the white college students from whom the composition was derived, could match these average measurements.[42]

In the process of gathering and recording anthropometric measurements, at least some medical experts came to focus on the connection between posture, exercise, and health. David Yosifon and Peter Stearns argue that, despite the relaxation of standards of etiquette in the early twentieth century and ever-increasing informality throughout the century, emphasis on posture and erect carriage intensified. Posture, they note, became a means to reinforce "traditional beliefs about character and discipline" in light of increasing anxieties about social change. It also provided a way to advance the professional aims of the emerging physical education movement. And it reflected the "growing attention to the body and concern about mechanistic efficiency."[43] Beginning in the 1880s and continuing into the 1940s and 1950s, a number of American colleges required, as part of the physical examination, that incoming students have a photograph taken of them in the nude in order to track their posture.[44]

In Canadian universities, anthropometric studies and posture tests appeared most prominently in institutions that established physical training programs and had sufficient resources to undertake these types of examinations. As we saw in chapter 1, under R. Tait McKenzie's guidance, the medical examination cards at McGill in the late nineteenth century requested detailed anthropometric measurements and a scaled-down version continued to be taken, at least for male students, into the 1920s.[45] At Toronto, the men's division of the university health service began taking such measurements in the 1920s and continued at least until the early 1940s.[46] It is unclear whether such work was done as systematically for female students at Toronto in the early part of the century. Certainly, however, the university required posture tests from at least 1947–8 until the early 1960s.[47] By the 1920s and 1930s, some universities used a silhouettograph – which provided a silhouette of the patient – in order to detect "abnormal posture."[48] Information on procedures at other institutions remains sketchy, but there is evidence that these practices occurred elsewhere. For example, UWO kept anthropometric charts in the early 1920s. And when UBC introduced voluntary physical education classes for women in the mid-1930s, the instructor charted the height and weight of, and performed posture tests on, at least some of the students.[49]

Physicians and physical directors who recorded anthropometric measurements remarked on such things as the increased weight, height, and chest expansion of both male and female students in a given year and compared one first-year cohort to the next.[50] It is generally difficult to know what physical educators and physicians in Canada did with these measurements. Certainly in some cases they used them to help sort students into the fit category versus those in need of remedial exercises. An occasional comment suggests some physical educators took a prescriptive interpretation of anthropometric data early on, attempting to have students' match the average measurements. In 1910 Scott Raff noted, "We have five little girls very eager to grow and by the rule of anthropometry four of them should have grown taller. They have been regularly stretched and the process has been life-giving we believe. We cannot force human muscles in a day or a month, so will report on these cases later on."[51] Health experts and university administrators also kept track of height and weight increases as an indication of the health of their students.[52] And they made a point of recording how favourably their own students' gains compared to those of students at other institutions. For example, in 1937–8, the physician at the University of Toronto wrote, "this makes our highest average … It may be interesting to note that our freshmen stand first in height as compared with those of eleven American Universities, and second in weight, and that the general upward trend in height and weight is very noticeable in the past sixteen years."[53]

Weight gain raised considerable discussion, particularly among female physicians. While dieting and slimming would start to make cultural inroads by the interwar years, physicians and nurses continued to focus on the importance of weight gain for female students. In the United States, Margaret Lowe notes that while some historians have documented women's dieting as early as the late nineteenth century, she in fact found that at the turn of the century, white college women believed weight gain "signified a healthy adjustment to college life."[54] Lowe argues that "by gaining flesh, they countered the notion that they were frail and that their bodies would 'break down' at college. Losing weight signalled trouble because of its association with some of the most common female illnesses, including neurasthenia, hysteria, and consumption."[55] Likewise in Canada, some early-twentieth-century health experts praised students' weight gain. In November 1914, for example, Marion Clark, the nurse at Victoria College, noted, "several have attained a weight never before reached. The least gained was 2 ½ pounds and most 9 and it was all gained in less than four weeks."[56] Physicians and nurses also consistently raised concerns about undernourishment. In January 1921 Dr Edna Guest found 30 of the 124 women examined, or 24 per cent, to be in need of extra nourishment.[57] In 1922 at the University of Toronto, Dr Edith Gordon similarly found "a surprising number of cases of undernourishment among the students."[58] Such comments continued into the 1930s. The nurse at Regina College, Saskatchewan, noted that students' weight was checked once a month "and if gains are not made, the reason is sought."[59] At UBC, too, the medical examiner noted concern about the number of underweight female students.[60]

Physicians and administrators were definitely aware of a changing culture around weight gain. In 1927, for example, the physician, nurse, and dean of women at Victoria College pondered the reason for the poor chest expansion of the students. The dean noted of the physician's finding, "I do not wonder you have found this because just look at the prevailing styles. Girls who used to have fine chests have become quite hollow – the up-and-down effect, with no breasts!"[61] In the early 1930s the medical officer at UBC blamed "the current fashion of semi-starvation or 'slimming' among the women." The officer went on to state, "this fashion which has become widely prevalent, may be a causal factor in the large amount of tuberculosis among women of this age group."[62]

Certainly by the interwar years, North American women's attitude towards weight had begun to change. The popular image of the flapper reinforced the link between youth and slimness. Equally, Lowe notes that "by the 1920s a heavy body pointed to the Old World – to the working classes and marginal immigrant groups."[63] Dieting thus denoted one's class status – a level of access to food that allowed one "the luxury to refuse food for aesthetic purposes."[64] Physicians were reacting to a very real cultural trend. Yet there is at least some evidence to indicate that some students responded well to the encouragement of weight gain, with underweight students often accepting the extra milk and eggnogs provided to them.[65] Students' willingness to gain weight suggests that beliefs equating health with weight gain may well have continued to resonate at least into the 1930s.

Physicians' concerns about weight and height went hand in hand with their attempt to evaluate and improve carriage and posture. Unlike in some American universities, posture examinations never became an integral part of most health service programs. Lack of personnel and finances seems to have been a prime reason. Yet physicians still considered the work of value. As late as 1953, W.A. Murray, the director of student health services at Dalhousie University noted,

> With the help of the five young women in the final year of the Diploma in Physical Education course, and one young woman from the fourth year of the Faculty of Medicine, a beginning was made on a study in posture using the line of gravity apparatus which was built some years ago for Dr Cates of the department of anatomy. This work proved most interesting, but was too time-consuming to permit the attention it merited.

Murray's statement thus confirmed the continuing belief in not only the usefulness of such work, but also the financial costs. He suggested that a graduate student in physical education turn attention to the issue.[66]

Physicians and educators believed this work to be important because they took increases in weight and height and evidence of erect carriage as indicators of physical health. That growth was in turn linked to mental development and improvement, moral fortitude, and for women, reproductive capability. In Canada, as in the United States, physical educators and physicians directly connected fitness and growth to academic success, and equally, lack of fitness to mental deficiency.[67] For example, using statistical information gathered during her examination of students, the medical examiner at McGill University reported in 1922, "considerable proportion of the students who failed to meet the requirements in this Department failed academically."[68] At the University of Toronto, Edith Gordon argued that "low-grade feeble-minded are always deficient in motor power and delicacy of coordination ... Growth implies something which becomes larger and better." She went on to state that it was when growth halts, when organs are not fully developed, that "the seat of disease" might develop.[69] Such ideas were not limited to universities but could be found within the education system more generally. Writing in the *Alberta Teachers' Association Magazine* in 1924, Captain Kennedy, the supervisor of physical training for the Edmonton Public School Board, emphasized the importance of good posture to future growth and development. The erect carriage was a visible demonstration of the elevation of "the human race from the lower animals." For Kennedy, as for many others, good physiology led to the evolution of the race, while sunken chests, rounded shoulders, protruding heads, and flat feet all marked physically and, ultimately, mentally and morally feeble children.[70]

In keeping with cultural beliefs of the time, physicians and educators had a tendency to blame individuals for their predicament. Examining the history of special education in Toronto, Jason Ellis notes that it was common to regard physical disability as something that, given the right training, could be overcome, thus placing the success or failure to do so on the individual.[71] At Victoria College, doctors attributed uneven development to a number of problems such as "carelessness or lack of proper exercise," "not standing up straight and by sitting in a twisted position," and "careless standing."[72] Equally, in 1922 Edith Gordon blamed students' low weight on their own carelessness in missing breakfasts.[73] In blaming slimming, physicians ignored the possibility that students' low weight might be connected to their financial position.

Students who were reluctant to improve themselves might find themselves berated. Edna Guest wrote to the dean of women at Victoria,

> When you have time I would like you to have a chat with Mary – and encourage her to take gym to correct a defective posture with slight curvature. She is very sensitive of not having had games and gym in her schooldays and also thinks because she is so tall she is too conspicuous when she does not do her gym well ... so she seems rather unwilling to try again. I told her she

was not a good *Canadian* for Canadians never admitted they *could* not do anything just because they did not want to![74]

Indeed, administrators and medical experts often used the guise of health to condemn the fashions and behaviour of an emerging youth culture and of female students' new-found independence. In October 1915, nurse Marion Clark attributed a number of colds and sore throats to "indiscretion, as I found from investigating the undergarments of some during the cold spell."[75] Dr Guest in particular waged a war against female students contributing to their own flat feet. In 1927 Guest reported that the students' flat feet were "for the most part, caused by badly chosen heels on their shoes ... I have tried to show the girls what is a correct shoe and to show them the ill-effects of a badly fitted shoe."[76] Several years later Guest was still trying to educate students to proper footwear, arguing, "We hope this will have some good effect in the future if not immediately. We feel it is of good educative value to start the girls talking about shoes and heels – it must then have a sure effect, even if their more or less juvenile ideas are not always in perfect agreement with our ideals."[77]

If individuals were responsible for their own predicament, then dispelling ignorance around health issues could solve many remedial problems. Indeed, if the aim of anthropometry was to measure growth and physical balance, and track physical improvement, it was also to show students where they needed to improve and how to do so. In the nineteenth century, Dudley Sargent focused on the uses of measurement to assess the results of his program of physical training.[78] Patricia Vertinsky notes, "Through his standardized charts (of referenced populations), students could 'see at a glance their relation in size, strength, symmetry, and development to the normal standard' and gauge their level of health and fitness accordingly. 'Study yourselves,' he exhorted, 'and most of all note well wherein kind nature meant you to excel.'"[79] One point of the posture assessments and the weight and height measurements was to indicate to students how they compared to the average and the ways in which they needed to change.[80] As we saw in chapter 3, the belief that students needed "lifting up" also formed a central component of educators' programs. While medical examinations assessed anywhere from 80 to 98 per cent of students as healthy, physicians worried about the need to bring all students up to Category A, and to ensure that students in that category did not backslide. Some students also emphasized the importance of this project. A 1923 column in the *Varsity* noted, "It is the matter of improvement that really concerns the University." This, the article continued, was something that could be achieved with "special, supervised exercises and intelligent advice." Indeed the writer noted, "61 per cent of those below A1 perfection have been brought up to that point and only 4 per cent went back."[81]

In the mid-1930s, the acting dean of women at Victoria College noted that the physical director planned the exercises so that they would be not only enjoyable, but also instructive. She continued, "The exercises were planned with one end in view, namely, the promotion of good posture. We are glad to report that the improvement in the posture of the classes as a whole was marked. A great many students were so interested that they came between the classes to discuss individually what could be suggested for their own particular posture defects."[82] While under the surveillance of university administrators, it was the responsibility of college staff to ensure students did not backslide, "not allowing the girl with flat feet to be lured back by a misguided fashion into ruinously heeled shoes again, nor the flat-chested girl or the many with poor posture or poor chest expansion to forget the few simple instructions which they have been given to correct those."[83] But the ultimate aim was to have students internalize health rules. Edna Guest wrote, "Thus I hope we are instilling into our girls, a knowledge of the ordinary rules to be followed if good health is to result – and in a way which without their realizing it, becomes a part of themselves, before they finally leave our care."[84] While some cajoled with a heavy hand, others did so more lightly. In her biography of Marion Hilliard, Robinson notes, "As part of her job Marion emphasized the importance of posture, weight control, and good-health regimes, and dreamed up end-of-the-year programs to make it fun. One such was the year 'Miss Annesley Hall' was chosen from among the healthiest physical specimens, and prizes were given for the ten girls who made the most progress during the year in overcoming health problems."[85]

While physicians and others often drew on, and reinforced, fears of evolutionary descent, in general their vision regarding the student body was more optimistic. Physicians, health reformers, and many administrators considered physical improvement, like mental, moral, and spiritual growth, as crucial for the survival and development of the race. Much of the thought of the time drew on cultural fears and anxieties about racial and evolutionary descent. In general there was widespread support for public health initiatives and education as methods to dispel ignorance and encourage racial improvement as well as for the segregation, institutionalization, and in some cases sterilization, of those unable or unwilling to follow instructions. Experts linked poverty, crime, perceived sexual immorality, even class position, to mental defect rather than the economic structure of society.[86] While some physicians, educators, and moral and social reformers worried about the effects of those they considered degenerate or feeble-minded on the health of society, many often took a more positive approach when writing or speaking about those they considered fit. David Churchill, in his study of bodybuilding and physical culture in Chicago at the turn of the twentieth century, notes that unlike eugenicist Francis Galton, Dudley Sargent believed that "individuals' physical and mental abilities were not just the result of a genetic inheritance, but could be learned and thus developed. Building the harmonious body was something that almost everyone could accomplish, even by individuals who did not have 'natural endowment.'"[87]

Despite their sometimes negative comments about students, physicians made a point to emphasize improvement.[88] This is clear in statements by physical educators and physicians at Victoria from the early twentieth century into the late 1930s. Emma Scott Raff, physical instructor at Victoria College, extolled the necessity of physical training not only for the benefit of the individual, but also "for the benefit of the race to which they belong."[89] Marion Hilliard argued, "Viewed from a moral and physical standpoint, the science of eugenics must be a factor in leading toward the goal of the best life."[90] Young women, Edna Guest believed, could be part of the solution to racial improvement. In a 1922 article on "Problems of Girlhood and Motherhood," Guest wrote that the student of today must study current social conditions "unbiased by custom." She must determine whether the laws of the country "will develop her people into the finest type or whether they will cripple them." Guest continued, "... she must fix her gaze in the distance on our personified God ... and rubbing any film from her eyes, write with a free and fearless hand the laws which will make for her a people perfect in mind and body."[91] If eugenic theory led physicians to fear evolutionary descent, liberal notions of progress could reinforce more optimistic ideas about the possibilities for racial improvement. If only ignorance could be dispelled, and students, like the rest of the population, could be enticed to follow health rules, both individual and societal improvement would ensue.

Young, healthy men and women, then, had a duty to maintain and improve their own health. The burden of responsibility for personal health lay with the individual. Yet as a national issue and concern, many administrators and health experts believed that a social institution such as the university should play a role in improving individual health.

Anthropometric measurements and posture tests would not only provide general statistical information on student health, but could also help individual students to understand how they compared to the average and what they needed to do to maintain or improve their health. With proper instruction, physicians believed, they could also impress upon students the links between individual responsibility and national duty.

Hygiene and Sexuality

Health experts focused not only on reshaping students' bodies through the lessons of anthropometry and physical culture, but also on instructing them on issues of personal hygiene and healthy living. Many universities provided voluntary and compulsory lectures on personal hygiene by the resident medical examiner.[92] Men heard topics with titles such as "Personal Hygiene," "Personal Hygiene and First Aid," or "Hygiene and Health."[93] Women listened to talks on "Personal Hygiene," supplemented by topics such as "Digestion and Dietetics," "Chest, Heart, Feet, Posture," and "The Nervous System and Emotional Control."[94] In 1938–9, for example, McGill's College Hygiene course for female students included subjects such as skin care; social hygiene (venereal disease); first aid; weight; mental health; menstruation; physiology of reproduction; the nervous system; heredity, the environment, and pre-natal care; nutrition; and public health measures.[95]

Little documentation remains on the content or nature of the talks given to students. Fragmentary evidence suggests that students learned basic health rules about personal hygiene, nutrition, and maintaining a balanced lifestyle. Margaret Lowe notes that in the late nineteenth century, women at Smith College attended hygiene classes stressing "moderate living habits that included cleanliness, sensible dress, balanced meals, daily exercise, and plenty of rest." They also learned some basic anatomy and physiology, such as the nature and functioning of the lungs and the parts of the skeleton.[96] In 1922, George Porter, the director of health services at Toronto gave a series of talks on "Personal Hygiene" to first-year men at University College. His four principles of health included work, relaxation, proper outdoor exercise, and proper diet. He argued that health could be maintained by not worrying and that the "greatest diversion against worry is work." Work needed to be balanced with relaxation, however, as "recreation kept up too long becomes dissipation." He recommended a mixed diet rich in dairy and vegetables as well as exercise "which takes you back to Nature as much as possible."[97]

While Porter focused on personal hygiene, others also stressed the importance of alerting students to the work of the public health movement. The women's branch of the department of physical education at McGill attempted to bring students' "attention to the work of Community Hygiene and her part as a responsible citizen in promoting this work."[98] Roy Fraser, professor of biology and bacteriology at Mount Allison University, noted in a 1939 article in the *Canadian Public Health Journal* that Canadian universities had devoted increasing attention to teaching health through classroom lectures on hygiene and physical training classes. He argued that this "puts most of its emphasis on personal hygiene and self-culture and not enough on community health and social responsibility."[99] At Mount Allison, students in arts or science took a course on "Personal Hygiene and Public Health," which in the public health section focused on "the general structure and functions of the national and provincial health departments. General studies in the annual reports of these departments are assigned, and the student must give particular study to the conditions prevailing in his own home district."[100]

In addition to these formal lectures, there is some evidence that deans of women and health experts gave talks or organized discussions in some way related to sexual knowledge and conduct relating to marriage and reproduction. Historians have little knowledge about the sexual practices of Canadian students in the first half of the twentieth century. Slightly more is known about the American context. Paul Axelrod notes, for example, that a 1938 survey of 1,300 American students found that 50 per cent of men and 25 per cent of women had had premarital sexual intercourse and 8 per cent of men and 4 per cent of women acknowledged being homosexual. While in the Canadian context there are certainly anecdotal reports of students engaged in practices such as necking and petting, Axelrod argues that in contrast to an American literature that sees the 1920s as a period of sexual experimentation, Canadian "campus sexual life was neither as loose as critics feared nor as pristine as officials pretended."[101]

Certainly, the war and post–First World War period witnessed an increasing openness towards public discussions of issues relating to sexuality, and in particular the role of sexuality within marriage. Victoria College provides a case in point. In the early 1920s, Margaret Addison, the dean of women, exposed students to a variety of speakers who covered the topic of sex hygiene and reproduction. She encouraged a visit from Emmeline Pankhurst who spent 1922 touring Canada on behalf of the Canadian Social Hygiene Council.[102] In conjunction with the deans of University and Trinity Colleges, she organized a university-wide lecture series by Violet Trench, a member of the British National Committee for Combatting Venereal Disease.[103] And in the 1920s and early 1930s, she asked the physicians employed by Victoria to offer lectures to "mature" students on "the origin of life" and "facts of life."[104] Addison's successor, Jessie Macpherson, provided such lectures herself. One female student at Victoria in the early war years remembered Macpherson as "a respected figure" who was "known campus-wide for her annual (S.R.O. [Standing Room Only]) lecture on sex."[105] Another, who graduated in 1950, remembered "Miss Mac" talking "in a matter-of-fact manner to an enthralled (and embarrassed) group of women about the facts of life and love."[106]

Health experts became strong proponents of students learning about sexuality and reproduction for trained professionals. In 1931 Guest expressed concern about the sexual knowledge of young men and women. She argued,

> Too frequently our boys and girls get knowledge from the street instead of from reliable sources, and equally do our modern girls in their late teens, our newly married girls and our young mothers get their knowledge from where they can pick it up ... Why should not our University – this University – lead the universities of the world who are attempting to educate women, by establishing an academic health course for Co-eds, which might associate itself with courses in Biology, Household Economics, Social Service, Psychology, in the University Extension courses ...[107]

In the interwar years, progressive student groups equally demanded such courses.[108] However, not all students were as eager to tackle the topic. Asked by health services to list the subjects for discussion that most interested them, female students at McGill did rank highly "heredity/ environment/pre-natal care," "the physiology of reproduction," and "social hygiene (venereal disease)" but placed all of these well below their prime interest, "the skin."[109] Still, marriage preparation courses would become a feature of many American campuses beginning in the 1930s and some Canadian ones in the 1940s and 1950s.[110]

What students learned from these talks and how useful they found them is less easily determined. Social hygienists at the time, for example, encouraged sex hygiene "as a cure for ignorance and a buffer against reckless impulses."[111] The early twentieth century witnessed an increased emphasis on companionate marriage and emotional and sexual fulfilment within that union.[112] Some talks reinforced marital relations – though not necessarily in a particularly useful way. In May 1915 Esther Clark, a student at Acadia University, complained to her mother,

> In the evening we went to Dr. Spurgeon's lecture of "Advice to married people & those who expect to marry." He told a lot of slushy yarns and gave some advice about choosing the right kind of husband or wife, about women knowing how to cook and men bringing home flowers and candy to their wives. But it really was hardly worth going to.[113]

Ideas about sexuality within marriage were also changing, particularly regarding parenthood. Helen MacMurchy, for example, did not believe in the use of birth control except for medical reasons and with medical advice.[114] She argued, "Those who marry but voluntarily refuse parenthood are robbing themselves of their greatest joy, and are failing to serve the highest interests of their country and their generation."[115] But ideas about birth control did not remain static. Whereas MacMurchy opposed birth control, Marion Hilliard advocated its use within marriage. This was a much more common attitude by the 1930s, as experts and society more generally came to see birth control less as a tool of radical change to improve women's position in society than as a means of maintaining stability.[116] Yet support for the use of birth control was still reasonably progressive at a time when some academics and medical experts continued to emphasize women's duties as wives and mothers and spoke out against the use of any form of contraception.[117]

Though social hygienists advocated sexual activity as a positive part of marriage, they believed that prior to that commitment, young people ought to exert self-control. That message was reinforced by church teachings and family expectations as well as by stories of those who had transgressed. The 1927 trial of Dr O.C.J. Withrow, who caused the death of a young woman from an affluent Toronto family by performing an abortion on her, was meticulously detailed in the local Toronto press. Although she was engaged, the young woman's demise was attributed to the couple's fast-paced life, with her father commenting "she was practically independent in her conduct ... she was fond of entertainment, motoring, dancing and so on."[118] Such comments echoed those of deans of women at the time concerned about the moral and physical consequences of exactly those types of activities.

In her 1938 book, *For College Women ... and Men*, Mossie May Waddington Kirkwood, dean of women at Trinity College, University of Toronto, supported the idea of the companionate marriage. She also recognized that young people were struggling with the issue of sexual intimacy prior to marriage. She reinforced the need for sex education, something that should start in childhood with instruction in plant and animal life. Yet she also warned against pre-marital sexual activity. While she rejected traditional views of marriage, she warned,

> Intimacy before marriage, especially in a society with many conservative members, will be a risk to self-respect that may quite over-balance the plea-sure experience. Promiscuity, or even intimacy with more than one indi-vidual, will dull the freshness and the beauty of the marriage relationship as involving the whole personality – that is, if we think of the marriage re-lationship as involving the whole personality. And this finally is what one does, when marriage and home are taken to represent an achievement of civilization. Marriage is not the mere satisfaction of desire. It is the assent-ing to life and a sacrament, the giving of body and mind to the mystery of existence, which lifts us up by using us.[119]

By the late 1930s, one topic which had become much less veiled was that of venereal disease (VD). Doctors began to learn more about VD in the late nineteenth and early twentieth centuries with the discovery that gonorrhea and syphilis were separate diseases; the 1905 identification of the microorganism that caused syphilis; and, in 1906, the creation of the Wasserman test for its detection.[120] In the nineteenth century, VD was perceived as a disease of immorality linked to prostitution. As physicians discovered its role in contributing to sterility, miscarriage, and neonatal blindness, eugenicists and social hygienists rearticulated it as a danger to not only the individual sinner, but also their innocent victims – wives and the unborn – and ultimately as a peril to the nation.[121]

The First World War brought a new awareness of the disease and greater public discussion. Military doctors estimated that 15.8 per cent of soldiers had VD, with 4.5 per cent of these infected with syphilis.[122] While health experts worried about soldiers' contact with prostitutes, they also began to realize that many young men entered the military infected, thus reinforcing the notion of VD as a broader societal issue. Medical experts and social hygienists also raised concerns about the return of troops to Canada.[123] In 1919, for example, they created the National Council for Combatting Venereal Disease. A federal-provincial cost-sharing program provided funds for free diagnosis and treatment of VD as well as activities such as the distribution of pamphlets, public lectures, and the creation of documentary films.[124] In the United States, concern about the spread of VD, along with the campaigning of prominent social hygiene organizations, led to federal funding of social hygiene programs in a variety of colleges and universities after the First World War.[125]

Concern about the presence of VD in society, along with the ability to detect syphilis, led to the introduction of testing for male students in many Canadian universities. Deeply held beliefs about class and respectability likely reinforced assumptions about the purity of middle-class womanhood. In addition, the attempt to preserve female students' modesty led to less invasive physical examinations. Thus testing remained limited to male students. The University of Toronto seems to have tested male students on a regular basis starting in the early 1920s, and McGill recorded cases of VD in the mid-1930s. A report of the health inquiry committee of the University of Manitoba recorded that in 1941 Dalhousie required a Wasserman test, Alberta performed one on suspected cases, while McGill provided one on demand.[126]

Medical officers found VD present on campus, though only in very low rates. In 1921–2, George Porter noted of students at the University of Toronto, "Those showing any evidence of diseases whose presence are generally traceable to immorality (Venereal Disease) are less than ½ of 1%."[127] Equally, in the late 1940s, the University of Alberta Medical Services Committee estimated that 1 per cent of tests for syphilis would probably show positive, although many of these would be false positives.[128] Despite contemporaries' claims regarding a high incidence of venereal disease in the general population, these rates correspond to the much lower ones gathered in the United States after the introduction of compulsory blood tests prior to marriage.[129] While the Wasserman test could catch cases of syphilis, Alan Brandt notes that detection of gonorrhea, a much more common form of venereal disease, was more difficult due to the necessity of performing a microscopic smear. Moreover, until the advent of penicillin, it could not be treated. As a result, he argues, health experts focused much less public attention on the latter disease.[130] University medical examiners were certainly aware of gonorrhea and reported small numbers of cases. However, detection occurred primarily through a visual examination. For example, the director of university health service at the University of Toronto noted, "It is pleasing to state that no case of syphilis has been found in our examination of the first three years of the student body. As for the other venereal disease (gonorrhoea), while doubtless here and there cases have occurred, no evidence of this disease has appeared during our examinations, and when it is recalled that the examinations are compulsory, that everyone comes up stripped before us it is evident that we have a remarkable freedom from venereal disease in our University."[131]

Despite low rates of infection on campus, the moral panic about, and public campaigns around, VD seem to have made it a more acceptable topic for public discussion by the late 1930s. Certainly the issue was raised with students earlier in the interwar years. Veiled references to it can be found in the 1920s. While in 1922 George Porter focused on "methods of promoting health," he also touched on the topic of "avoidance of disease" – likely a euphemism for venereal disease.[132] By the late 1930s, however, references to VD were more explicit. As we've seen, female students in the required college hygiene course offered by the health service at McGill University discussed the topic.[133] During the war, the UBC health service created a health pamphlet library. In reference to students' use of the library the director commented, "… it is particularly gratifying to note that many more students are becoming conscious of the dangers of Venereal Disease and how to avoid them."[134]

University officials targeted male students in particular as in need of reminders about the dangers of VD In 1945–6 the department of physical education at McGill sent a circular to all male students warning them to stay away from prostitutes, "an extremely dangerous source of contagion, with its consequent mortification and misery."[135] The emphasis on prostitutes as the source of contagion was common to other university and municipal authorities. In 1944–5, for example, authorities at the University of Montreal supported an Anti-Venereal Disease Campaign organized by the Montreal Chamber of Commerce, in cooperation with the Province of Quebec Health and Social Welfare Department, to have municipal and provincial governments close all brothels permanently because of the spread of venereal disease in Montreal and other North American cities.[136] University authorities recommended abstinence, not protection, as the means to avoid disease.[137]

If a student did happen to contract a venereal disease, however, medical experts emphasized how imperative it was that he seek out proper medical attention. The McGill circular, for example, warned students that "if, through indiscretion, exposure to infection should occur, under no circumstance whatever must there be a delay of even a few hours in securing properly controlled and scientific treatment. Immediate treatment is absolutely essential if the dreaded inroads of the disease are to be prevented." It continued, "THE 'QUACK' MUST BE AVOIDED AT

ALL COSTS." Rather, professional treatment such as that provided by the student health service should be sought.[138]

Conclusion

Health experts advanced the cause of student health through admonitions that mixed morality, sanitarianism, and the new germ theory. A healthy and moral living environment, good personal hygiene, an erect carriage, general fitness, and healthy sexual practices – all these, educators believed, constituted the basis for creating and maintaining healthy students and future citizens. This work was carried on within the powerful ideological framework of race betterment. Physicians, physical directors, and university authorities generally focused on improvement and uplift. But they always worried about halted growth or worse, moral and racial descent.

Within universities, administrators placed the responsibility for growth – intellectual, physical, moral, and spiritual – on the student. While the university had a duty to create favourable conditions for development, ultimately the student was responsible for ensuring that he or she took advantage of the opportunities provided. Mossie Mae Waddington Kirkwood, dean of women at Trinity College, stated in 1938, "What the student puts into his college course will determine the values he gets out of it, and that is what repays the country and repays the private benefactor – the fine type of university graduate who emerges. The university stands for a way of life, and for obligations more than rights."[139] University administrators might resort to compulsion to ensure that students fulfilled their obligations to themselves and society, but they hoped that students would take up the lessons learned and as graduates continue to follow them on their own.

As can be seen with Kirkwood's statement, ideas about health were not the sole preserve of physicians. Medical doctors performed medical examinations, diagnosed disease, and suggested treatments. Moreover, university administrators listened to medical authorities. Yet the lines of expertise remained blurred. Doctors and physical educators waded into moral debates such as students' fashions or their keeping of late hours. Equally, deans of women used medical language to bolster moral concerns. In blurring these lines, deans and physicians showed their commitment to a common aim: creating conditions for healthy living and shaping the body in order to allow for the emergence of a student's character.

Many of the issues raised in this chapter continued to animate educators and health experts in the years after the Second World War. Yet in the first four decades of the century, some of the rhetoric had already begun to recede. In the early twentieth century, there was a trend away from the collection of anthropometric measurements.[140] By the 1940s, commentaries on the moral nature of the living environment would become more rare. And while venereal disease remained a concern, the discovery and widespread availability of penicillin after the war meant that some forms, such as gonorrhea, could now be treated.[141]

Two new issues – tuberculosis and mental health – would come to dominate the discourse of health experts, and indeed were already beginning to do so in the 1930s and 1940s. These new issues would shape, and reflect, the organization of medical practice. They also reveal the changing ideology regarding character formation within the university and society at large – developments we'll return to in chapters 7 and 8. Yet there is one more aspect of the growing concern about student health that must first be considered: the new occupational and personal opportunities it provided to female professionals.

5

Female Students' Health and the Creation of New Occupational Opportunities for Women

As university administrators established residences, created programs in physical training, introduced medical examinations, and set up infirmaries, they found that they needed individuals to oversee these new areas. As a result, positions opened up that in particular provided enticing work opportunities for women. Historians have documented the employment of academic women.[1] But there was another group of emerging professionals on campus – members of the non-academic staff, such as deans of women, doctors, nurses, physical-training instructors, and dieticians.[2] Together they comprised a small, but significant, presence on the university campus. This chapter focuses on women's professional work at Victoria College, University of Toronto, supplemented by the experience of women at some of the other universities under consideration.[3] It examines the kind of space they created for themselves and the female students under their care.

The Personnel

From the 1900s to the 1940s, Victoria employed a number of women to fill key positions within the women's residence, Annesley Hall, and its various annexes. Many have already appeared in these pages. Deans of women were Margaret Addison, 1902–30, with Marjory Curlette serving as acting dean from 1917–18; Dr Norma Ford, 1931–4; and Dr Jessie Macpherson, 1934–63.[4] The university hired four doctors through this period: Lelia Davis, 1902–10; Helen MacMurchy, 1910–13; Edna Guest 1920–32; and Marion Hilliard, from 1932 to the early 1940s. The roster of women who filled the positions of physical-training instructor, nurse, and dietician, changed fairly regularly. Prior to the war, some of the more prominent physical-training instructors were Emma Scott Raff and Mary G. Hamilton and, in the mid-1930s, Dorothy Jackson. Nurses included Marion L. Clark, 1913–17; Gladys E. Phelps, 1925–32; and Alison Maitland, 1932–41. Housekeepers/dieticians were Mina Richardson, director of the household, 1904–13; Helen G. Reid, dietician, 1913; and Jessie Elliott, house director and dietician for the years 1913–20 and 1922–41.

These women generally had significant credentials. Margaret Addison received a BA from Victoria College in 1889, the sixth woman to do so at that institution. After graduation she taught mathematics and chemistry at the Ontario Ladies' College for two years. She then obtained her high school teaching certificate from the Toronto School of Pedagogy, after which she taught French and German at Stratford Collegiate Institute and later at Lindsay Collegiate Institute before taking up her position at Victoria.[5] Marjory Curlette graduated from Trinity College in 1900 and had been principal of Westbourne School in Toronto.[6] Norma Ford received a PhD in Entomology from the University of Toronto in 1923 and in that year became the first female faculty member in the department of biology.[7] Jessie Macpherson received her BA from the University of Toronto in 1923. She acted as the girls' work secretary for the Ontario Religious Council as well as director of the Canadian Girls' In Training Camp Council in Ontario prior to her appointment at Victoria College.[8] In 1945, she became the first female faculty member in the department of philosophy at the University of Toronto.[9]

All of the physicians had graduated from the University of Toronto: Lelia Davis in 1889, Helen MacMurchy in 1901, Edna Guest in 1910, and Marion Hilliard in 1927. They all had local family practices and in addition held a variety of other posts. For example, while Lelia Davis acted as medical examiner at Victoria, she also held that position at the Margaret Eaton School from 1904 to 1907 and was lecturer in histology at the Ontario Medical College for Women prior to its closure in 1906.[10] MacMurchy, hired in 1910, was the first woman appointed to the department of obstetrics and gynaecology at Toronto General Hospital. From 1902 to 1905, she taught anatomy at the Ontario Medical College for Women, and from 1904 to 1906 was instructor of anatomy and physiology as well as examining physician at the Toronto Conservatory of Music. She helped found Women's College Hospital in 1911, and acted as medical inspector of Toronto schools in 1910–11. In 1920, she was appointed to the Federal Department of Health's Child Welfare Division.[11]

MacMurchy's successor, Edna Guest, not only acted as physician to women at Victoria from 1920 to 1932 but was also the first medical adviser for women at McMaster in the 1920s.[12] Guest completed postgraduate work at Harvard, interned at the Women's and Children's Hospital in Boston, and then held the position of professor of anatomy and assistant in surgery at the women's medical college in Ludhiana, India from 1912 to 1915. During the First World War, she had charge of a base hospital in Corsica and saw active service in France. She was appointed head of the special department of venereal disease at Women's College Hospital in 1919 and became chief of surgery there in 1926. In 1940–1, she became president of the Federation of Medical Women of Canada.[13] Guest's successor, Marion Hilliard, joined the staff of the Women's College Hospital in 1928, specializing in obstetrics and gynecology and becoming chief of that department in 1947. She became well known for her publications on women's health, work popularized through several books as well as articles in *Chatelaine* magazine. In 1955–6, she held the position of president of the Federation of Medical Women of Canada.[14] Thus Hilliard, like the other female physicians hired by Victoria College, had a wide range of medical experience.

The physical-training instructors employed at Victoria equally became leaders in their field. As we saw in chapter 3, Emma Scott Raff had a significant impact on the field of physical education through the creation of the Margaret Eaton School, at which most of the other instructors at Victoria worked. Hamilton went on to be a leader in the camp movement, as did Dorothy Jackson, a member of the department of physical education at the University of Toronto.[15] Many of the nurses also had a fair degree of training. Marion Clark received her diploma from Clifton Spring Sanitarium in 1904 and her RN certification from New York State. In 1914, Gladys Phelps also graduated from Clifton Spring Sanitarium, receiving her RN certification from New York State in 1915 and from Ontario in 1925. She held the post of resident nurse at Cornell College, Iowa, from 1920 to 1923 and superintendent of the Wellesley College infirmary from 1923 to 1925.[16]

Unlike most of the deans, physicians, and physical-training instructors, the first woman who oversaw the daily running of the residence and dining room had few formal credentials. Mina Richardson had been a teacher in Peterborough for fifteen years and in addition had run her mother's household, which included a servant and some boarders. In her letter of introduction, Richardson informed Addison that if she received the appointment she would complete "the Housekeeper's Course in Domestic Science so as to be fully competent to fill the position."[17] When Richardson retired in 1913, the committee of management searched for a trained dietician, settling on Mrs. Helen G. Reid. Reid's successor, Jessie Elliott, who remained at Victoria for most of the period from 1913 to 1941, was a graduate of the faculty of household science.

Obtaining Work

Employment opportunities became available to these women in the early twentieth century when university authorities saw the need to staff newly built residences and ensure the morality and health of students. Those positions then reopened for a variety of reasons: doctors tended to resign as they became more senior within the hospital system. Some nurses and dieticians left due to upcoming marriages. A number of women vacated positions as a result of illness. Other women resigned to discharge their responsibilities to sick family members. And some women remained with the college for many years, vacating their position only when they retired.[18]

Women obtained positions at Victoria in a variety of ways. Physicians tended to be recommended by their predecessors. For example, Lelia Davis put forward the name of her friend Helen MacMurchy.[19] Hilliard had helped Guest perform the student medical examinations for several years and had filled in for Guest for a year prior to her own appointment. The dean of women also approached local experts for advice. While a number of dieticians applied for the vacant position in 1913, the residence committee of management settled on a recommendation made by Annie Laird, head of the faculty of household science.[20] That faculty had its origins in initiatives by Methodist women connected to Victoria and was located next to the residence building. Moreover, Laird had a number of personal connections with Victoria's administrators.[21] The subsequent dietician, Jessie Elliott, was known to Victoria administrators, having first worked at Victoria as a housekeeper and then obtained training in the faculty of household science. Other women heard informally about the opening of a position and then approached officials. For example, in 1904 Mina Richardson wrote to Margaret Addison, after hearing from an acquaintance whose daughter boarded at Annesley that the current director of the household had announced her engagement.[22]

The women hired often had some personal connection either to Victoria itself or to the Methodist (or after 1925 United) Church. Emma

Scott Raff had the support of leading Methodists connected with Victoria. Margaret Eaton, of a Methodist family, gave both her name and some financial support to Scott Raff's school of physical culture. Nathanael Burwash, president of Victoria from 1887 to 1913, and his wife, Margaret, not only socialized with the Eatons but were close friends of Scott Raff's father. They both supported Scott Raff's work financially. In addition, from 1906 to 1918, Nathanael Burwash was a member of the board of directors of the Margaret Eaton School. So too, for a year in the mid-1920s, was R.P. Bowles, Burwash's successor as president of the college. Moreover, Margaret Burwash belonged to the Victoria Women's Residence and Education Association the year that it hired Scott Raff, while Nathanael Burwash sponsored her application.[23]

Margaret Addison was similarly well connected. She had graduated from Victoria College. She was the first president of the alumnae association, established in 1898, in part in order to raise funds for the creation of a women's residence at Victoria. She was well acquainted with Margaret and Nathanael Burwash. While teaching in Lindsay, Addison and other local women formed the Lindsay Ladies' Physical Culture Association. Through her contact with Margaret Burwash, Addison secured Scott Raff to provide a number of lessons each week.[24]

Although having less illustrious connections, some of the other women also had personal ties to Victoria. Helen MacMurchy not only had Lelia Davis's endorsement but was friends with Margaret Addison.[25] Marion Hilliard had lived in residence as a student at Victoria from 1920 to 1924. She had the support of Edna Guest, the previous medical attendant, and was friends with Jessie Macpherson, the dean at the time of her appointment. Macpherson and Hilliard had attended the University of Toronto at the same time and had both been active in campus athletics as well as the Student Christian Movement.[26] Mina Richardson, who heard about the vacancy of the housekeeping position through the daughter of a friend attending Annesley, was a Methodist and ran a Sunday school class. She also had a deceased brother who had been a minister in Toronto. Marion Clark, who obtained the position of residence nurse in 1913, was a cousin of Mrs. A. E. Lang, a member of the residence committee of management. Clark also knew Mary Rowell, instructor in French at Wesley College, Winnipeg, who promised to write to her sister-in-law, Nellie Rowell, also a member of the residence committee of management. In addition, Clark's brother-in-law, James Elliott, a professor of philosophy at Wesley College, was an old friend of Addison's and wrote to the dean on Clark's behalf. Gladys Phelps, who was hired as a nurse in 1925, also knew Addison personally.[27]

In general, then, women usually obtained positions through their connections to administrators or employees of the university, their personal relationships to the institution as alumnae, their membership in the Methodist or United Church, or some combination of these. Personal relationships thus facilitated these women's access to employment, which in turn provided them with opportunities to fulfil professional goals and ambitions. Once established, professional women drew on their connections to fill new positions, thereby providing opportunities for like-minded women. While some women benefitted from their relationship with prominent men, it is clear that female networks and kin ties played a key role in women's obtaining employment.

Salaries

Once hired, non-academic women generally received a significant salary. By the early 1920s, the deans, medical advisers, and the senior physical-training instructors connected to Victoria College and the University of Toronto earned roughly between $1,800 and $2,500 a year, nurses received $75 to $100 a month for the school year, and dieticians were paid $100 a month. Deans, nurses, and some physical-training instructors and dieticians also received free room and board.[28] These rates seem to approximate those at Canadian and leading American institutions.[29] By the late 1930s and early 1940s, the salary for the University of Toronto medical adviser, whose duties included the supervision of Victoria students, ranged anywhere from $3,000 to $5,000, depending on level of experience and seniority.[30] That of physical-training instructors, nurses and dieticians, had increased modestly by $200 to $500 annually, with the senior physical-training instructors at Toronto and elsewhere earning $2,400 to $3,000 a year; dieticians, $125 a month; and nurses, $100 to $120 a month.[31] Not surprisingly the salary scale matched the administrative hierarchy of the institution. Deans of women and doctors received the most, followed by physical-training instructors, dieticians, and then nurses. All of the former received significantly more than maids or janitors did.[32]

The rates for the deans, physicians, and physical instructors seem comparable to those of at least some academic women at the time.[33] According to the 1931 census, this placed them in the top 3 to 4 per cent of female wage and salary earners. Dieticians too fared well, placing within the top 17 per cent of female wage earners, while nurses fell just below. In comparison to male salaries and wages, these occupational groups also did well. Deans, medical advisers and physical-training instructors placed at the lower end of the top 20 per cent of male wage earners. At just over $900 a year (plus room and board) for nurses, and $1,200 for dieticians, these women fell into the same category as male skilled workers and clerical workers, who earned between $950 and $1,450 and who comprised the top 40 per cent of male wage earners.[34] Well-credentialed and experienced, many of the non-academic staff under consideration earned a good wage or salary.

However, while these women earned a significant income for the time, they also experienced gender inequities. Historians have demonstrated that professional women, like female workers more generally, held subordinate positions to, and received less income than, their male counterparts. In the late 1920s, the director of women's physical training at the University of Toronto earned $1,000 less than the male gymnasium director.[35] Similarly, in the late 1930s and early 1940s, female medical advisers earned between $2,000 and $3,000 less than the directors of the university health service.[36] It is clear that because women held subordinate positions to men they also earned less. It is possible, however, that there may have been greater gender parity in the case of men and women holding lesser positions, something historians examining other occupations have discovered.[37] For example, in the mid-1920s, the University of Toronto hired both a male and female physical-training instructor for work among female students at a rate of $1,200 each.[38] Similarly, in 1948–9, the health service employed four male doctors at $1,800 each for eight months and two female physicians, one for nine months at $2,250 and one for seven months at $1,750.[39]

While gender inequities clearly existed, both women and men profited from the creation of new occupations related to student welfare. For women in particular, these new occupations formed part of the broader growth of women's professional and white-collar work within universities, as these institutions expanded.[40] It marked too what Peter Baskerville has referred to as a "silent revolution," beginning in the late nineteenth century, of women's increasing participation in their own business affairs.[41] In general, both within the academic stream and outside it, women held positions of lower rank and pay than men. At the same time, considering women's opportunities at the time, these positions also offered a handful of women significant income and financial stability.

Conditions of Employment

As well as seeking women with excellent professional credentials, university administrators stressed the need for employees of good character. What they sought were not just efficient administrators, doctors, nurses, and dieticians, but also female role models. Here religious participation proved key. A liberal Protestant atmosphere pervaded the college. Chapel, though not mandatory, was a feature of daily life. Administrators expected students to attend church on Sunday. Grace was said at dinner. And a significant number of students attended the meetings of the YWCA and later the Student Christian Movement. The members of the residence committee of management made their religious expectations explicit when they hired Marion Clark as nurse in 1913, in part, because they felt she could "contribute to the evangelical side" of residence life.[42] So too did Margaret Addison, who described one of the duties of the dean in the following way: "Through a council of her staff and through her own personal efforts, to keep a Christian spirit which will make the residents believe in the possibility of the existence of the Kingdom of God upon earth now."[43] Equally, Edna Guest had impeccable religious credentials, having been a medical missionary in India from 1912 to 1915.[44] As a student, Marion Hilliard was president of the medical students' branch of the campus Student Christian Movement.[45] And both Emma Scott Raff and Mary Hamilton "strongly endorsed tenets of Christian social reform."[46]

Religious requirements were limited neither to Victoria nor to the interwar period. In the early 1950s, the form letter created by administrators at University College for applicants for the position of dietician included questions such as "Church affiliation if any and do you attend?" and "How much do you smoke? Drink?" One applicant appropriately answered that she attended the United Church and neither drank nor smoked.[47] Similarly, historians have documented the way in which nurses' status and legitimacy was built on an ideal of feminine respectability based on middle-class Anglo-Christian ideals. During training, they lived in hospital residences with strict rules and regulations, often much stricter than those in university residences, and in which Christian rituals formed part of the daily routine.[48] As a result, they would have been accustomed to the rhythm and nature of residence life.

Beyond their own personal moral attributes, university officials expected their employees to provide moral and intellectual leadership and to help oversee residence life. Nurses, for example, were not only responsible for the supervision of the infirmary and sanitation of the residence but were also expected to "guard the health of the student." This included visiting students' rooms every day, watching students' weight, ensuring students took exercise, overseeing students' personal hygiene, and teaching them "the laws of health."[49] They, along with doctors, formed part of the dean's council, meeting together with dons and the dean of women to discuss and advise on the running of the residence.[50] As we saw in the last chapter, doctors often joined forces with the dean of women, giving, to the more mature female students, special talks on such issues as "the origin of life," venereal disease, and eugenics.

University administrators also required that these women be of upstanding character because many lived full-time in residence and thus had significant contact with, and influence over, students. Physicians spent the least amount of time on campus. They performed medical examinations in fall, would return if called, and gave some lectures. Deans, nurses, and dietitians spent considerably more time in residence. The fact that they both lived and worked on site had specific implications for both the nature of their working conditions and their private lives.

For all of the women under consideration, employment brought a fair amount of independence. When Marion Clark applied to be a nurse she was in her forties. She had been helping her sister out for two years, looking after her child. Prior to her arrival at Victoria, Mina Richardson was gainfully employed as a teacher but also living at home, looking after her sick mother.[51] For women such as Clark and Richardson, work in a residential institution provided freedom from both family obligations and dependence on family members.

Yet if employment offered financial and familial independence, it also involved a significant lack of privacy and free time. The residential setting made it difficult for staff to separate on-duty and off-duty time. This was particularly true for the dean of women, who oversaw the running of the entire institution. Yet administrators also expected staff to contribute to activities beyond the narrow definition of their job description. In 1907, for example, the residence committee of management requested that Mina Richardson, the housekeeper, and Emma Scott Raff, the physical-training instructor, both of whom lived in residence, "share equally with Miss Addison the responsibility of sitting up at night for late comers."[52] Scott Raff attempted to extricate herself from this duty, reporting to the committee of management that her doctor forbade her to work after 6 p.m. Her efforts, however, came to naught.[53]

Similarly, nurses had no regular hours. Like private-duty nurses, they had a half day off every week as well as alternate Sundays off.[54] The dean of women, in consultation with the medical adviser, could grant the nurse an occasional long weekend "when she shows fatigue."[55] The nurse was also "allowed leave from the infirmary at times other than her prescribed time off, provided that someone else is on call in the building, and that the nurse be easily available."[56] Nurses may have gradually gained greater freedom. For example, in 1945–6 the nurse at the University of Manitoba had twenty-four hours off each week as well as the occasional evening away from residence.[57]

Given the long hours required of many of these women, and the fact that they often lived in residence, it is not surprising that administrators also expected that they remain single. At Victoria, this was not a written regulation so much as a commonly held assumption. In the 1920s, for example, two nurses and a dietician worked for several years at Victoria, but resigned prior to marriage.[58] The impulse to hire only single women became much stronger during the economic depression of the 1930s. During an interview in the 1970s, Mossie May Waddington Kirkwood revealed that she felt obliged to resign as dean of women at University College as a result of the hostility towards married women holding jobs.[59] The tendency in the interwar years to employ only single women and the hostility that even some single women encountered as workers was common on campus and off, in Canada and throughout much of the Anglo-British world.[60]

While employment on campus generally remained restricted to single women, during periods of labour shortage, administrators made some accommodation for female heads-of-household and their families. For example, when they employed their first dietician, Helen Reid, they found rooms for not only Reid, but also her two daughters. Similarly, Miss Morris, dietician from 1920 to 1922, had responsibility for her elderly mother. In order to secure Morris, university administrators provided both women with room, board, and laundry at a rate of nine dollars a week.[61]

Although employment at Victoria provided women with some independence and financial stability, staff members still held their positions at the behest of the university with little recourse if they ran into difficulties. When, in 1914, Helen Reid found herself at odds with both Margaret Addison and many of the female residents, she lost her position.[62] Margaret Addison in turn found herself in difficulties several years later. In 1920, Victoria undertook a reorganization of the administration of

Annesley Hall. Although promoted to dean of women, for a couple of years Addison was forced to vacate her residence rooms, which she had occupied for seventeen years.[63]

At the same time, loyal employees could find themselves rewarded for their extra efforts. During epidemics, for example, some of the heaviest responsibility for caring for students fell on the shoulders of residence staff, such as the dean of women and the head housekeeper. University officials did at times recognize the additional burden placed on these women. After the first outbreak of influenza in 1918, the dean of women received three weeks' vacation to recover. Similarly, Miss Elliott, the house director, who had been short of help during the epidemic, and who had had to attend to all the cooking herself, was given a bonus of twenty-five dollars, this at a time when her salary was approximately a hundred dollars a month.[64] As with any other job, then, the beneficence or truculence of senior administrators could significantly affect non-academic staff.

Women's Networks

If employment at Victoria did not offer complete independence, it did allow female administrators and health experts a means of carving out a space for themselves and other women on campus. They did so by creating women's networks on a number of different levels: in the residence, on campus, and through national and international organizations. Within residence, professional women encountered others of like mind. At Victoria, the dean was responsible to a female committee of management, which brought her into contact with the Methodist elite of Toronto. She also worked in close association with the physicians and instructors in physical education and thus regularly met and interacted with other prominent professionals living in the area.

In addition to figures such as the dean or physician, administrators at Victoria also employed dons to oversee the various houses of the residence system and to act as role models. These included university graduates, often early in their careers or finishing up graduate degrees.[65] These positions widened the network of female intellectuals on campus. For example, Clara Clinkscale held a position as don from 1913 to 1915. A 1912 graduate who had been top of her class in mathematics and physics, Clinkscale held the position of don while teaching at a local private girl's collegiate school. In 1918, Mary Rowell became residence head. A graduate of 1898, she had been dean of women and instructor in French

at Wesley College in Winnipeg. In 1919, she became the first permanent
female member of the department of French at Victoria. Beginning in
1921, Gertrude Rutherford held the position of general head of Annesley Hall, resigning in 1923 to become travelling secretary for the Student
Christian Movement of Canada.[66]

In the mid-1920s, students at Victoria had dons such as Ruth Jenkins,
a fellow in the department of classics; Constance Chappell, who had
taught at Christian College, Tokyo; and Dorothy Forward, who graduated at the top of her class in biology and held a fellowship in botany at
the University of Toronto. Similarly, in the early 1930s staff and students
came into contact with Kathleen Coburn, a graduate student and future
faculty member in the department of English; Jean Fraser, an instructor
in the department of biology; Rose Beatty, a YWCA secretary; Dr Florence Smith, a member of the staff in the department of English; Kathleen Hung, a teacher at Harbord Collegiate Institute; Blanche Snell, a
teacher at York Memorial Collegiate Institute; and Dorothy Bishop, a
graduate student in the department of history.[67]

The relationship between dons and the professional women at Victoria is generally unknown. Although grateful for the work, Kathleen
Coburn found herself enforcing rules she didn't agree with. But she
also formed a lifelong acquaintance with Addison. Still, much like the
students, the dons remained in training. In 1932 the dean of women,
Dr Norma Ford, wrote,

> We are hoping that the work involved in a donship may give to each woman
> such experience and poise as may enable her to step into positions of
> greater responsibility elsewhere. To meet this end the dons will share some
> of the responsibilities with the dean and warden, such as the formal duties
> of presiding at dinner and pouring coffee afterwards, of taking prayers, of
> chaperoning various college parties, etc.[68]

Clearly, Ford saw the position of don as one that could provide learning
experience and leadership skills to recent graduates. At the same time,
it offered deans and others contact with emerging female scholars and
young professionals.

Through residence work, and an interest in women's issues, professionals at Victoria College became acquainted with their counterparts
at other colleges on campus. Deans of women met to compare notes on
their institutions and suggest solutions to campus problems. For example, concerned about the lack of athletic facilities available to women on

campus, professional women, along with faculty members, established a Women's Building Committee in 1928. Proponents of women's athletics had, for some time, raised concerns about lack of opportunities for physical activity on campus. As far back as 1914, Margaret Addison, Mary Hamilton, and Ivy Coventry, the first directress of athletics and physical training at the University of Toronto, among others, had discussed the need for courses in physical education.[69] The opening, in 1919, of Hart House, an athletic and social facility reserved for men, reinforced the discrimination female students faced. Women would not gain their own, modern, gymnasium until 1959. Even then, it compared poorly to the Hart House facilities.[70] Yet, despite the lengthy, and what must have been discouraging, process of advocating for women's facilities, through the years the Women's Building Committee included prominent academics, deans and athletic directors such as Jessie Macpherson; Mossie May Waddington Kirkwood; and Ivy Coventry; along with Marion Ferguson, dean of women at University College; Clara Benson, a member of the faculty of household science; and A.E.M. Parkes, secretary-treasurer of the University of Toronto Women's Athletic Association.[71]

Deans and physicians at Victoria also forged other university networks. They participated in the activities of the University Women's Club, founded in 1903. The members of the club organized social events, lectures, and reform activities. For example, they investigated the local conditions and wages of women workers and discussed housing and employment possibilities as well as the need to improve women's educational opportunities.[72] Margaret Addison and Helen MacMurchy both attended club meetings. Indeed, in the early decades of the century, the group often met in the women's residence at Victoria.[73] Through membership, Addison and MacMurchy socialized with other campus women such as Clara Benson, Edith Gordon, and Mabel Cartwright, a graduate of Lady Margaret Hall, Oxford, and dean of women at Trinity College from 1903 to 1936. Membership also brought them into contact with prominent graduates such as Edith Elwood, an 1896 graduate of Trinity College, a founding member of the club, and, from 1905 to 1914, head worker at Evangelia House, one of the local settlement houses.[74]

These women also helped create, and participated in, alumnae associations. Addison, for example, cofounded the Victoria Alumnae Association. These types of associations proved forceful tools in women's efforts to establish equal space on campus. While building and working through separate women's organizations, as was common at the time, they fought any notion that women should receive an education that was separate from, and possibly inferior to, that of men. Thus in 1909, when the University of Toronto Senate established a committee to investigate the possibility of creating a separate women's college, Toronto women banded together, creating the United Alumnae Association in order to fight the proposal. Members included Margaret Addison, Marjory Curlette, Helen MacMurchy, Mabel Cartwright, and Clara Benson.[75] Similarly, women at McGill used their alumnae association as a vehicle for women's issues, from pressuring various departments to admit women to creating alumnae scholarships.[76]

In addition to their campus activities, many of the non-academic staff and their acquaintances also joined off-campus professional organizations and associations. In 1922, Margaret Addison travelled to Chicago with Mary Bollert, dean of women at UBC, to attend the meetings of the National Association of Women Deans, an American professional society for deans of women established in 1916.[77] In 1924, Helen MacMurchy and Maude Abbott, a leading medical researcher in Montreal, founded the Canadian Federation of Medical Women.[78] Hilliard became president of the federation as well as both vice-president and president of the Medical Women's International Association.[79] Similarly, the women with whom the staff interacted on campus were leaders in their own field. Annie Laird was a founding member of the American Dietetic Association in 1917, the Ontario Dietetic Association in 1926, and the Canadian Dietetic Association in 1935. Clara Benson was a founding member of the Canadian Institute of Chemistry in 1919.[80] Women at other campuses created similar professional organizations. Ethel Cartwright, for example, helped found the Women's Amateur Athletic Federation of Canada and became the first president of the Canadian Massage Association.[81]

Many of the women employed at Victoria also provided leadership and inspiration through their United Church–related youth activities. A number played active roles in the YWCA at the national and international level.[82] In 1927, prior to her appointment as dean, Jessie Macpherson was director of the Canadian Girls' In Training Camp Council, which included among the staff leaders her friend Mary Rowell.[83] At different times, Addison, Guest, and Hilliard all attended the United Church's annual student conferences held in Muskoka. In one of her reports, Guest noted her disappointment at being unable to accompany Margaret Addison to the meeting that year. She argued, that "to do the best educative medical work with our modern young teen age students, one must know their minds as well as their bodies, and these conferences more or less planned and managed by themselves, and held in the midst of the wild and free Muskoka beauty invite the frankest expression of what is in their minds ..."[84]

Hilliard also brought her influence to bear at other campuses. In 1940–1, she attended a Student Christian Mission in Winnipeg. Doris Saunders, the dean of junior women at the University of Manitoba, reported, "I was particularly impressed by the delight experienced in the talks of Dr Marion Hilliard to the women students on the Broadway campus. The desire they expressed for more knowledge of a medical and ethical kind suggests that these talks might, with advantage, be followed by others given by Winnipeg women doctors."[85]

Some women also joined their Local Council of Women. Lelia Davis addressed an early meeting in Toronto, speaking to 3,000 women on the topic of "The Conditions of the Unemployed," which ultimately resulted in the opening of a Civic Employment Bureau.[86] Edna Guest became vice-president of the National Council of Women.[87] Deans and physicians elsewhere also became prominent members of their locals. For example, Ethel Hurlbatt, warden of Royal Victoria College, McGill, from 1906 to 1929, along with other influential graduates, became involved in the Montreal Local Council of Women's protests against the 1914 decision of the Quebec Supreme Court refusing to allow Annie Langstaff to sit the bar exam.[88]

The creation of, and participation in, women's campus organizations such as the Women's Athletic Association, the Building Committee, the University Women's Club, alumnae associations, as well as other off-campus professional and religious organizations, forms part of a broader North American pattern of women's associational life that dates at least to the early nineteenth century. By the late nineteenth century, women's and religious groups, infused by Christian idealism, began to develop international networks to bridge national divides and support each other in common aims.[89] The women under consideration likewise participated in these international associations and gatherings, in the process forging connections with women at other campuses. In 1912, Addison attended the World YWCA's conference in Swanwick, England, and represented the United Alumnae of the University of Toronto at the Congress of the Universities of the British Empire.[90] One of the sessions at that congress was on "The Position of Women in Universities." Addison addressed attendees at that session at the urging of Ethel Hurlbatt, who had spoken earlier in the program.[91] In 1922, Addison attended the World YWCA's conference in St. Wolfgang, Austria, at which she was a voting delegate along with both Nellie and Mary Rowell.[92] She also attended the meetings of the International Federation of University Women in Paris. Similarly, as president of the Canadian Federation of University Women from 1926 to 1928, Mary Bollert attended the meetings of the International Federation of University Women held in 1924 in Paris, in 1929 in Geneva, and in 1932 in Edinburgh.[93] Allie Vibert Douglas, dean of women at Queen's University from 1939 to 1959, was also active in the International Federation of University Women.[94] Moreover, as Leila Rupp notes, involvement in one group often brought women into contact with the work of other groups. For example, in 1925 the International Council of Women created the Joint Standing Committee of the Women's International Organizations to bring together a number of groups, such as the World YWCA and the International Federation of University Women, to advocate for a female appointee to the League of Nations.[95] Thus by participating in one organization, women often became aware of the larger international women's movement.

Educated women not only forged professional networks, but also developed supportive personal relationships. Addison and Bollert travelled together. Scott Raff and Hamilton became close friends and drew into their circle Dora Mavor, a graduate of the Margaret Eaton School who would become a leading Canadian actor and theatre director. Mavor not only helped Hamilton create an outdoor theatre at her girls' camp in Algonquin Park, but also assisted with theatrical productions during summers from the 1930s to the 1950s. Through her camp work, Hamilton formed friendships with other female camp operators such as Mary S. Edgar and Ferna Halliday.[96] Similarly, Annie Laird travelled regularly to Europe and the United States in the company of her sister, Elizabeth Laird, a physicist at Mount Holyoke in the 1920s and 1930s, to attend conferences and keep apprised of work in nutritional sciences.[97] Jessie Macpherson and Kathleen Coburn bought a small island in Georgian Bay, where they built a cottage and summered together.[98] Others developed lifelong partnerships. For example, Marion Hilliard lived with Opal Boynton, a social worker. Dorothy Forward, a don at Victoria College in the mid-1920s, later shared living accommodations with Elizabeth Allin. Both were members of the department of physics at the University of Toronto from the 1930s to the 1960s. Some of these relationships were platonic and others romantic, but all provided these women with both financial and emotional support.[99]

Supporting Female Students

Female students often benefitted directly from the formation of women's campus networks. Within residence, professional women acted as mentors for, and supervisors of, the young women under their care. The residence hall was much more than a place to sleep and eat. Administrators believed residence life could contribute to the moral and intellectual formation of residents.[100] Addison, for example, aided women's intellectual development by bringing in speakers of local, national, and international prominence, such as the head of Toronto's Women's Court, Dr Margaret Patterson; social reformer J.S. Woodsworth; suffragist Emmeline Pankhurst; and birth control activist Dr Marie Stopes.[101] In doing so, she encouraged in students an awareness of public events, local social conditions, current intellectual trends, and their future economic and professional opportunities.

Professional women also supported students in other ways. For example, not only did a number of these women at Toronto fight for better athletic facilities, they also took a direct role in promoting women's athletics. Female patrons of the Women's Athletic Association, such as Scott Raff and Addison, fostered a competitive spirit by providing athletic trophies for winning teams in a variety of sports.[102] Similarly, Dr Edna Guest provided the women's athletic board at McMaster University with a trophy to be awarded to a female athlete.[103] At the University of Toronto, deans of women and academic women, such as Mossie May Waddington Kirkwood and Clara Benson, acted as faculty advisers on the Women's Athletic Association Directorate.[104] For others, such as A.E.M. Parkes, Ivy Coventry, and Edith Gordon, support for women's athletics flowed naturally from their employment at the university.[105] These women nurtured programs for students such as Marion Hilliard and Jessie Macpherson, presidents in the 1920s of the tennis and gymnasium clubs respectively, both of whom in turn became leading members of the campus and wider community and of various professions.[106]

Professional women also created a variety of scholarships. Hilliard established one for needy students at Victoria College, while Edith Gordon did so at the University of Toronto.[107] This type of action was true of women elsewhere. Indeed, one of the ways that academic women and university graduates supported female students in the early twentieth century was through the creation of scholarships. For example, the Canadian Federation of University Women, founded in 1910, quickly established a travelling scholarship for study in Britain, which allowed numerous women to embark on studies that they would not otherwise have been able to pursue.[108] Similarly, Wilhelmina Gordon, a member of the department of English at Queen's University in the interwar years, together with Mary Bollert, adviser of women at UBC and instructor in English, established the Imperial Order Daughters of the Empire's War Memorial Scholarship, which aided students pursuing graduate degrees in Britain.[109]

In creating scholarships, supporting athletics, and developing lecture series, professional women at Victoria and elsewhere sought to enrich students' lives and extend their social and intellectual opportunities on campus. In doing so, they acted as role models and offered support. Historian Karine Hébert has shown that as female students at McGill and the University of Montreal gained entrance into these institutions in 1884 and 1908 respectively, their integration into student activities was slow and their full integration as students rather than "co-eds" remained incomplete as late as the 1960s.[110] Many of the professional women employed by Victoria College and other institutions had themselves attended university, knew first-hand the difficulties female students faced, and aimed to encourage their educational endeavours.

Visions of Womanhood

If the women considered here developed networks with one another to pursue political aims, enhance job opportunities, and encourage female students in their studies, they did so within specific bounds. British and North American administrators hired physicians, deans, and physical educators for the very conservative roles of monitoring and protecting the health and morals of female students and shaping womanhood. The professional women under consideration perceived the university as the last chance to correct and catch problems unseen by a school system that failed to inspect and train students physically or educate them regarding health matters. They also saw the university as the final site in which to mould young women who, they believed, were not yet fully formed – mentally, physically, or spiritually.

Yet shaping womanhood was never simply a conservative endeavour. The women hired envisaged students as playing a role in individual and social improvement and regeneration and perceived it as their responsibility to ensure that students would be able to undertake the duties of citizenship. Progressive ideals counterposed conservative realities. For example, on the one hand, Addison boldly introduced a form of self-government into residence life in 1906. On the other hand, she was responsible for her charges and felt the weight of that responsibility. In 1905 she, along with the deans at Trinity and University Colleges, felt there was too much campus socialization and thus petitioned the university to limit campus social functions.[111] Similarly, professional women supported women's athletics and physical culture, but did so within existing norms that reinforced notions of female difference.

In the 1920s and 1930s, professional women also saw women's primary responsibilities as being those of mother and volunteer. They continued to emphasize late-nineteenth-century notions of female difference and women's nurturing instinct.[112] As historians have found, the importance of health and education was often stressed in relation to motherhood and citizenship. In 1923, Edith Gordon, medical adviser to women at Toronto, gave a talk to teachers on "Physical Training for Girls." She argued that physical education was more important for girls than boys, because girls were the "future mothers of Canada."[113] Most of the administrators and health experts also emphasized female difference. Wendy Mitchinson notes of Marion Hilliard that she worked within the "medical world she inhabited" and "the limits provided by that perspective." Hilliard, like many other men and women at the time, understood women as being defined by their bodies, saw marriage as a natural goal, and accepted the patriarchal household.[114]

Yet professional women's ideas about marriage and motherhood in these decades also underwent change. Paul Axelrod notes for the 1930s that while the ideal of "the successful housewife and mother" remained dominant in the interwar years, it counterposed the model of "the accomplished professional or businesswoman."[115] This shift in rhetoric could already be seen in student newspapers in the 1920s. In that decade, students still debated women's role in society, and newspaper articles still reflected unease with the notion of the educated woman, in particular on the part of male students. Yet increasingly, some articles endorsed women's rights to a career over motherhood.[116] The public discourse of some professional women also reflected this shift. In the interwar years, Geneva Misener, professor of classics at the University of Alberta and an adviser to women students, argued that women should combine marriage and professional development.[117] Alison Mackinnon argues for the Australian context that by the 1930s women began to "challenge the belief that marriage meant abandonment of paid work, support for husband's careers, and dedication to child-rearing."[118] This occurred in Canada too. In 1931, when the University of Toronto board of governors expressed disapproval of hiring married women, the Canadian Federation of University Women, the University Women's Club, and the various alumni associations all protested the policy.[119] In the early 1930s, Mabel Thom, president of the Canadian Federation of University Women opposed the dismissal of married women from the labour force. The Canadian Federation of Business and Professional Women equally opposed discrimination on the basis of marital status.[120] In the late 1930s, Mossie Mae Waddington Kirkwood wrote of women's financial and emotional need for work outside the home.[121] In her book, *For College Women ... and Men*, she focused one chapter on "Women's Right to Work," advocating equal pay for equal work and repudiating discrimination against women working. Kirkwood emphasized men and women's equality as human beings and as such the need for both to work, broadly defined, be it as homemaker or in paid employment. She argued, "Work releases energy, absorbs body or mind or both, gives deep satisfaction to the worker when the work promotes or serves the purposes of life in any way, gives hope for the future, makes life significant."[122] Such views gained increasing resonance. Although Hilliard argued in the early 1930s that women needed to choose between medicine and homemaking, by the 1950s she recognized the increasing numbers of married women in the workforce and supported their right to be there.[123] Moreover, if Hilliard's public pronouncements lagged behind those of some professional women, she was still progressive in her views. In her study of professional women in Manitoba, Mary Kinnear found that even as late as 1961 only 4 per cent of professional women married.[124]

These professional women, then, recognized societal emphases on women's roles as mothers yet never offered up marriage and motherhood as the only option available. At Victoria, they opened students' eyes to the range of occupations available to them, thereby offering a vision of economic independence.[125] Despite the links made by experts between overall female health and reproduction, professional women also equated female health with career success. Some physical educators emphasized the importance of physical training in order to "earn wages"[126] or more vaguely, as a "value to a citizen in whatever part of life he or she treads."[127] Similarly, female doctors recommended to younger women the need for "a strong mental and physical constitution" to sustain career performance.[128] In other words, a robust womanhood would see women through their life's work.

Conclusion

Why did professional women exude such mixed messages? The answer lies in the reality of their own professional lives and work, which were marked by both independence and social constraint. Victoria offered employment to a handful of female health professionals. It offered significant degrees of financial independence, personal fulfilment, and community networks. In creating women's networks and supporting women's activities these women in turn increased the space for women on campus. Yet they also faced constraints. Although many opportunities in higher education and the professions opened up to women, historians have shown that female students and faculty continued to face discrimination – from unequal access to social and athletic facilities as students, to the need on the part of most graduates to choose between career and marriage/motherhood, to lower pay and limited advancement as faculty.[129] Non-academic women on campus faced similar difficulties. In addition, their employment depended on adhering to the moral codes, both written and unwritten, of the university. Moreover, if this was a space that allowed a woman a room of her own at a time when many did not have that opportunity, that room came with a price – lack of privacy, the obligation to remain single, to be in good health, and to exhibit moral rectitude.

The mixed messages also reflected the structure of employment. The women under consideration obtained their positions because of general beliefs within the university that female students needed special care and protection – work appropriate for women. In her research on the education and careers of American female scientists, Margaret Rossiter refers to this as a territorially based form of sex segregation.[130] At the same time, there was also a hierarchical work structure, though unlike in the academic setting, one that gave some women power over others. The dean, physicians, and physical instructors spoke on women's issues from a sense of their expertise and authority. Nurses and dieticians ensured the daily workings of the residence and while their views and opinions could shape attitudes towards a particular student or the running of the household more generally, they offered few public statements. Thus women worked within structural constraints that shaped their beliefs and attitudes.

Still, despite certain constraints, these women were able to use existing notions of respectability, bolstered by their claims to expertise, to carve out space on campus for themselves. Historians in the United States have written of the rich worlds created by and for women in women's colleges.[131] This situation did not exist in Canada, where institutional survival required co-education. Yet there were places where that separatist strategy could be found. Wendy Mitchinson notes, of Toronto's Women's College Hospital, where most of Victoria's attending physicians practised, that it provided "a refuge – a supportive environment in which women physicians could practise and feel accepted."[132] The Margaret Eaton School allowed physical educators a similar space. Household science opened up an academic field to women while settlement houses offered women employment and community engagement.[133] Equally, women's residences at places such as Victoria, Trinity, and McGill, could be counted among such centres.[134] Within a residential college, some women could forge careers, often supported and promoted by other women. Moreover, in a large city such as Toronto, women could piece together a world for themselves by moving between these various institutions as well as building and participating in local, national, and international organizations.

Historians of women and higher education in Canada have argued that in the first half of the twentieth century academic women occupied a marginal position within universities. Indeed, historical work has focused on women's limited impact and isolation within these institutions.[135] For example, Mary Kinnear writes, "For all their actual shared experience, the women on faculty at the University of Manitoba before 1970 had very little to do with one another. There was no overt solidarity, political or social. There were no formal or informal associations beyond the personal gatherings of a few friends."[136] Alison Prentice's work on academic women in physics at the University of Toronto indicates that they had much the same feeling of professional isolation as those women studied by Kinnear.[137] Yet the lives and activities of non-academic women suggest that they may have had a different experience. This is not to say that non-academic women did not feel their secondary status within universities. One is left only to imagine what the personal impact must have been on a dean such as Alice Vibert Douglas at Queen's who, as Katie Pickles notes, trained as an astrophysicist but as dean spent some of her time "counting out towels."[138] Or indeed, how Addison, or any other dean, for that matter, felt as a fifty-year-old woman living in a residence room surrounded on each side by eighteen-year-olds? Some of these women experienced acute pain at being excluded from academe or passed over in favour of men. According to Addison's biographer Jean O'Grady, Addison felt the denial of a position on Victoria's academic staff to be "the greatest defeat of her career."[139] Still, it is also possible that their position on the margins of academia provided some of these women with the space to forge their own careers and lives.

In a 1931 talk to students, Hilliard enthusiastically recommended medicine to women, arguing that female doctors were no longer pioneers but had fully broken into the field.[140] Despite Hilliard's optimism, the movement of women into universities and new professions remained a radical, often daring, act, albeit one that provided those who did so with a significant amount of intellectual, financial, and emotional control over their own lives. Moreover, by creating and participating in women's and professional associations, both faculty and staff created solidarity among women, and worked to increase educational opportunities for themselves and others. Historians have begun to point to the importance of women's clubs and organizations to the creation of nineteenth-century national and international women's movements.[141] It seems also a fruitful venue for understanding women's activism in Canada after women gained the vote. By creating and participating in a variety of associations, non-academic and professional women played a significant role in extending the venues in which women could play an active role in public life.[142]

Professional women's vision of women's place was always constricted – shaped by contemporary ideas about respectability and limited by existing concerns, among women and men alike, about women's role in society. Non-academic women accepted many of the constraints on their own and other women's lives and, indeed, played a part in creating and perpetuating some of those constraints. Yet they also believed strongly in their responsibility to shape women into educated citizens who would be ready to fulfil their role as mothers, perhaps as professionals, and certainly as community leaders within organizations on the national and international stage. The administrative and health positions that opened up in the first decade of the century for the conservative task of overseeing the activities, behaviour, and development of female students thus provided a means to support women's education. In addition, the connections that women made through their positions at Victoria College allowed them to create, and contribute to, a variety of women's networks. Indeed, Victoria College and its environs provided an enclave where a female space flourished.

6
Changing Contexts and Programs, 1930s to 1960s

Female health professionals' ability to carve out new careers and spaces for themselves, depended, like that of male physicians and physical educators, upon their general adherence to new assumptions about the importance of health to moral, spiritual, and intellectual development. In addition, female professionals relied on notions about their particular insight into the special and separate needs of female students. Yet even as such beliefs gained ground, significant change was occurring within the university that would affect the nature of the institution and challenge the ideas of many educators about the purpose and aims of education. This chapter examines some of the institutional changes developing within universities generally and health services and physical training more specifically. The subsequent two chapters focus on the ways in which new health priorities both reflected and aided the specialization and fragmentation of knowledge occurring within the research university, and on the ideological shift that accompanied and supported an emerging multiversity.

General Institutional Change

The end of the Second World War marked the beginning of two decades of expansion and growth.[1] While universities suffered from deteriorating facilities, small staffs, and low salaries caused by over a decade of depression, war, and immediate post-war inflation, they would emerge from the war with a stronger presence within Canadian society. The Veterans Charter, which subsidized veterans' tuition, housing, and general rehabilitation, helped infuse the university with much-needed financial resources. A growing belief in the importance of universities to the economic and cultural success of Canadian society resulted in the initiation of massive provincial and federal grants during the period. And once the veterans graduated, enrolments remained high, sustained first by the prosperity of the post-war period and then, starting in the mid-1960s, by the entry of the first wave of baby boomers.

Universities not only increased in size, but also were transformed in nature. In the first four decades of the twentieth century, the idea of the university as a moral community had been maintained in the liberal arts curriculum through the belief in the cultural and moral influences of courses in English literature and Western civilization. It continued to flow through the work of social scientists steeped in the ethics and beliefs of liberal Christianity. At denominational colleges, it remained influential through required courses in religious knowledge and chapel attendance. It resonated, too, in the pronouncements of university presidents – in their university reports, their convocation speeches, their myriad public addresses. It even informed extra-curricular activities – through the ideals of sport and through religious clubs that continued to play a prominent role on campus. And the moral community remained potent within residence life, and, where university authorities could exert pressure, in boarding houses.

But while the Christian vision of the university held sway well into the twentieth century, it was also undergoing a process of erosion. Indeed, it had never been the only voice on campus. Small numbers of radical professors spoke out against the religious and political status quo embraced by most administrators and faculty at their institutions. Evangelical Christians stood apart from the social gospel message of more liberal groups. Jewish and Catholic students established their own spaces. And as these groups grew, and as the faculty and student body became more diverse, administrators subtly changed their language to become more inclusive. Moreover, as societal mores changed, authorities like deans of women and residence councils had to continually liberalize their rules in order to maintain control over residence life. In addition, university officials found that they could exert only so much moral pressure on students who boarded and on off-campus culture more generally. Thus while many administrators and faculty perceived the university as a shaping force within society, it was also being gradually and subtly reshaped by new beliefs and values.

While at mid-century universities were still relatively small and intimate places and thus able to maintain a Christian moral culture, academic life had been undergoing a significant transformation for some
time. The ideal of research and a culture of utility had begun to make
inroads through the first half of the twentieth century. This was a process
that occurred gradually and in fits and starts. The emphasis on research
took hold within German institutions in the mid-nineteenth century, a
phenomenon that would infuse the American educational scene and
lead to the establishment in the late nineteenth century of some of the
great American research centres, such as Johns Hopkins and the University of Chicago. At the turn of the century, Canadian students began
to undertake post-graduate work at those and other similar institutions,
and brought back to Canadian universities many of the ideals and aims
they had learned there.

The culture of research encouraged disciplinary development and the
attempt by academics within a variety of fields to create or improve professional status. The old curriculum, centred around a select number of
subjects, quickly expanded in the twentieth century to include various
social science disciplines, as well as more practical vocational and professional subjects. In some fields, academics attempted to attain new legitimacy by distinguishing themselves from their predecessors, as was the
case in the 1960s when in the scientific study of religion, departments
of religious studies came to replace theology-based courses in religious
knowledge. The same would happen at a slightly later date as kinesiology,
the scientific study of human movement, replaced activity-based departments of physical education. Moreover, the second half of the twentieth
century witnessed the creation of a whole host of institutions, schools, and
professional programs to meet the changing needs of modern society.

The development of the modern research institute was a protracted
process that occurred at different rates both across and within Canadian
universities. This was equally the case within social scientific disciplines.
Nancy Christie and Michael Gauvreau have demonstrated both that social scientific methods permeated the work of social reformers and that
the moral impulse of the social gospel continued to shape the beliefs
and work of social scientists in the interwar years.[2] Yet the emphasis on
knowledge derived from social scientific methods, the growth of new
fields, the specialization and differentiation of disciplines, all aided the
erosion of the idea that the purpose of learning was to lead to knowledge
of God. Learning increasingly came to be perceived as important not for

understanding the Christian world but for the sake of new research and new knowledge itself.[3]

Thus, through the first three-quarters of the century, universities were undergoing change on a variety of levels. By the 1960s, they had grown in size. The reorientation towards research had become clear. A host of new disciplines and new ideological emphases emerged. Scientific and social scientific methods, with emphasis on disinterested objectivity, dominated researchers' approaches to their subjects. While Christian beliefs and attitudes remained, explicit references to Christianity were increasingly muted, and the force of regulations based on traditional moral values gradually weakened. The nature, shape, and purpose of the modern university had yet to be determined, though elements of what Clark Kerr, president of the University of California system from 1958 to 1967, referred to as the multiversity could already be seen. All of these factors had particular effects on, and were reflected in, the development of health and physical education programs. Moreover, in their own ways, these programs played an important role in the process of reshaping the modern university.

The Expansion of Health Facilities and Insurance Programs

War and post-war necessities led to the expansion and consolidation of pre-existing medical facilities. For example, in 1940, administrators at the University of Toronto, unable to cope with the needs of the 1,700 man – strong University Training Centre Battalion, enlisted the help of the university physician to reorganize the health services.[4] These services were given a boost by returning veterans. The Department of Veteran Affairs not only paid the health service fee for student veterans but made arrangements with the director to ensure that the health service would act as a screening clinic: treating minor ailments; placing the infirmary at the disposal of veterans with minor illness; and referring those with more serious illnesses to the local veterans' hospital.[5] This expansion in services, at least for veterans, was matched by a process of consolidation as medical staff established university-wide infirmaries for men and women that would eventually replace the individual college infirmaries.[6]

Other institutions also began to improve their facilities during the war years. While francophone universities in Quebec did not institute physical training programs, during the war and immediate post-war years they too set up basic health service programs. By 1944, Laval offered all students access to a health service and required that they undergo a medical examination.[7] In October 1945, the student government at the University of Montreal organized a medical service. This included a medical exam for first-year students performed by the municipal department of health, a permanent office staffed by a nurse, and access to a physician. By December 1948, all students received a full medical exam and had access to the student government doctor without fee.[8]

Post-war improvements occurred at many universities. Mount Allison undertook major upgrades to its facilities in 1946.[9] The University of Manitoba, which had struggled financially in the interwar years to provide services equivalent to those of many other institutions, secured a permanent nurse for the women's infirmary and created a treatment room in the men's residence in the immediate post-war period. In 1953–4, it also added an athletic injury service.[10] Similarly, Acadia developed a formal student health service in 1948, McMaster did so in 1951, and Queen's followed suit in 1964.[11]

Established programs also increased significantly in scope. In 1943, the University of Alberta built an infirmary separate from that in the residences. By 1954–5, its health service employed eight part-time physicians, two full-time nurses, and three part-time nurses.[12] By 1955, UBC's university health service consisted of both an out-patient department and a twenty-six bed hospital.[13] A decade later, it employed two full-time and five part-time physicians, ten full-time and three part-time nurses, one full-time lab technician and an X-ray technician, a part-time psychiatric consultant, and two full-time resident psychiatrists.[14]

The expansion and consolidation of health services provided students with greater medical facilities. This happened as governments increased funding to universities and as the student population rose. Yet it also occurred simultaneously with a general expansion of the welfare state and in particular the development of private and public hospitalization and medical insurance. The latter would prove key to the financing of health services.

Despite the largely middle-class composition of the student body, at least some young men and women found it difficult to cover medical bills. Periodic reports suggest that this was not an issue new to the 1940s and 1950s. In 1922, for example, *The Varsity* published a letter to the editor complaining that the University of Toronto health service provided only annual medical examinations, with few students receiving further medical attention. The writer noted that most students lived on a limited budget while others had to "work their way through college, without any financial assistance whatsoever." The student complained, "This makes it very hard for the average student to pay for medical treatment." He continued, "I know of a case, that of an Arts' student, last year, who could not possibly pay a doctor for a visit … He was, therefore, forced to apply to the General Hospital for free medical treatment. This was refused to him and he was told to go to work that he may earn money to pay a doctor."[15] The situation was much the same at UBC over a decade later. In 1938–9, physicians performing the medical examinations discovered that almost 55 per cent of students required follow-up sessions. While 71 per cent of these reported back to the health services after being treated by a private physician or dentist, the director of health services noted that the others had been unable to do so due to their precarious financial status.[16]

At the University of Manitoba, the poor financial situation of at least some students provided the rationale for demands for students to have greater access to medical services. While students at UBC and Toronto clearly had access to some facilities, this was not the case at the University of Manitoba. In 1936–7 the dean of men attempted to convince university administrators of the need for medical personnel to be available for consultation for both resident and non-resident students. "Such a system," he argued, "would meet the difficulty occasionally found in which a student who should be under medical care, but who is in difficult financial circumstances, hesitates to call a doctor whom he may not be able to pay in a reasonable time."[17] In 1941, a sub-committee of the University of Manitoba Student Union that was looking into health schemes noted,

> … many students are financially unable to afford the added costs incurred when an illness necessitates a stay at a hospital or at home. The expenses of doctor's attendances, medicines, drugs, surgery, etc., are more than usually beyond the average student's means, and a bout with anything more than a trifling complaint will often by reason of financial circumstance force a student to remain out of University a year, in order that his limited finances may be recouped.[18]

Such concerns continued in the post-war years. A 1964 incident at the University of Alberta is illustrative. In that year a student in a boarding house woke up with severe pain in his side. He went to the emergency ward at the university hospital but was told that he had to go to the student health service first. When he arrived at the health service he found that there was no physician available until the afternoon. He made an appointment and returned home. His landlady advised that a doctor be called who then admitted the student immediately to hospital where physicians performed an emergency operation.[19] The advisor of men later inquired into the incident and received a response from J.W. Wallace, the executive director of the University of Alberta Hospital, stating that "out-patient services (including Emergency) are not covered as a benefit under the hospitalization plan. In the past a number of university students have found themselves faced with hospital bills because they came to our Emergency Department for treatment before reporting in to the Student Health Service."[20]

Prior to the 1930s, medical services and hospitalization plans generally tended to be private university schemes supported largely through the pooling of student fees, though of course the university often covered many hidden costs, such as the establishment of infirmaries or lump sum payments to local hospitals. In addition, the medical services were often limited in nature, with students lacking ongoing access to a physician through the year. Still, in a period prior to private or provincial medical or hospitalization insurance, this system of universities creating their own private form of insurance seems to have dominated. Moreover, it had the advantage that, as the medical fund improved, the university could offer additional services. At the University of Alberta, for example, surpluses in the 1930s allowed for increased benefits to cover the cost of surgical fees in case of emergency operations.[21] By 1941, its medical services committee had a surplus of two thousand dollars invested in bonds. This money was dedicated to covering unusual costs, such as an epidemic, or to help improve facilities. Some of it, for example, was used to equip a thirty-bed infirmary.[22] In investigating the possibility of establishing a medical health fund, the student union sub-committee at the University of Manitoba favoured that type of option on the grounds that "when a suitable reserve has been established, the insurance could be withdrawn, the fee lowered, the benefits increased and the reserve invested in trust securities."[23]

Students often played a role in the establishment, or further development, of health services, particularly at places where these lagged behind other institutions. In the early 1940s, the University of Manitoba student union did significant legwork in identifying the types of insurance possibilities available and making recommendations to the university.[24] During the same period, University of Toronto students belonging to Campus Co-operative Residences undertook a survey of the state of health services at twenty-seven North American universities, which then formed the basis of a public critique of those provided at the University of Toronto; facilitated the establishment of an alternative and more extensive fund for its members; and permitted the Co-op to lobby the student union to request that the board of governors extend the existing services at the university.[25]

Students' concerns regarding medical costs reflected increasing North American anxieties about payment of medical bills. The first health insurance schemes developed in Europe and Britain at the turn of the twentieth century aimed to cover wages workers lost due to sickness.[26] Examining the American context, Paul Starr argues that by the 1920s, particularly for the middle class, the financial cost was no longer the wages lost but rather the cost of medical treatment. "Estimates at the end of the 1920s," he notes, "now showed that medical costs were 20 percent higher than lost earnings due to sickness for families with incomes under $1,200 a year and nearly 85 percent higher for families with incomes between $1,200 and $2,500."[27] Both physicians' fees and hospital costs began rising as a result of the increased quality of services doctors and hospitals were able to provide as well as physicians' growing monopoly of power. As a result, individuals, families, and health reformers in the 1920s became increasingly aware of the consequences of rising medical costs.[28]

In the interwar years, few options existed other than that of creating one's own fund, in part because private health insurance carriers had yet to discover how to make medical insurance a profitable enterprise. Here, developments at the University of Western Ontario are illustrative. In the early 1930s, the university established a medical board, consisting of three members of the faculty of medicine and several other staff members, charged with visiting ill students in residence, boarding houses, and in their homes. Members of that board sought out an insurance company willing to provide student medical insurance. Only one, Union Insurance Society of Canton, Ltd., represented by J.A. Nelles and Sons of London, proved interested. The Society agreed to charge three dollars per student and to pay out expenses up to a maximum of two hundred dollars. However, the company did not put enough restrictions on usage. It collected $2,500 in fees but paid out $5,300 in claims. In 1931–2, it submitted a modified scheme in which each student would pay five dollars but could claim no more than seventy-five dollars. This reduced the expenses of the insurance company significantly, though it still received

only $12,701 in premiums, compared to the $12,968 it paid out in claims.
The company declined to continue the experiment the following year,
though another one did take up the challenge at higher rates.[29]

Western's experiences illustrate the difficulties of securing and maintaining private insurance in the 1920s and 1930s. By the post-war years,
and particularly by the 1950s, this would become a more common option. Indeed, in the early 1940s, insurance brokers began to approach
some universities. The move to a private carrier was not, however, as-
sured. In 1941 the student government at the University of Montreal
turned down a proposal which would have seen student fees increased by
eighteen dollars – this compared to the five to eight dollars paid by students at other institutions who belonged to a university-run health fund.
The student union and university officials had a similar reaction to a
proposal put forward in 1950 by Les Services de Santé du Québec.[30] Similarly, despite their experimentation with private carriers in the interwar
years, in the 1940s authorities at Western opted for the creation of their
own health service where students could obtain treatment or advice.[31]

An alternative option that emerged in the post-war years was a physi-
cian-run medical service plan.[32] By 1950, administrators at the University
of Saskatchewan, for example, had made arrangements with Medical
Services (Saskatoon) Incorporated (MSI) so that students could have
access to physicians belonging to MSI as well as coverage for some X-ray
and surgical benefits. The university combined this with the provision
of access to a free campus clinic offering "minor surgical and medical
attention."[33]

Although university authorities and students were reluctant to embrace private medical insurance schemes, they often opted for private
hospitalization plans. While Western set up its own clinic in the post-war
period, it adopted a hospitalization plan with London Life Insurance.[34]
Yet students quickly found that insurance companies benefitted inordi-
nately from such plans. In 1956, Don French, president of the Pre-Med
Society at St. Francis Xavier University, condemned the students' Blue
Cross hospitalization plan. Having investigated the scheme for the student union, French found that while the union had paid eight thousand
dollars to Blue Cross, students collected only one thousand dollars in
claims. Over the course of a four-year period, he estimated that the difference between the amount paid out and the benefits collected came
to around $29,000. French concluded, "This money might have been
used to the benefit of all the students on some project such as a Students
Union building."[35] In the late 1960s, administrators at Acadia University

encountered a similar problem with private carriers. The director of the health service noted, "three medical insurance groups submitted plans and costs for taking over and administering an all-inclusive student health service at Acadia. By careful scrutiny of these plans it was clear that the cost in insurance fees alone would be at least twice that of our present system."[36]

The pressure for universities to develop their own hospital and medical funds would lessen only once provinces began to implement hospitalization plans in the 1940s and 1950s and, by the late 1960s and early 1970s, medical coverage.[37] Still, in the 1960s, medical coverage in particular remained an issue. While no statistics exist for medical coverage among students, within the general population, enrolment in medical plans certainly increased, from 6 per cent in 1945 to 53 per cent in 1961. Yet that left 47 per cent uninsured, and of those insured, 9 per cent were not covered for in-hospital professional services, and almost the same number lacked comprehensive coverage.[38] While significant numbers of students did gain coverage under provincial hospitalization plans, these too left gaps. For example, in the 1960s, out-of-province students often remained uninsured, with university officials needing to maintain emergency funds for them or arrange for coverage with a private carrier.[39]

Despite continuing gaps in medical coverage, however, medical insurance would, by the 1960s, help infuse cash into health services and create a commitment to providing medical treatment on campus. In some cases the expansion of health services had already begun during the war and immediate post-war period, as administrators responded to the needs of the war effort and the care of veterans. Growing public belief in the importance of welfare provisions likely also informed administrative decisions to expand campus health provisions. Yet the increasing availability of hospital and medical insurance also made such provisions possible. As a result, not only did health facilities become a familiar feature of Canadian campuses but, increasingly, they would also be able to provide more comprehensive coverage.

Changes within Physical Training Programs

As campus health services grew in size and scope, they also became more specialized and focused on their own priorities. This had particular consequences for those places where health services had developed in tandem with physical training, spurring the differentiation of health

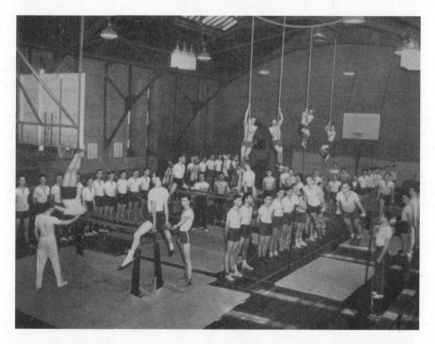

6.1 Gymnastics class, Hart House Gymnasium, University of Toronto, n.d. T.A. Reed, *The Blue and White: A Record of Fifty Years of Athletic Endeavour at the University of Toronto*. Toronto: University of Toronto Press, 1944, p. 50.

services from the latter field. For example, during the war years, health services and physical education at the University of Toronto became separate entities.[40] At McGill in the 1940s, the attending physician for Royal Victoria College and the University Medical Officer for Women remained responsible to the head of the department of physical education, but by 1950 administrators at McGill had similarly seen fit to separate health services and physical education.[41] The separation of the two fields recognized the growth of, and increasing specialization needed to run, each area as well as the diverging professional interests of personnel and changing priorities within each program. Moreover, during the war and post-war years, physical education underwent its own process of specialization, with the creation at many universities of physical education

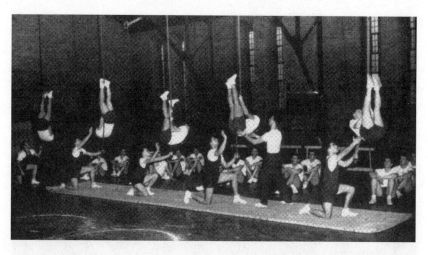

6.2 Gymnastics class, Hart House Gymnasium, University of Toronto, n.d.
Bruce Kidd, personal collection.

as a degree program and, in many cases, its elevation from the status of
a department to that of a school or faculty.[42]

Within physical education, change occurred not only at the bureaucratic and institutional level, but also within the physical training
program. At many universities, gymnastics and corrective exercises in
combination with sports and games remained central to the core program. Yet even in the interwar years, physical educators, influenced by
contemporary educational theories had begun to introduce new methods into their programs. For example, the natural movement gained adherents. Individuals such as Jesse Feiring Williams and Thomas D. Wood
at Teachers' College, Columbia University; Clark Hetherington, who
held positions at a number of institutions including New York University
and Stanford; and J.B. Nash at New York University began to re-articulate
the aims and ideals of physical education in light of the increasingly influential progressive educational work of academics such as G. Stanley
Hall, John Dewey, and William Kilpatrick.[43] Never an ideologically unified movement, progressive education encompassed a variety of strands
arising from the intellectual and social changes of the late eighteenth
and nineteenth centuries: the influence of romanticism; the child-centred ideas of Jean-Jacques Rousseau, Johann Pestalozzi, and Friedrich
Froebel; the reduction of family size; liberalization of Protestant ortho-

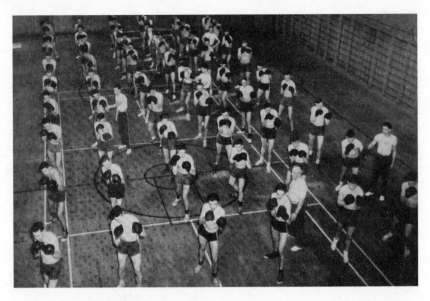

6.3 Boxing class, Hart House Gymnasium, University of Toronto, n.d. Bruce Kidd, personal collection.

doxy; and the impact of religious and secular reform movements. All of these contributed to changing views of childhood that placed greater emphasis on child rearing, early learning, and childhood innocence rather than sin, and encompassed new ideas about teaching and learning.[44] Progressive educators advocated, among other things, training in activities useful to everyday life; a child-centred approach; a focus on the whole person; the importance of the physical health and emotional well-being of the child; attention to a variety of learning styles and range of abilities; the notion of the teacher as guide rather than instructor, and the child as an active rather than a passive learner; and an enthusiasm for expertise and scientific methods in teaching and learning. They emphasized the need for vocational training such as shop and domestic science; access to subjects such as art, music, and health and physical education; and teachers' attention to students' emotional life through awareness of mental hygiene.[45]

Informed by progressive ideals, proponents of the natural movement introduced new influences and priorities into physical education.

Dorothy Ainsworth notes a de-emphasis on gymnastics in American women's colleges, in favour of activities such as "sports, swimming, and dance."[46] Health enthusiasts perceived swimming as therapeutic, a method of cleansing the body and providing a life skill that could promote good citizenship.[47] In Canadian universities, as elsewhere, swimming gained particular favour as part of the compulsory program. As early as 1921, Toronto introduced, for male students, compulsory swimming basics, with those unable to swim doing a half hour in the pool and then the requisite half hour of physical training.[48] Similarly, by at least the end of the 1930s, men at Acadia engaged in swimming throughout the year.[49] This activity would spread during the 1940s and 1950s. Beginning in 1943–4, women at the University of Toronto had to pass a swimming test, which consisted of "entering the water head first and keeping afloat for five minutes."[50] If they failed that test, then they were required to take swimming as their elective.[51] UWO instituted swimming as part of its required program in the 1940s.[52] By the mid-1950s, the University of Saskatchewan had instituted a swimming test while by the mid-1960s, Mount Allison required female students to complete twenty hours in the pool.[53] Indeed, at some places in the post-war period swimming requirements replaced those of gymnastics.[54]

At the same time, universities began to offer more options. In 1945–6, the director of physical education for women at UBC offered only one class in "keep-fit or traditional gymnastic exercise." In her annual report, she noted that this was done on purpose in an attempt "to overcome the rather rampant antipathy to this type of physical activity which had developed as a result of the required War Work Programme in operation on the campus during the previous three years."[55] Instead of a structured and prescribed program, UBC offered female students options such as "grass hockey, basketball, volleyball, archery, fencing, badminton, tennis, golf, swimming," a variety of forms of dance, and "a class in basic rhythmics using such small hand apparatus as clubs, balls and skipping ropes."[56] The director of athletics and physical education for men at the University of Toronto made a similar comment in 1947–8:

> The syllabus for the required gymnasium work in Physical Education has been changed greatly during the past seven years. The emphasis now is on making the work both interesting and instructional. The tedious "P.T. classes" comprised of pure calisthenics are a thing of the past. Conditioning exercises, self-testing activities, self-defence games and competitions on the gymnasium floor and out of doors, make up a large part of the curriculum.[57]

Instructors at other institutions also attempted to offer more numerous options. In 1940–1 at the University of Saskatchewan, the women's requirement of one hour of fundamentals was balanced by a choice of basketball, swimming, track, tennis, or hockey.[58] These options had increased by the mid-1950s to include "badminton, dancing, advanced or ornamental swimming, golf and figure skating."[59] Similarly, men could take "tennis, golf, badminton, volleyball, basketball, gymnastics, wrestling, curling, hockey, square-dancing and swimming."[60] At Dalhousie University, the first hour of the weekly required program consisted of instruction, according to the season, in "field hockey, tumbling, apparatus, archery, badminton, basketball, volleyball, square dancing and social dancing." The second hour involved participation in an elective sport, in intermural competition, or in varsity athletics. This included activities such as "tennis, field hockey, archery, badminton, swimming, basketball, ice hockey and ping pong."[61] In 1955–6 at Acadia University, the required work consisted of swimming, marching, tactics, tumbling, folk dancing, country dancing, gymnastics, and games.[62] By 1968, the program had expanded to include "swimming for one term, and a choice of participating in two activities which for the men were badminton, basketball, conditioning, football, handball, soccer, squash, and tennis – and for the women, badminton, basketball, modern dance, field hockey, figure skating, squash and tennis."[63]

In addition to providing students with access to a greater number of sports and introducing them to new activities such as swimming, physical educators at some institutions also began to focus on skills and tests. Doing so required decreased emphasis on established practices. For example, Roberta Park notes that as early as the first decade of the twentieth century in the United States, the Society of College Gymnasium Directors had begun advocating a reduction in time spent gathering anthropometric measurements.[64] The related endeavour of posture correction certainly remained into the post-war period. Yet David Yosifon and Peter Stearns note that even there, cultural beliefs linking posture to character began to recede in the 1940s and had virtually disappeared by the 1960s. As they did so, doctors' campaigns to improve posture, which had always been based more on social than medical grounds, lost sway.[65]

Although the massive programs of measurement and quantification of body parts fell out of favour, physical educators began to turn to new, more modern, tests, to measure and evaluate overall fitness and health.

Park notes for the United States that strength tests began to gain favour in the early part of the century. Despite seeming at odds with the emphasis on activities, active learning, or the natural movement emphasized by many progressive educators, such tests fell within an emerging strand of the progressive movement that focused on testing as a means of educational reform.[66] Increasingly instructors came to focus "on tests of heart function, fatigue, and physical efficiency" as well as "reaction time, accuracy, and endurance."[67] By the end of the 1930s, Acadia included physical ability tests and motor ability tests in its physical training program.[68] During the war, educators at McGill explored the usefulness of the Harvard step test as a method of determining "organic and functional efficiency."[69] In the 1950s, M.S. Yuhasz, working in the physical education measurement laboratory at UWO, developed the Western Motor Fitness Test and, in collaboration with John Faulkner, the Western Motor Ability Test.[70] By 1960, all UWO students were being tested in not only aquatics, but also motor ability.[71]

Over the course of the 1940s and 1950s, then, physical educators gradually began to introduce new emphases and priorities into their programs. Influenced by a variety of elements of the progressive education movement, physical educators began to shift away from formal gymnastics and drill towards more practical programs or activities relevant to life; offered an increasing number of options; and experimented with new forms of testing. In addition, during this period at least some physical educators worked to establish their field as a discipline equal in status to other academic areas, with its own administrative structure, program, and degree-granting rights. Over time, the aims of physical educators to professionalize their field would elevate the status of the discipline. Yet that would not come without some cost to activity-based physical training programs.

The Impact of Institutional Changes on Women

The institutional and ideological transformations occurring within health and physical training had a particular effect on women's role on campus. The bureaucratization and consolidation of services routinely placed female health professionals, who had headed their own department, under male directorship. This process accelerated during and after the Second World War. For example, during the war, the University of Toronto established a department of physical education by amalgamating existing personnel at Toronto with staff from the Margaret Eaton School, the latter becoming members of the department under male directorship.[72] Similarly, the University of Toronto's consolidation of its college infirmaries into a university-wide system eliminated the position of college physician, which at some places, such as Victoria College, had supported women in the advancement of their careers. Within the broader University of Toronto health services, the female physician was subordinate to the male director. This was a phenomenon that occurred equally in other areas within North American universities.[73]

At the same time that women's health and physical education programs at some institutions became amalgamated into and under one general student program, physical educators interested in the instruction of sport began to find that within departments or faculties of physical education, "activities" were increasingly devalued in favour of more scientific research. Beginning in the 1960s, though more prominent in subsequent decades, research specialists would come to dominate most institutions with a degree program.[74] While this affected all instructors engaged in activities, women tended to be more involved in the practical side of physical education as opposed to the scientific study of the body, and as a result this shift had a particularly negative effect on their place within the field of physical education.[75]

While the activities side of physical education faced devaluation, female students gradually experienced greater freedom in the physical training programs available to them.[76] Elements of the physical training programs remained gendered, particularly gymnastics, dance, and body building. In 1945–6 Jean Sleightholme, the instructor at UBC, noted, "rhythmic activity is particularly attractive to women." Female students there also had access to folk and modern dancing.[77] In the early 1950s, the University of Alberta taught both men and women skills in volleyball, basketball, and body mechanics, but men also received instruction in tumbling, apparatus, and conditioning exercises while women were taught badminton and dancing.[78]

At the same time, some new approaches to training had begun to appear. In 1945–6, for example, UBC offered square dancing and ballroom dancing to men as well as women and co-ed classes for a small number of students in advanced tumbling and apparatus.[79] At the University of Toronto, square dancing had become co-educational by the mid-1950s.[80] By 1960–1, UWO had dropped traditional offerings to women such as "correctives" and folk dancing. It now offered most activities to both men and women. These included aquatics; recreational

activities such as badminton, tennis, golf, squash, handball, and archery; team sports such as volleyball, soccer, and basketball; personal
defence; gymnastics; and fitness and weight control. Only wrestling was
limited to men.[81]

Thus, while programs remained gendered in the post-war years,
men and women increasingly had access to similar types of activities
and sports. As the range of options increased, however, the general regard for the place of physical activities on campus was in decline. The
professionalization of physical education and attempts to raise the status of the academic programs became tied to research, particularly to
theoretical and scientific methods. The specialization of the field and
educators' attempt to establish a footing within the research university,
however, resulted in the sidelining of the practical side of the program –
a phenomenon that, at least in the short term, seems to have had a particularly negative effect for female physical educators.

Conclusion

The 1920s and 1930s witnessed the spread of physical culture and health
services in Canadian universities. Propelled by the belief that the university played an important role in character formation, infused by a
spirit of social and moral reform, adhering to new ideas about the power
of the social sciences to improve humanity and the important role of
public health in building a better society, many university administrators and medical officers across the country embraced at least the ideal
of physical training and access to medical care, if not always the reality.
In many places, the impulses of the late nineteenth and early twentieth
centuries would carry into the 1940s and 1950s. Indeed, war reignited
concerns about the fitness and health of male citizens in particular, an
issue carried over into the post-war reintegration of veterans and reinforced later with the start of the Cold War. The latter also gave credence
to longstanding beliefs about the important role the university could
play in bolstering the values and ideals of Western civilization as well in
preparing university students as the future leaders of the nation. Despite
the structural changes occurring within Canadian universities and the
process of specialization and differentiation of health services and physical education, social and cultural concerns about youth and the stability
of the nation reinforced the need for a strong and fit citizenry.

The changes occurring within the fields of health services and physical education both reflected and helped facilitate broader trends within

the university as well as the process of professionalization. As individual disciplines developed and institutions increased in size and scope, those employed by, and attending, universities experienced a process of specialization and fragmentation not only of knowledge but in the workings of their institutions. Historians have documented this process in relation to curricular developments. Yet insight into the process can also be gleaned through an examination of the development and impact of new health priorities. It is to this that we now turn.

7

Shifting Health Priorities – Tuberculosis and Mental Health

Just as the infrastructure supporting student health services began to change, so too did the emphases shaping the work of those services. In the early decades of the twentieth century, health programs tended to focus on the environment, on the detection of physical defects that could be rectified through physical training, on vaccination, and on issues of moral concern such as sex education or control of venereal disease. Beginning in the 1930s, but more so in the 1940s, health experts turned to new concerns – ones that increasingly relied on specialized medical detection and treatment by health experts rather than by members of the broader university community. They came to focus first on tuberculosis and, as that disease came under control, turned their attention towards mental health. Despite the very different nature of these illnesses, an analysis of health experts' approach to them helps illuminate some of the transitions occurring within medicine at mid-century that would reshape future practice.

Eradicating Tuberculosis

Prior to the First World War, physicians believed tuberculosis to be caused by a combination of bacterial infection, individual predisposition, and social and economic circumstances. Adhering to hereditarian beliefs, they perceived some individuals to be more susceptible to the disease than others. To those affected they prescribed a mix of rest, fresh air, and good diet in order to strengthen the body. Georgina Feldberg notes that "medical texts and advice manuals suggested that exercise, proper climate, good diet, wholesome living, general hygiene, outdoor work, and reasonable caution in regard to contact with consumptives would effectively check the spread of the disease."[1] Anti-tuberculosis health workers also attacked the disease's social causes, such as poor housing, overcrowded living conditions, badly ventilated and lit indoor spaces, and low wages. Equally, they investigated the methods of selling milk, campaigned against practices such as spitting and the use of shared drinking cups, and focused on dust and flies as carriers of disease.[2] In their reaction to the disease, health and social reformers, often one and the same, understood consumption as both a reflection of an individual's constitution and the consequences of rapid urbanization and industrialization.

During the interwar years, physicians began to turn away from the pre-war focus on poor living and economic conditions as a means to eradicate tuberculosis and towards an emphasis on eliminating the germ. Katherine McCuaig sums up this change in attitude as follows: "In the pre-war period it had been a disease that affected the individual but that had its causes rooted in the community; in the post-war period, the causes were seen to be rooted in the individual, and the community was affected."[3] She argues that rather than focusing on improving living conditions, those in charge of tuberculosis campaigns used "'preventive' methods such as travelling and stationary clinics, examinations of suspect groups, and isolation ..."[4] In addition, in the 1930s attention shifted to "specific occupational or racial groups that were particularly prone to infection – contacts, teachers, students, industrial workers (for example, miners), psychiatric patients, nurses, and aboriginals."[5] By the 1940s, public health workers had begun to undertake "mass surveys of the whole population."[6]

The shift in emphasis towards bacteriology can be seen in the efforts to counteract tuberculosis on campus. In the United States in the interwar years, tuberculosis was the leading cause of disease among college students. Heather Munro Prescott has found that surveys among university students revealed high rates of infection – as high as 50 or 60 per cent in the northeast and 80 per cent in the South – findings that spurred concern about the disease and led many university administrators to institute mandatory tuberculin testing.[7] With tuberculosis being the leading cause of death in Canada for those aged fifteen to forty-five, Canadian health experts also worried about the disease. Surveys of school children undertaken in the early 1920s had already revealed that Canadian rates of infection matched those in the United States.[8] University administrators began to institute some testing of students for tuberculosis in the early- to mid-1930s, though it tended to be limited to suspected cases identified during the medical examination, to a particular segment of the student population such as female residence students, or to larger numbers if special outside funding was provided. Systematic and continuous mass surveys of university students became more common in the late 1930s and early 1940s, beginning with first-year students and expanding beyond this group as resources allowed.[9]

The statistics gathered on first-year female students at the University of Toronto and on all new students at UBC indicate that in the late 1930s roughly 43 per cent of new students tested positive for tuberculin.[10] However, high rates of reaction to tuberculin testing did not translate into high numbers of active cases. The number of individuals with an active infection was usually well below 1 per cent of the student body, in fact, often below 0.5 per cent.[11] At the University of Toronto, authorities found in the 1940s that its rate of active cases was generally the same as that of the population at large.[12] Some chest surveys performed on university students also indicate declining rates of reaction. Statistics gathered at the University of Toronto for first-year female students indicate a positive reaction rate to the tuberculin test of 43.6 per cent in 1937–8, 30 per cent in 1938–9, 28 per cent in 1940–1, and 20.3 per cent in 1944–5.[13] This decline in reaction rates at the University of Toronto matches broader provincial patterns. In Ontario, for example, the mortality rate from tuberculosis, which had been at 71 per 100,000 in 1921, had fallen to 27 per 100,000 by 1940.[14] Similar trends existed elsewhere.[15]

With findings that indicate low rates of active disease within the student population as well as declining rates of reaction, why did health experts continue in the 1940s and 1950s to focus extensive attention on tuberculosis? Ironically, declining rates of reaction made tuberculosis a more significant problem, as those who tested negative were more susceptible to the disease if they came into contact with someone who was infected. Moreover, where doctors had believed that occurrence of tuberculosis in adults was due to the reactivation of an infection contracted as a child, surveys of student nurses undertaken in the early 1930s revealed "the danger of *exogenous* infection."[16] Indeed, nurses with a positive tuberculin reaction but whose chest X-ray showed no infection were less likely to contract tuberculosis than those with a negative tuberculin test. As a result, as the number of young people testing positive declined, risk of infection seemed to increase. The main counter to this problem was the identification and isolation of the contagious – something that could be achieved only through mass surveys.[17]

In the 1930s, and more so by the 1940s, universities spent considerable time and energy identifying the infected. On American campuses, Heather Munro Prescott notes, "surveys indicate that the proportion of colleges with TB prevention programs increased from 10 percent in the early 1920s to more than 60 percent by the mid-1950s, and that funding for college health programs increased substantially during this period."[18] By the 1940s and 1950s, tuberculosis testing in Canada had not only become a significant portion of the work of health services at the start of each school year but was also considered a key element of its activities. In 1942–3 the director of the UBC health service noted that "the control of Tuberculosis remains one of our chief functions."[19] Similarly, five years later the director of the university health service at Toronto reported that, "this phase of our work is considered to be one of our greatest contributions to the health of the student body."[20] Not only did universities check students but in certain cases they re-checked them. In 1948, four students in the sophomore law class at UBC tested positive for tuberculosis. Although it turned out that none had an active infection, the university ordered all law students in that year to be rechecked.[21]

French- and English-Canadian universities attacked the problem of tuberculosis in different ways. In the early twentieth century Albert Calmette and Camille Guérin, of the Pasteur Institute in Lille, France, developed a tuberculosis vaccine based on a weakened live bovine bacillus. Due to the testing methods and the form of the vaccine, English-Canadians, like their American counterparts, remained sceptical of the reliability of the BCG (Bacillus Calmette-Guérin) vaccine. While some surveys were carried out in Quebec, physicians there relied more heavily on vaccination. Influenced by practices in France, Quebec authorities began testing the BCG vaccine on infants in the 1930s and 1940s, approving its use among school children by 1949. In contrast, medical experts in English Canada adopted the survey method, using the BCG vaccine for high-risk groups such as tuberculosis-negative medical and nursing students.[22]

Large-scale chest surveys became possible in part due to technological advances. While the tuberculin test allowed for identification of possible cases of tuberculosis, those with a positive reaction required a follow-up X-ray in order to determine if the disease was active. Widespread use of X-rays became possible only in the early 1940s with the invention of cheap miniature X-ray films. After purchasing a machine, administrators at the University of Toronto estimated that it had reduced the cost of chest plates from one dollar per student to twenty-five cents.[23]

In general, tuberculosis screening was made possible only through the resources put into this work by voluntary and government agencies. Mc-Cuaig notes that in the 1940s, the Christmas Seals program paid for 75 per cent of the cost for the mass surveys carried out by the Ontario Department of Health.[24] Indeed, organized by local tuberculosis societies, it "paid for travelling and stationary clinics, mobile x-ray units, public health nurses ... tuberculin, BCG, and x-rays of general hospital admissions."[25] Provincial health departments then provided the medical and technical personnel.

Universities relied on both voluntary and government agencies in order to accomplish their screening of students. Acadia provides a good example. In 1928, faculty and students founded the Acadia University Tuberculosis Council, with Dr DeWitt, the university physician, as president. It organized the annual Christmas Seal sale and forwarded the money raised to the Nova Scotia Tuberculosis Association, which then aided the department of health to undertake testing. At the university, local physicians performed the tuberculosis test, and students found to be positive were then sent to the Nova Scotia Sanatorium for an X-ray. By 1948 the department of public health had purchased a mobile X-ray unit, a significant amount of the funds for which had been raised by the Nova Scotia Tuberculosis Association. The mobile unit visited the provinces' universities, taking X-rays which were then read at the sanatorium.[26] University health services relied on that unit. In 1954–5, for example, when the mobile unit was unable to provide services to students at Acadia, the university physician had to confine his work to new students and those needing to be rechecked.[27]

Other institutions relied equally on this type of support. For example, the Tuberculosis Division of the British Columbia Provincial Board of Health and the BC Tuberculosis Society, through its Christmas Seal fund, enabled free testing and X-rays for students at UBC. The Alberta Department of Health provided testing for students at the University of Alberta, while the mobile unit of the Sanatorium Board of Manitoba did so for students at the University of Manitoba, the Ontario Department of Health for students in that province, and the Ligue Anti-tuberculeuse for students at the University of Montreal.[28]

Mass tuberculin testing and chest X-rays for positive reactors continued well into the 1960s. Yet death rates were significantly reduced between the late 1940s and early 1950s after the introduction of several chemotherapies.[29] For a number of years before its closure in the mid-1970s, the chest survey at the University of Toronto recorded no active cases.[30] By the mid-1960s, university health services no longer worried about a disease that earlier in the century had been a killer for young people.

The campus focus on tuberculosis formed part of a larger Canadian campaign, from the 1930s to the 1970s, to eradicate the disease. It is important not only in and of itself, but also for what it can tell us about the transformation of medicine during this period. In many ways, the early history of tuberculosis fits within the moral and environmental concerns of health experts and educators. It was a disease linked to heredity, to poverty, and to moral weakness, and one which experts believed could be countered through education, healthy living, and the creation of strong bodies and minds. Yet from the university records examined, it was not one that dominated the concerns of educators in the first few decades of the century. This may be due in part to the fact that prior to the First World War for general physicians it was difficult to diagnose and impossible to treat. They could identify only advanced cases of tuberculosis, and they offered as a solution only the removal of infected students from university and their transferal to a sanatorium. It was not until the 1930s, and more prominently in the 1940s, that tuberculosis became a priority for health service personnel – a point at which physicians could actually diagnose and isolate patients much earlier in the progression of the disease and thus also prevent others from contracting tuberculosis.

Both the perception of being able to provide a service, and the actual ability to do so, were key to the development of health services on university campuses. Physical examinations, vaccinations, medical tests, and health instruction, for example, were integrated into the health services system as physicians perceived these as offering solutions to various health issues of concern to educators. These procedures also became a means of extending the authority of experts. Heather Munro Prescott argues that members of the American Student Health Association "saw the tuberculosis threat as a way of justifying increased support for college health services."[31] Indeed, she suggests that "college physicians used the threat of the 'white plague' to both legitimize their professional efforts and justify a more prominent position for themselves within the college environment."[32] In Canada, too, experts were able to draw on the resources of provincial departments of health and voluntary societies to increase the scope of university health services.

At the same time, the nature of the work increasingly shifted health care from the purview of general university staff to medical practitioners. The reports on tuberculosis are located in those of the directors of university health services rather than those of physical educators or deans of women. Historians writing about tuberculosis have noted this process, with the campaigns against the disease removed from the hands of moral and social reformers to those of medical practitioners.[33] Investigations into, and treatment of, tuberculosis required specialized personnel as well as significant resources. While many of the first university physicians undertook student medical examinations as part of their general practice, the completion of mass chest surveys required greater time, resources, and administrative infrastructure than that available to a general physician. Moreover, as knowledge about tuberculosis increased and the availability of new technologies improved, diagnosis shifted from the general practitioner to a series of specialists such as radiologists and laboratory technicians.[34]

The growing attention paid to the eradication of tuberculosis thus illuminates a transformation occurring within university health services in particular and medical practice more generally. For a variety of reasons, health became increasingly professionalized, specialized, and over time, the preserve of medical experts. In addition, the large-scale nature of testing for tuberculosis, the increasing reliance on specialists, and the provision of funds by private and governmental agencies aided the growth of university health services and the commitment to provide such services by university officials. In this sense, the focus on tuberculosis laid the groundwork for the specialized services required in the 1950s and 1960s to contend with the newest concern: student mental health.

Mental Health

Even as medical experts focused attention on tuberculosis in the 1930s and 1940s, calls could be heard to expand the work of university health services beyond the physical body and towards mental health. Concern about students' mental health was not new to the post-war years. Indeed, physicians and deans made references to various forms of mental stress through the period of this study. However, what they meant by mental health and the terms they used to describe it changed significantly. So too did the perceived way of dealing with the issue.

In the early decades of the century physicians and educators referred to mental health problems in terms of "nerves" or "neuralgia." At Victoria College cases of "strain," "troublesome nerves," "nervous breakdown," and "neuralgia" appeared relatively frequently, roughly one case every couple of years.[35] The diagnosis of "nerves" or "neurasthenia" developed in the mid- to late-nineteenth century as an attempt to distinguish those suffering from madness as opposed to the "vagueness of apparently ordinary mental functioning."[36] Neurasthenia was believed to affect both men and women and, according to George M. Beard, the physician who coined the term in 1869, manifested itself in a wide variety of ways: "insomnia, dyspepsia, heaviness of limbs, palpitations, sick headaches, bad dreams, hopelessness and impotence."[37] Physicians attributed it to overwork, especially to mental labour, in men, and to reproductive problems in women.[38]

At Victoria College, where reports regarding student health are most revealing, doctors, nurses, and administrators used terms such as nerves or neuralgia to refer to a broad set of problems with significantly different solutions. They generally applied such concepts to students considered in need of extra rest and greater supervision. Depending on the degree of illness, students might be placed temporarily in the infirmary for some quiet time, sent home for a short break or, in more extreme cases, sent home for a significant portion of the year, sometimes never to return.[39] Mainly, however, they used the terms to refer to milder cases of students having trouble coping. Sometimes university officials attributed strain to too much socialization. This was the case for a fourth-year student in 1909. The dean of women reported that "she has never been robust and the preparation of the wedding of a friend and the presidency of a college society together with the work of the fourth year proved too much for her. She will probably complete her year in 1910."[40] At times, health experts attributed strain to overcrowding in residence. In December 1914, after one student who occupied a room with two others was put in the rest room, the nurse wrote: "I hope the time may soon come when it will not be necessary to have three girls in one room as it involves a heavy strain on the girls."[41] Similarly, in 1921–2, Dr Edna Guest recorded that during the medical examination,

> each girl was talked to individually, and told the need for real rest lying down for [a] half hour after lunch, and [a] half hour before dinner and bed at 10:30 pm. Individual cases needing extra rest were given detailed instructions – and one particularly nervous girl who might otherwise have been sent directly home, has been brought to the Infirmary for a month's special supervision.

Guest also attributed strain to other medical conditions. For example, in the same report she noted that she had found thirty-five girls who needed their eyes tested or retested – a finding she considered important for, as she wrote, "so very many nervous break-downs in the spring are the direct result of over-strained eyes, and eyes whose glasses are not quite right."[42]

While the records at Victoria are much richer regarding the health of female students, there are indications that male students, too, suffered from strain and nerves. In 1933–4, the dean of men noted that "two students in residence are unable to write their examinations from nervous troubles. Not only have we the problem of the student who will not work enough but of a small number who are inclined to study too hard."[43] Similarly, in 1936 the dean of men at the University of Manitoba noted that one student had had to withdraw due to a nervous breakdown.[44] While the evidence for male students is slim, it appears that administrators applied the term "nerves" fairly specifically to students unable to cope with their studies. This was also the case for female students, but strain was also attributed to their inability to regulate their involvement in extra-curricular activities.

Rise of North American Psychology

At Victoria College, references to terms such as "nerves" or "neuralgia" appeared most prominently until the 1920s and began to thin out thereafter, gradually replaced by the concept of neurosis.[45] This corresponds to a broader North American pattern resulting from the rise of psychology as a discipline and the gradual rethinking of the nature of mental health. Mental hygiene, the attempt to investigate, identify, and prevent mental illness and promote mental health, developed as a formal movement in the early twentieth century. American progressives in fields such as psychology, psychiatry, and social work joined together in 1909 to form the National Committee for Mental Hygiene and established the influential journal *Mental Hygiene* in 1917. In Canada, the rise of psychology was slightly slower. Those concerned about mental health created the Canadian National Committee for Mental Hygiene in 1918. By the 1920s, both McGill and Toronto had independent departments of psychology. But while psychology courses became more common at Canadian universities through the interwar years, most institutions did not have an independent department until the 1940s. Still, as Mona

Gleason notes, during the interwar years psychology began to gain influence, making inroads into schools through psychological testing, counselling, and diagnosis. It became central to teacher training programs. And psychologists, asserting their expertise, established child guidance clinics. They also solidified their professional status through the creation in 1939 of the Canadian Psychological Association.[46]

At the same time, psychologists themselves began to popularize their ideas, "promoting themselves to the general public as experts" through their work in schools, with teachers and parents, in newspaper and magazine columns, the publication of guides and manuals, in public lectures and radio broadcasts.[47] In the 1930s and 1940s, psychologists' and psychiatrists' authority increased as "psychoanalytically-oriented practitioners won a middle-class clientele and a wider popular and intellectual audience."[48] Psychology and psychiatry gained influence during the Second World War as practitioners applied their knowledge to military personnel selection. Large numbers of men were rejected from service and others discharged from duty due to psychological disorders. Paul Starr argues that in the United States experts both used military discharge statistics to argue for the need for greater psychiatric services, and bolstered their authority by claiming success in treatment.[49] The perceived need for counselling services for military personnel continued after the war. In Canada, for example, the Veterans Charter included provisions for the establishment of such services to oversee veterans' adjustment to university life.[50] In addition, psychologists and psychiatrists gained prominence as mental health became incorporated into post-war reconstruction plans, first with the creation of a mental health division within the Department of Health in 1945 and then the infusion of significant research funds for mental health work through the 1940s and 1950s.[51]

Part of the growth in psychology occurred as a result of a gradual rethinking of mental illness in the early decades of the twentieth century. In Canada, psychology gained momentum in part due to its close connection to the Canadian National Committee for Mental Hygiene (CNCMH). Early proponents of that organization drew public awareness in particular to the problem of mental deficiency, reinforcing eugenic theories linking mental development and inheritability. Members of the CNCMH included well-placed and influential professionals and university people, giving prominence to the CNCMH as an organization. And the CNCMH played a significant role in providing funding for applied psychological research.[52] By the late 1920s, however, some psychologists had begun to distance themselves from the hereditarian beliefs articulated by the founders of the CNCHM, which left little role for psychological practice, and instead began to embrace environmental explanations for mental development that understood the mind as malleable and mental illness as treatable.[53]

As part of the shift from the belief in mental illness as a hereditary disease to a greater emphasis on environmental causes, experts began to replace the language of "nerves" or "neurasthenia" with that of "neuroses." That shift was accompanied by a change in meaning. "Neuresthenia" was generally attributed to a handful of individuals, to a weakness inherited by a few that was often linked to a deficiency in character. "Neuroses," psychologists believed, could develop in anyone. Indeed, they argued that it was likely that everyone might at some point find themselves under some form of mental strain.[54] In turning their attention to methods to identify, treat, and prevent individual adjustment, a handful of psychologists carved out the sub-field of personality development. The shift in language, then, marked a reconceptualization of the field from the more narrow parameters of mental illness to the all-encompassing topic of mental health. In the process, Kurt Danziger argues, psychologists attempted to establish "the claim of Psychology *as a discipline* to special and privileged knowledge about the *entire* range of human affairs."[55]

The idea that all might be affected by mental disturbance developed at the same time as interest in child and adolescent development. In the first half of the twentieth century, psychologists began to focus in particular on adolescence as a period of crisis and turmoil. By the 1950s, that notion had become firmly set. Writing on "The Problem of Adolescence" in *Student Medicine*, the journal of the American College Health Association, Graham Blaine, a psychologist with the university health service at Harvard University, wrote that adolescence should be considered "a period of 'normative' crisis." Regarding the male students at his institution, Blaine argued, "many conflicts beset the growing child as he goes through this strange transitional period which lies between childhood and adulthood."[56] These could be categorized into four main areas: "first, the conflict between independence and dependence; second, the problem of the formation of identity; third, the problem of performing academic work; last, the conflict over sexual orientation."[57] Blaine noted, "Because there is so close a resemblance between what might be termed normal adolescent behavior and emotionally disturbed, truly symptomatic behavior, it is important for physicians and parents to have as clear a picture as possible of what adolescence is like."[58]

As psychologists became concerned about childhood and adolescent development, they turned to schools as a natural site of application for new theories and developments in the field. This paralleled progressive educators' promotion of school social services – from public health nursing, nutritional services, instruction in health and physical education, mental testing in the early part of the century, to psychological, psychiatric, and counselling services from the late 1930s on.[59] As the statement by Blaine indicates, psychologists, like the university community more generally, perceived university students to be in the later stages of adolescence. Moreover, at least some psychologists argued that because university students often lived away from home and without intense parental supervision, they might even be at greater risk of maladjustment than children.[60] Such reasoning enabled them to promote the idea of the importance of university students' access to the services of psychologists.

Promoting Mental Health on North American Campuses

In the 1920s, some American colleges and universities began hiring psychologists and psychiatrists to provide counselling and, in some cases, teach courses in mental hygiene.[61] Heather Munro Prescott notes that "mental hygiene experts in colleges and universities argued that young adulthood was the last opportunity to detect and prevent mental illness."[62] Advocates of college mental hygiene programs believed that the university had a responsibility to provide such services. L.J. Thompson, a physician at Yale, speaking at the 1927 conference of the American Student Health Association, stated,

> There are many students with habits of thought, reaction and emotional responses that might never develop any serious mental illness, but at the same time these habits might be a lasting handicap to them after they have left college. It seems logical to state that the college owes the student some instruction about his emotional problems and about how to adjust to life in general after he leaves college.[63]

Thompson believed that larger colleges should employ at least two psychiatrists, a social service worker, and a psychologist.[64] At the same conference, Robert Legge, a physician at the University of California, Berkeley, argued that "one of the most important health functions of a University Student Health Service and a Department of Hygiene is the promotion of the study and teaching of Mental Hygiene." He continued,

> In the health services of our universities today, every medical director sees cases of inferiority complexes of various types, perversion, and mental deterioration. The administrative offices are constantly dealing with students who are queer and erotic, those who cannot concentrate in their studies, the immoral, and others with peculiarities, a result of mental and behavioristic abnormalities. Therefore, mental hygiene is particularly related to administrative hygiene in a university health program.[65]

Students did not only arrive at university with mental problems but might develop them as a result of their very entry into the university. In a 1935 article in *The Lancet*, R.W. Bradshaw, a physician at Oberlin College, worried,

> The individual finds himself removed from his familiar home environment where he has made satisfactory adjustments emotionally, where he has been accustomed to family protection, where defense mechanisms have been developed to take care of most of his conflicts and where danger from physical as well as biological enemies has by experience been reduced to a minimum. Snatched from this familiar haven and placed in an entirely new environment, perhaps an entirely new climate, where unaccustomed physical dangers present themselves, where strenuous competition of intellectual, social and physical activities challenge him to exert every ounce of energy, he finds his old defense mechanisms ineffectual. The adjustment to this unusual environment and the experience of life and work in it give rise to many pathological, physical and mental conditions.[66]

Concern about the mental health of young people gained further ground in the post-war years. In 1946 a group of American psychiatrists established the well-funded and influential Group for the Advancement of Psychiatry (GAP), which gave weight to the belief that "prevention and public awareness were the best ways to combat the problem of mental illness" and advanced the need to target children and adolescents in particular. This belief was reiterated in the 1947 report by President Truman's Commission on Higher Education as well as by various university presidents who emphasized the importance of mental hygiene.[67] A 1951 report of a student health survey conducted in the late 1940s at

Oxford University confirmed the need for concern about student mental health, pointing to the high level of minor psychological problems among students. Indeed the report noted that 50 per cent of absences from class were due to mental disturbance or nervous breakdown and that the suicide rate among men was five times that for the same age group in the general population in England and Wales.[68] In the 1950s, Dana Farnsworth, director of health services at Harvard University, a former member of the GAP and former president of the American College Health Association, worked tirelessly to expand campus mental hygiene facilities across North America.[69]

In Canadian universities, which had fewer resources than many American ones, the inclusion of psychologists and psychiatrists in student health occurred at a much slower pace. University reports suggest that in the 1920s and 1930s some universities had the resources to send a few students to consult with an expert in mental hygiene.[70] Speaking of the aims and purposes of compulsory physical examination at the 1936 Congress of the Universities of the British Empire, H.J. Cody, president of the University of Toronto, noted,

> ... by calling in the aid of the psychiatric experts the medical director is able to make deductions as to the mental state of particular men; and very frequently these are raised from depression to good health in a way which could not be possible but for a compulsory medical examination.[71]

The ability of universities to provide for such work was, however, limited. The principal of McGill University noted in 1931 that "more time has been devoted to the examination period, thus affording an opportunity for the discussion of personal problems. Dr W.T.B. Mitchell, director of the Mental Hygiene Institute, has rendered very valuable consultative assistance, but it is obvious that the numerous problems involved require more attention than is possible under existing conditions."[72]

A few institutions implemented psychological testing, if only for a brief period of time. For example, the University of Saskatchewan did so for a period of several years during the 1930s, due largely to the influence of S.R. Laycock.[73] Hired in 1927 as a member of the College of Education, Laycock specialized in child and adolescent psychology, and, in particular, adjustment and mental testing. In the mid-1930s Laycock was able to convince university authorities to schedule a psychological test that would accompany the medical examinations held during Freshman

Welcome Week.[74] Between 1934 and 1938 he administered tests to entering students. His findings over the course of this period indicated that the test identified a correlation between intelligence and class marks and could be used to identify and help students with "mediocre records but high ability," aid faculty committees regarding student dismissals or probation, and assist in determining course selections as well as selections for entry to university, honours courses, or graduate work on the grounds that those of "low test ability almost never do high grade work."[75] University officials, however, do not seem to have continued the tests once Laycock completed his study.

Thus, beginning in the 1930s, but more frequently in the subsequent three decades, university health experts began to call for greater resources devoted to counselling services and mental health.[76] Indeed, mental health was seen as being equal in importance to physical health, both for the student and in the activities of health services. The director of the University of British Columbia health service noted in his 1940 report, "the purpose of the Health Service for Students is to supervise the physical and mental health of the student from the time of admission to University until graduation, so that as the student takes his place in the outside world he will not be handicapped by physical defects or mental breakdown during the period in which he is adjusting himself to his career."[77] Similarly, the dean of junior women at the University of Manitoba argued in 1945 that the university should help provide

a sense of health and well-being. In order to get the most out of her course, a student should be relatively free from emotional disturbances of an acute kind, neuroticism, and, of course, organic troubles. While the undergraduate period is precisely the time when major emotional experiences do occur, an opportunity to discuss problems arising from these has many times lifted a weight, or pointed a path.[78]

Not everyone was supportive of the intrusion of psychologists into students' lives. Muriel Roscoe, warden of Royal Victoria College, was much less keen than other university officials on the probing nature of psychological investigation. In 1946–7 Dr Frederick Hanson, psychiatric consultant with the McGill Student Health Service, undertook an investigation into "the prevalence and importance of emotional instability and psychiatric disorders among students entering McGill." He

developed a test questionnaire distributed to 650 first-year male students in engineering and sciences in order to help discover and clas-
sify students in need of "treatment for existing psychiatric disorders"
and provide "preventive therapy." After this first round of testing, health
services personnel decided they needed to survey a larger pool of students in order to determine if such testing should become regular practice. The female students at Royal Victoria College, already subject to a
physical exam, must have seemed like the ideal test group. Percy Vivian,
chairman of the department of health and social medicine, wrote Roscoe requesting that the test be given to entering students, after which
it would be scored by Dr Hanson and his associates. Findings would be
noted in the student's health record and the results brought to the student's attention.[79]

After examining the questionnaire, Roscoe refused the request, even
for a select group of senior students, on the grounds that "this questionnaire, prepared for men, and obviously more mature than our women
students, would raise many questions and could do a good deal of dam-
age. I am sure that it would have a lot of unfavourable reaction from
parents."[80] The questionnaire asked medical questions, such as "Do you
have headaches, faint, or suffer from stomach trouble?" Looking for
signs of depression, mental imbalance and paranoia, it probed students'
emotional state with questions ranging from "Do you get all nervous and
shaky when approached by a superior?" to "Are your emotions usually
dead?" "Do you usually feel cheerful and happy?" and "Do you often
get into a violent rage?" Perhaps more seriously for Roscoe, this survey
contained questions such as "Have you ever gotten into serious trouble
or lost your job because of drinking?" "Have you been arrested more
than three times?" "Have you ever taken dope regularly (like morphine
or 'reefers')?" and, number 99 of 101 questions, "Is the opposite sex
unpleasant to you?"[81]

While Roscoe worried about the probing nature of the survey and
the fact that it raised issues that students might not have thought about
prior to being asked such questions, others worried about the place of
psychology within the emerging hierarchy of medicine. In 1946, a few
students at the University of Toronto began advocating for the creation
of a student counselling service on campus. The department of psychology backed their demands for such a service. However, the director of
the health service was less enthusiastic. In his report to the president
he noted,

Our policy is set forth in the following paragraph which occurs in our instructions to Staff Physicians. "Many American Universities have a 'Campus Psychiatrist' or 'Psychologist' to whom the student may go direct for consultation or be referred by Student Councillors, or Vocational Guidance Staffs. It is felt that such a service is not only undesirable but dangerous. If a student is worried, maladjusted or in such a nervous condition that his health is affected, it is a Health Service problem and he should be seen by one or our Staff Physicians who will go into the problem thoroughly and give such advice as is indicated. If the case requires a skill in psychological medicine or neuropsychiatry which is beyond that expected of a good general physician, he will then arrange for a psychiatric consultation through the Director or Assistant Director."[82]

Ultimately, those worried about the infiltration of psychology into student health would find themselves out of step with the modern turn towards such services. In 1941, leading administrators, Christian activists, and psychologists came together to discuss the issue of the impact of university life on students in Canada. Funded by the Edward W. Hazen Foundation, an American institution that commissioned leading scholars to write about religion in higher education and sponsored faculty conferences on the same topic, the gathering brought together educators not only involved in personal counselling but concerned about the place of religion in higher education.[83] The report that emerged from the conference advocated the adoption of the type of student health services in American universities that dealt with students' emotional problems and provided guidance.

While students were not involved in that conference, they soon took up the call. That trend would become more apparent in the United States in the mid-1950s and in Canada in the early 1960s. In 1954, some members of the National Student Association in the United States helped plan, and participated in, the Fourth National Conference on Health in Colleges. In his opening address, Dana Farnsworth, director of health services at Harvard University, noted the importance of student involvement in developing campus health services.[84] In 1963, the National Federation of Canadian University Students (and its successor, the Canadian Union of Students) initiated a conference at Queen's University on Student Mental Health that was co-sponsored by the World University Service of Canada and the Canadian Mental Health Association. Participants included psychologists, psychiatrists, directors of student services, members of university health services, directors of admissions, deans of men and women, university chaplains, student counselling services, and student leaders.[85] The conference acted as a forum for discussion regarding the perceived causes and consequences of the emotional and mental health of students as well as the responsibility of the university in helping students to adjust to their environment. The resulting report recorded that "... it was generally agreed at the Conference that one of the urgent needs was the provision of more highly individualized counselling and psychiatric services on campus, and for those services to be coordinated with other aspects of the university experience."[86] And in 1966–7, one of the central aims of the president of the students' representative council of the Regina campus of the University of Saskatchewan was the creation of a psychological counselling service.[87]

Some of this pressure paid off. In the post-war years, universities gradually added psychiatric consultation to their general health services.[88] At some institutions, mental health issues became integrated into the compulsory health lectures. In 1948, a year after engaging a psychiatric consultant, the University of Toronto Health Services, with the help of the department of psychiatry, provided lectures on topics such as "Effective Study and Work Habits," "Social Tension on entering University," "Worry, Neurosis and You," "Resentment, Anger, Hate," and "The Psychology of Examinations."[89] The University of Alberta established Student Advisory Services in 1950, renamed Student Counselling Services in 1959, offering personal, general academic, and vocational counselling as well as study skills training.[90] By 1952–3, UBC not only had a department of personnel and student services but gave all first-year students educational and evaluative tests, after which students could receive counselling based on results. In 1954, the university established the UBC counselling service.[91] In 1966, Acadia created the position of student counsellor, filled by David B. Barnes, a faculty member. Barnes advised students on academic, occupational, behavioural, social, marriage, personal, and emotional issues. He also administered "reading and interest tests" to new students, the results of which "were sent to the Deans for their use in helping students register" as well as "to select students for the remedial reading program."[92]

Such services often developed in an ad hoc fashion. Dr Peter Rempel of the University of Alberta noted at the 1963 Queen's Conference on Student Mental Health that "three agencies primarily concerned with the welfare of the student have grown up independently, the health service, the department of psychiatry and the counselling service. The counselling service has five full-time psychologists. We make referrals to the health service or to psychiatry when indicated. In turn, we get cross-referrals from both of these."[93] Yet by 1966 a survey of forty-nine campuses indicated that twenty-two, or 44.9 per cent, had a psychiatrist available for student consultation.[94]

Advocates of services for student mental health recognized that while services were needed to contend with students with serious mental illness, increasingly they were dealing with "transient or situational cases." In other words, psychologists and psychiatrists were being asked to help students cope with the transition to university. Dr G.E. Wodehouse of the University of Toronto noted that many cases involved "financial crises, family conflict, lack of motivation, competition for job placement at the end of it all, competition for academic standing merely to get through, or into a particular course, examination deadlines, the readjustment of ideas and philosophies concerning religion, relationship with their peers, girlfriends, families and teachers. This area is our therapeutic programme."[95] The president of UBC commented in his 1952–3 report that "… counselling has become an essential service in the university community. At best we live in a complex and an uneasy world; the period of adjustment between high school and university is seldom an easy one, and many of our students require advice based upon the best principles that are available to us."[96] Student counselling thus not only became a matter of serious consideration on the part of mental health advocates but was seen increasingly by administrators as a central component of the work of the university.

Conclusion

The growing concern about student mental health seems on the surface to have little to do with that regarding tuberculosis. Indeed, anxieties about the former began to appear only as the latter had begun to wane. And certainly the attempt to eradicate tuberculosis and the search to identify and treat mental illness have their own distinct histories. Yet the attention devoted to these issues also points to broader patterns reflecting both earlier concerns and new methods and priorities.

In many ways, the attention directed towards tuberculosis and then mental health reinforced late-nineteenth- and early-twentieth-century approaches to student health that were focused on preventative care and the need to encourage all students to develop to their full physical potential. At the same time, the increasing focus given to those areas highlights the changes that had already begun to appear at the turn of the century and that were marked by a gradual shift in emphasis from eradicating environmental causes of disease to promoting individual health. Paul Starr argues that in the United States, new public health measures such as the introduction of medical examinations, the concern about venereal disease, and the attempt to control tuberculosis, focused attention on personal or individual hygiene. This process began with the introduction of medical examinations for insurance purposes, which invariably showed that "very few people were healthy and normal" and thus reinforced the belief in individuals' need of medical attention by their physician.[97] Similarly he argues that with tuberculin testing and the discovery of infected individuals who were healthy, physicians could have advocated the need to prevent infection by improving living and working conditions rather than through individual health exams and hygiene.[98] Instead, they focused attention on individual health and away from broader social reforms. This trend was reinforced with the turn to mental health.

One of the effects of increasing medical authority involved a process of differentiation between experts and lay people. Activities such as social hygiene, civic improvement, and the creation of sanitariums, which had their roots in a broad social reform movement, gradually gave way to direction by experts. Similarly, in some places in the 1940s and 1950s, health services were becoming differentiated from physical education. That process can also be seen in the way in which deans of women and physical educators ceased to lead discussion on medical subjects, while doctors made fewer pronouncements on general living conditions. The earlier pattern, whereby authorities at a place such as Victoria College worked together to ensure the moral, mental, spiritual, and physical health of students, gave way to a separation of roles. This occurred neither quickly nor completely. Yet gradually, comments by deans and physical educators on medical issues became muted, and comments by doctors and nurses on what might be termed moral or social issues, such as women's late nights or lack of proper footwear, became less common.

This process of differentiation both aided, and was a product of, the elevation of medical authority. In health services, as in physical education, educators and medical experts aimed to carry out their work on a scientific basis. Health care, like other aspects of the research university, was becoming increasingly specialized. This development had more than a simply bureaucratic effect; it marked, too, a new way of thinking that would promote different understandings of, and approaches to, student formation.

8

From Character to Personality: Changing Visions of Citizenship, 1940s to 1960s

In the late nineteenth century and the early decades of the twentieth century, educators envisioned the role of the university as contributing to the final stages of a young person's moral, physical, spiritual, and intellectual formation. No matter the individual distinction that a student might attain in his or her studies or extra-curricular activities, it was the achievement of character that educators perceived as reflecting the true quality of one's alma mater. A nebulous concept to be sure – at its core rested the notion of individual contribution and sacrifice to the greater social whole.

The language and ideals of character would, however, increasingly fall out of step with some of the new beliefs and values emerging in the twentieth century. Over time, educators began to adopt the discourse of personality that psychologists so readily promulgated. The gradual shift from the use of "character" to that of "personality" was not simply a shift in terms. Rather, it represented a more fundamental change in societal values and beliefs regarding the nature, meaning and development of self. In contrast to the emphasis on self-sacrifice inherent in the concept of character, the new discourse of personality focused on self-realization – the development of an individual's specific characteristics and traits in order to provide that individual with the greatest chance of fulfilment and success.

In this chapter, I focus on the shift in discourse from character to personality by examining the rhetoric of educators, particularly as expressed in the two conferences already referred to, the 1941 gathering on the influence of the university on student life, and the Queen's conference on student mental health in 1963. I then elucidate the way in which the adoption of the new discourse of personality was part and

parcel of broader societal developments such as the process of secularization, changing concepts of citizenship, and the growing emphasis on
the importance of "expressive individualism." This turn to the discourse
of personality and the interest in human adjustment, I argue, both reflected and contributed to ideological shifts within North American
culture.

The Shift in Discourse from Character to Personality

By the 1930s and 1940s, health experts, physical educators, and university presidents had all begun to employ the language of personality. Initially they did so by intermixing older ideals of character with the newer
language of psychology. For example, in 1938–9, S.A. Korning, associate
professor of physical education at Dalhousie University, described the
aims of that institution's program in physical education as follows:

> The physical education achieved in games and other activities is valuable
> as a development of personality, in that the physical exercises give to the
> practisers not merely physical development, but also the development of
> valuable qualities of will and character. The designation "physical educa-
> tion" is in reality too narrow, because in teaching the participants how to
> use the body and how to master it, the physical exercises have the effect
> of cultivating the whole personality. This is not physical education, but an
> education by physical means.[1]

Korning, then, interchanged the terms, equating the cultivation of personality directly with the development of will and character.

Other educators simply replaced the term "character" with that of
"personality." In 1934–5, Robert Falconer, former president of the University of Toronto, stated, "The university is at once a source of individual
culture and of public service. It deepens and enriches personality, and
through the enriched personality of its members it can be a servant to
the whole nation."[2] Similarly, in his 1935–6 annual report, the principal
of McGill argued that "while a university exists as a training ground of
skillful workers it must remember that the first need of society is the production of men and women not merely stored with factual knowledge
but trained to think and to judge: men and women moreover whose
personality is physically, intellectually and spiritually developed to the
utmost capacity."[3] In these cases, leading university administrators adopted the new, and more up-to-date language of personality, yet used

it in a manner similar to the way in which the term "character" had been employed in previous decades.

This type of slippage between the ideals of character and the language of personality was not uncommon. The 1941 conference on the impact of university life on Canadian students is illustrative. Drawing on the new psychological theories of the time, participants identified adolescence as a key period in the process of maturation, but one wracked by turmoil and crisis. They perceived this process not as a problem for one or two students, but for all students. The conference report laid out the problems encountered by students in universities within that context. It stated that because students arrived at university in late adolescence and not as fully formed adults, the purpose of liberal education should be to address the whole person – the social and physical side as well as the intellectual. Participants wanted students to become adults who could think critically about contemporary problems and issues, who would be able to find their place in their chosen profession and become active in the community, and who completed sexual adjustment within "a happy marriage." Finally, students needed to figure out how to integrate learning, work, family life, and their contribution to society into a broader purpose of life.[4]

The report blamed parents and the school system for not doing more to ensure adolescent adjustment, but did not leave the university unscathed. In particular, the report emphasized the need for the insertion of progressive methods into educational practice. It criticized teaching practices that treated students "not as thinking, self-reliant beings but as automatons."[5] The relationship between teachers and students needed to change: "Instead of a bored professor reading or dictating notes in a classroom, to an equally bored group of students, the university class must be a co-operative group of students and teachers."[6] The report continued, "It remains for the university to realize that the whole student comes to the university – not just his mind – and to take the responsibility of developing the whole student as an integral person in all aspects of his being."[7]

This emphasis on progressive educational methods was reflected in the rhetoric of physical educators of the time. A 1940 memorandum on physical education at McGill stated that in implementing a physical education program, the university intended to create not a "dull weekly routine of 'physical jerks' but exercise students will enjoy."[8] Maurice Lewis Van Vliet, a physical instructor at the University of British Columbia, wrote in an article on physical education in wartime, "We plan to promote opportunities for mental expression, encourage creative thinking and develop personality, and do not believe in training our young people to memorize a few set exercises ... University students should not be forced to educate the physical but should be educated through the physical."[9] Thus physical educators, like members of the university community more generally, soaked up the rhetoric regarding the importance of progressive educational methods.

Perhaps not surprisingly, given the nature of the 1941 conference, participants linked the methods of progressive education to the need for development of a faith-based philosophy of life, primarily assumed to be Christian. Indeed, they intertwined liberal education, democracy, and Christianity. A liberal education, based on the methods of progressive education, would result in "active citizenship," a central linchpin of democracy.[10] "In addition," the report continued, "democracy, which is merely a secular expression of Christianity, means *reverence for personality*."[11] Thus, the report concluded, "The integrating value of fellowship with, and devotion to, any great cause is beyond question. 'Thy *faith* hath made thee whole' contains profound psychological truth. Many students discuss intellectual ideas literally all night – and yet their lives are split and uncoordinated. To have integration of personality is surely the supreme goal of developing values in the university."[12] In envisioning the university as moulding students who could contribute to national development, conference participants assumed in general that personality development would accord with the values and ideals of a Christian nation.

It is clear from the report that the language of personality had penetrated academic circles by the early 1940s. In the post-war years, that language, along with an increasingly explicit emphasis on mental health, would come to dominate the discourse of physical educators and university administrators. In considering the creation of a compulsory program in physical education, a senate committee at McGill University noted that "the Department of Physical Education considers the student to be a young, vigorous active total personality, with all his functions cooperating harmoniously for buoyant, healthful living."[13] Keith King and Angus Gillis, co-directors of the physical education department for men at Dalhousie University, argued in the early 1950s that while physical education helped develop "vitality and neuro-muscular skills" crucial "for the proper functioning of an individual in this modern, tense world," it was also "an essential agent for the development of the proper attitudes and the intangible factors required for wholesome living." They went on to state, "there is no other activity that offers the opportunity that Physical

Education offers in learning such intangible factors as safety, living with others, and respect for authority ... Our aim is to help the University build a wholesome, well-rounded citizen."[14]

W.A. Stevens, director of physical education for men at the University of Toronto, drew on the emerging language of mental health in order to bolster his physical education program. He commented that physical education could be a panacea for mental problems:

> Our kind of society has placed severe demands upon emotional and nervous stability. To live fully today, the individual must be able to get along with others, control his emotions, and find outlets for self-expression. More people have more leisure time today than ever before, and many need guidance in using their leisure hours constructively. Physical education is a way of education through physical activities which are selected and carried on with full regard to values in human growth, development, and behaviour. It is an integral part of the educational experiences available to all students at this University.[15]

Zerada Slack, director of physical education for women at the University of Toronto, noted in a report to the president in the early 1950s, "It is the aim of modern Physical Education for women to make some contribution to the development of the student as a whole person; it contributes, that is not only to her organic health but also to her expanding personality."[16] Near the end of the decade she wrote, in an article in *Health* magazine, "Physical education is a service programme which has as its aim the development of mentally, emotionally and organically sound citizens through skills, games and physical activities."[17]

Indeed, by the early 1960s the aims and purpose of physical education, at least as articulated at the University of Toronto, had become fully entwined with creating and ensuring mental health. In 1961 the president struck a Committee on Athletic Programs in order to assess campus athletic needs. A sub-committee on "the medical aspects of physical exercise in relation to health and well-being" developed a report aimed at elucidating the "Values in Athletic and Physical Education Programs." The report argued

> that (i) individual-type sports have a good effect on health and general well-being and are desirable for participation in later life; (ii) all forms of athletics and physical recreation provide a relief from normal tension and

the routines of academic study; and (iii) the program of competitive sports and games provides an opportunity for students to meet, compete, and make friends with other students on the campus. It was the consensus of the Subcommittee that all of these factors contribute in one way or another to good mental health.[18]

Many of the ideas of physical educators found expression in the 1963 conference on Student Mental Health. Much of that conference reiterated the ideas and themes expressed at the 1941 Hazen conference: the need to understand the student's college years as part of a final stage of adolescence; the important task of identifying the elements of stress leading to a potential identity crisis; and the role of the university in creating the conditions conducive to the development of well-adjusted personalities.[19] Yet adjustment focused relatively singularly on individual development. Dana Farnsworth, director of the university health service at Harvard University, noted that the aim of a university health service was "to develop persons who are intellectually self-propelled."[20] He understood student adjustment to consist of "... the capacity to react in a reasonably adequate fashion to anything which comes along."[21] Graham Blaine, also at Harvard, perceived the role of the university to be helping students "towards self-expression, towards being himself ..."[22] M. Jean-Charles Bouffard, director of student affairs at Laval University, noted, "La fin concrète que toute université doit pour suivre est l'éducation supérieure de l'homme, de l'homme en son entier, afin de lui permettre d'acquérir la science et la technique exigées par sa profession, de développer pleinement sa personnalité et tout ce qui lui permettra de jouer dans la vie le rôle que la société attend de lui."[23] And J. Wendell Macleod, director of medical education of the Canadian Universities Foundation, noted, "... we foster the growth of each student to his full capacity."[24]

The emphasis on personality development that occurred during the 1940s and 1950s thus marked a transition in educators' understanding of the aims and purposes of the university in students' formation. Earlier in the century, physical educators and health proponents had perceived body shape as a representation of one's masculinity or femininity. They equated character with the creation of manhood and womanhood, emphasizing common qualities such as honesty, loyalty, self-control as well as distinct ones such as, for men, leadership, initiative, courage, and for women, unselfishness, obedience, and cooperation. The acquisition of such traits was perceived as part of a process of integrating inner development into a Christian philosophy of life. The aim of that inner force was subordination of the self in the service of others, and ultimately of the nation. Self-denial and self-sacrifice were key components in character formation: sacrifice to one's team, one's family, one's community, one's country.[25]

In contrast, the aim of developing personality was more narrowly focused on self-realization. Educators highlighted the importance of bringing out and shaping the characteristics and traits of the given individual, to find what he or she was successful at, and provide that individual with the greatest chance at adjustment and success. They spoke and wrote of creating a "total personality," developing the students "as a whole person" and building a "well-rounded citizen" in the effort to promote, among other things, "healthful living," "safety, living with others, and respect for authority," and "creative thinking." Inner harmony would facilitate societal cooperation. Moreover, inner development would allow an individual to fulfil his or her full social potential. In contrast to emphasizing fulfilment through self-sacrifice inherent within the concept of character formation, the discourse of personality emphasized that fulfilment would come through individual development. And instead of a Christian philosophy of life, there was now no one way to find inner harmony, to develop one's place in society, or to complete one's development – the practical implications of which required the recognition of difference within physical education programs.

The Impact of the Turn to Personality

Why did the concept of personality gain influence and what was the impact of this turn of events? Educators' adoption of the concept of personality and their attention to student mental health intersected with three other developments occurring on campus and within society more generally: a process of secularization; the changing concept of citizenship; and a turn towards "expressive individualism," the result of a growing sense of alienation among youth from the values and ideals of mainstream society. Each of these developments helps to explain why educators turned to the concept of personality and how it was perceived as a useful tool to explain and understand the process and aims of student formation. They also illuminate the way in which that concept gained popularity alongside other significant social, cultural, and intellectual changes.

Educators' move away from the attempt to help students develop a Christian philosophy of life and towards an emphasis on the individual finding his or her own place in society is tied to the process of secularization within the university. Character had a particular meaning and history rooted in middle-class Christian ideals. While the force of that Christian vision remained strong in the 1940s and 1950s, it was also undergoing a process of erosion. Thus it was possible for a social scientist such as S.R. Laycock, trained as a Methodist minister and raised in a culture imbued with progressive ideals, to emphasize personality adjustment while embedding personality within traditional moral strictures of the Christian middle-class family. Equally, ministers and theologians – and here Falconer and Cody, university presidents but also ministers, are good examples – could reinforce traditional moral strictures by drawing on the latest, most progressive ideas such as that of personality development. The shift in language, then, did not indicate a rupture from religious-based moral beliefs to secular ones. Rather, at least for a time, there was a fluid transition in values and ideals as academics drew on both Christian beliefs and social scientific methods.[26]

At the same time, the language of personality could be used in different ways by different groups. In interchanging the terms, students, university presidents, and physical instructors were not misusing them. In the American context, Heather Warren argues that mainline Protestants regularly switched the terms in the 1920s and 1930s.[27] Ian Nicholson comments that, among psychologists, the very popularity of the term "personality" arose from its "freshness and flexibility," its ability to "maintain an ethical emphasis" in the modern world without the "full weight of Christian ethics."[28] The vagueness of the term probably helped make it popular. As Nicholson states, "To some, the language of personality signaled science, the body, measurement, and all that was modern and right about academic psychology. To others, personality spoke of time-honored truths, personal freedom, spirituality, and a respect for individual human dignity and subjectivity."[29]

Yet if the very vagueness of the concept of personality enabled its widespread adoption in the early part of the century, over time it came to have a meaning reasonably distinct from the idea of character development with which it was often initially entwined. The concept of personality, which embraced the idea of malleable rather than fixed traits, reoriented psychologists' focus from mental illness to mental health and adjustment through counselling. Nicholson points out that "the character ideal was all about realizing selfhood by internalizing the values of a supposedly permanent moral order."[30] But the concept of personality embraced the idea of human diversity and adaptability, the idea of an adaptive self or "a self that exists independently of moral frameworks."[31]

What is apparent in the 1963 conference is the clear separation of adjustment from the creation of a Christian philosophy of life. The secular nature of this conference is significant, and indeed, was remarked upon at the time. In his summary comments Graham Blaine stated, "I was surprised that in a country which is so deeply religious this did not come up as a topic in the general discussions."[32] Between the 1941 and 1963 conferences, a period of just over twenty years, the topic of students' emotional health shifted from one embedded within explicit Christian language to one in which Christianity was not mentioned. This was a gradual process. For example, while the 1941 report was couched in Christian moral language, it attempted to leave room for non-Christians. The 1920s and 1930s had witnessed a growing international outlook within the Protestant churches, evident in the report in a passing reference to the need to help students develop *a sense of fellowship with and devotion to whatever the student finds to be the life-principles of the universe.*"[33] Still, if participants acknowledged Canada's religious diversity, they still very much assumed a Christian society. By 1963, as Graham Blaine stated in his summary comments, "The ticklish matter of what we may call moral responsibility was not raised."[34]

This process can equally be seen in the aims of some physical education programs. To give one example, while the 1957–8 *Calendar* for St. Francis Xavier emphasized the role of physical education "to develop standards of conduct," that for 1966–7 noted that the "program is devised to promote physical fitness as well as general knowledge and development of skills in many sporting activities."[35] This separation of the teaching of moral values from explicit Christian beliefs and doctrines formed part of a broader societal shift occurring in the 1950s and 1960s.[36]

While the 1941 conference placed significant emphasis on attempting to help students develop a Christian philosophy of life, in 1963 participants focused on individual development and readjustment. G.E. Wodehouse, director of health services at the University of Toronto, noted that the cases his staff saw included "financial crises, family conflict, lack of motivation, competition for job placement at the end of it all, competition for academic standing merely to get through, or into a particular course, examination deadlines, the readjustment of ideas and philosophies concerning religion, relationships with their peers, girlfriends, families and teachers." To these he offered a "thera-peutic programme."[37] Fixing personal problems, then, emerged as the focus of the conference. Certainly moral imperatives remained: students were to learn "wholesome living," "safety," "living with others," "respect for authority," and to be "well-rounded citizens." Within a Christian na-tion, these terms could all be understood in a broad Christian frame-work. But the explicit Christian moral language that had appeared around the term "character" disappeared.

Indeed, the concept of creating "an" ideal citizen who had assimilated his or her individual development into "a" broader philosophy of life receded. No longer, according to Graham Blaine, was the task of faculty the "moulding" of the student "by someone who has pre-conceived ideas about how young people should behave," but rather aiding students "to-wards self-expression, toward being himself."[38] Pierre Dansereau, dean of the faculty of science at the University of Montreal and chair of the conference, noted, "We do not train students for good citizenship or to fit themselves to an existing social pattern. No, we get together to criticize this pattern."[39] In the conference proceedings, neither Wood-house nor any of the other participants addressed or offered solutions to the problem of students' place in society or their responsibilities and duties to that society. It would be up to each student to figure out how he or she should best undertake self-development and how to link self-development to their contributions as national, and global, citizens.

As the process of secularization made inroads within campus culture, new ideas about the nature and meaning of citizenship were also begin-ning to take hold. These ideas would help faculty and students challenge traditional notions about their role and place on campus. They were also ideas that meshed with, and reinforced, a corresponding emphasis on self-realization.

The transformation in the concept of citizenship that had clearly be-gun to take place by the mid-twentieth century involved a rearticulation of the needs, duties, and rights of citizens. Mid-nineteenth-century liber-als promoted the concept of citizenship as embodying a claim to indi-vidual rights, such as the right to vote, to own property, or to live from one's own free labour. In the early- to mid-twentieth century the growing belief in the need for a welfare state extended this definition to one of social citizenship, the idea that states owe citizens a certain level of social security, such as a basic standard of living and access to health care and education.[40] This concept of citizenship as involving rights and entitle-ments included a redefinition of the relationship between citizen and state. Examining the 1930s, Lara Campbell notes that in terms of social services, they marked "a shift from a charity model of welfare provision to one based on an articulation of rights," a redefinition of unemployment that no longer viewed it as an individual moral failing but rather recognized "structural problems in the capitalist economy" and "a level of state responsibility for the economic welfare of men, women, and children."[41]

The language of rights became more prominent after the Second World War and has become increasingly entrenched since the 1960s.[42] Writing about the history and contemporary relevance of this rights revolution, Michael Ignatieff argues that while this new conception of citizenship has continued to emphasize individual responsibility and duty to the state, the idea of individual rights has stressed the notion "that each of us is an end in ourselves, not a means to an end."[43] It is, in other words, a version that endorses the "values of individual autonomy."[44] The increasing emphasis placed on human rights, along with the secularization of society, has resulted in a variety of intellectual changes. For example, in conjunction with the ideals of progressive education, the long-term impact in the public schools since the 1960s has been the emergence of what sociologists Scott Davies and Neil Guppy refer to as "the new morality." It "is now about exposing students to a fuller range of contemporary controversies, beliefs, and ideals, and encouraging them to make informed choices. It is less likely to portray certain and unambiguous truths." Moreover, it encourages students to "criticize society, question dominant values, and illuminate social problems."[45]

That viewpoint could already be seen developing in universities in the years after the Second World War. Indeed, the broad shift in a concept of citizenship emphasizing duties and obligations to one of rights and entitlements is reflected in faculty and students' re-envisioning of their role within the university in the 1950s and 1960s. While historians have focused on the late 1960s as a period in which the professoriate and students demanded change to their institutions, academics had already begun in the 1940s to point to the tensions inherent within the older and newer conceptions of the nature and purpose of the university. The 1941 Hazen conference report, for example, highlights academics' desires for the resources to expand their institutions and create research possibilities as well as their lament at the loss of intimate and teaching-focused institutions, such as the ones from which they had emerged. On the one hand, the report criticized the financial stringency of many institutions, the lack of resources for research and the development of graduate programs, the need for faculty participation in governance, and the difficulties being encountered by some universities in reconciling their religious origins with more secular orientations.[46] On the other hand, it decried the negative effects that educators saw emerging within their own institutions: the increasing lack of intellectual and moral coherence of the university, the separation and specialization of knowledge into narrow fields of learning, and the limited guidance provided to students.

Criticism of the nature of the university and the methods of university teaching became more prominent through the 1950s and 1960s. At the 1963 conference, Neil Morrison, dean of Atkinson College, highlighted the authoritarian nature of universities which ran counter, he claimed, to the kinds of ideas faculty attempted "to teach about freedom of speech, personal and social responsibility, individual behaviour and the democratic process."[47] Morrison's ideas were reflected in the group discussion that highlighted the authoritarianism of some teachers' approach and their focus on providing knowledge narrowly in their area of expertise. One student noted the need for "balance between the responsibility of the faculty member as someone who teaches and grades, and as someone who relates as another human being."[48]

During the war and immediate post-war period, many academics perceived these problems to be ones that could be solved through reform of their institutions. Drawing on ideas of progressive education, participants in the 1941 conference emphasized the importance of more interactive learning and participation in education. In the 1950s and 1960s, the professoriate became increasingly vocal about the need for participatory democracy in the workplace.[49] Both administrators and faculty also attempted to improve the educational experience through the creation of small seminars and tutorials rather than large lectures, placing resources towards first-year teaching, and encouraging participatory education.[50] By the late 1960s, students had begun to take up many of the issues articulated by some faculty in the post-war years. In particular, they echoed faculty demands for participatory democracy, arguing for a student voice in the running of departments, faculties, and governing boards as well as a greater role in their own education.[51]

At the same time, students began to articulate their own place on campus as one befitting adults. While administrators through the first half of the twentieth century generally understood the university as *in loco parentis*, by the mid- to late-1960s that conception of the university was under challenge. Students also began, in greater numbers, to look beyond the campus to involvement in issues in their community and on the national and international stage.[52] The Vietnam War in particular galvanized at least some students to conceive of their role in university not only as student-citizens, or as citizens in the making, but as fully-formed citizens with the ability to influence political affairs in ways that might counter the status quo.

The shift in language from character to personality, along with the rearticulation of citizenship as embodying rights, may also have had significant implications for the reconceptualization of women's place on campus. Character was about the creation of manhood and woman-hood. At least on the surface, personality was more gender-neutral, and focused on creating individuals and citizens.[53] In their emphasis on de-veloping personality, educators used language that did not differentiate between men and women but rather focused on students. This change in language obviously did not institute gender equality. In the 1950s, traditional gender roles remained prominent.[54] On campus, men and women had unequal access to athletic facilities and their programs re-mained different. In residence, female students continued to be seen as in need of protection, while female professionals on campus assumed roles subordinate to those of men. Moreover, the shift to a more superfi-cially gender-neutral language could also allow sexism to become more hidden. At the same time, over the decades women had made gains on campus. While women continued to face restrictions on their behav-iour throughout this period, they also experienced a gradual liberaliza-tion of rules and regulations as well as greater integration into many extra-curricular activities.[55] Equally, Karine Hébert has shown that by the 1950s at McGill University, designations for campus women such as "freschette" or "co-ed" were increasingly replaced by that of "student."[56] The shift in language from "character" to "personality" is also a subtle reflection of this shift. The language of personality had the potential to subsume womanhood under the rubric of personhood. Educators' use of this new discourse can thus provide one clue as to how women may have begun to conceive of themselves as deserving of the full rights and privileges of student life – something they would begin to fight for more overtly in the late 1960s.

Within the university, then, the rights revolution became articulated by faculty and students as the right to full participation within the struc-tures of the university, and by many students as a right to be treated as adults and to fully participate in community and world affairs. Both faculty and students re-envisioned their place within the university as bearers of rights and entitlements rather than as groups at the mercy of boards of governors, presidents, administrators, and faculty members. That reconceptualization was due not only to the transformation in ideals of citizenship, but also to the growing adherence to the concept of personality and the influence of the rhetoric of progressive education. As we saw earlier, educators from the 1940s on had begun to embrace the idea that self-development, or the development of the personality, could be accomplished only through learning methods aimed at developing students' creativity and self-expression. By extension, development could not be encouraged through regulation and command but by active citizenship, with students participating in their learning and in the institutions in which that education took place. Thus the intellectual current of progressive education, psychology, and social citizenship that had been gaining favour over the course of the first half of the twentieth century both reflected and advanced the course of the transformation occurring within universities in the 1950s and 1960s.

By the 1960s, the move towards rights and entitlements was accompanied by an emphasis on "expressive individualism." Examining the context of the progressive movement in Ontario after the Second World War, Scott Davies argues that progressive educators had long held to beliefs that individual satisfaction and constant self-development were ends in themselves, beyond actual achievement. But in the 1960s, this became "animated with a new emotive force," promoting the idea that students be judged less by external standards than by "a more subjective understanding of learning." In the educational reforms of the late 1960s, learning was to be understood as a much more individualistic and subjective process.[57] Such notions clearly fit with the idea of the democratically run classroom and university. It also reflected a growing anti-authoritarianism and sense of alienation among youth.

The idea of individual alienation from society and community began to enter popular discourse in the 1950s.[58] In 1962–3, the director of student health services at the University of Toronto reported, "One of the more common aggravating features frequently mentioned was that of the 'bigness' of our universities, the loss of personal contact between student and faculty, together with the increasing impersonality and lack of identification on the part of many students."[59] In the mid- to late-1960s, students expressed a sense of alienation from their universities as their idea of the university experience and the reality of that experience clashed. Patricia Jasen has illuminated the way in which administrators and faculty in the 1950s and 1960s emphasized the importance of the liberal arts curriculum in training students for active citizenship and promoted the notion "that higher education was, by definition, financially and spiritually rewarding for both the individual and society at large ..."[60] Yet students' experience, she notes, was something altogether different. Those entering university in the late 1960s found overcrowded classrooms instead of intimate seminars, professors focused on research rather than teaching, courses that seemed irrelevant to modern issues, and disciplinary rigidity rather than flexibility of learning.[61] While faculty and administrators attempted to respond to such concerns through new academic initiatives, the reality of the sudden influx of the first wave of baby boomers led to problems of overcrowding that aggravated the situation and produced a crisis of legitimation.

While some students experienced a sense of alienation caused by their attachment to an idealized vision of the university, analysis of student unrest and countercultural activities indicates that many students expressed their discontent in psychological terms. Writing in 1975, for example, sociologist Kenneth Westhues argued that both the political and countercultural arms of the student movement "were agreed on the goal of an alienation-free society, a society of equality and freedom."[62] He notes that the ideas of the counterculture travelled through mediums such as rock music and the underground press. The lyrics of the former "stressed the importance of choosing for oneself, of maximizing the freedom of both partners in love relationships, of being autonomous in the conventional world, and of living spontaneously and honestly." The latter expressed values that "were expressive as opposed to instrumental; the emphasis was on being oneself and loving others, not on getting ahead and striving for success."[63]

By the late 1960s and 1970s, a visible shift in values and beliefs had occurred within North American society. On university campuses and beyond, many young people focused on "finding themselves." Rejecting the perceived conformity of their parents and the communities in which they had been raised, radical youth attempted to define and formulate values and beliefs appropriate to the new world they envisioned. As writings at the time illuminate, these included being true to one's self, respecting difference, and searching for authenticity. The attempt to realize one's true self existed alongside a political project that, while expressed in a variety of forms, had at its roots the search for greater equality for all. Indeed, as one historian has strongly argued, that search for authenticity infused the radical politics of the late 1960s.[64]

Some historians have argued that such ideas were forged in the culture of the 1950s middle-class child rearing in which parents, influenced by the new psychology promoted in the books of Doctor Spock and other child advice literature, emphasized values of "independence, self-expression, permissiveness, and democratic relations."[65] This is no doubt true. Yet none of this was due simply to the rise of psychology as a discipline. Rather, this discourse drew on the intellectual currents that had been developing since the nineteenth century, the ideas of Marx, Nietzsche, Freud, and existentialism. It was part and parcel of a very gradual process of secularization, never complete, but that encouraged acceptance of different and new philosophies of life. It was informed by the new social scientific methods applying natural laws to the study of society in the attempt to uncover the means of achieving social efficiency. And it was due to new beliefs regarding the rights of individuals and the obligations of the state to its citizens. The turn towards a form of expressive individualism thus occurred at the confluence of a variety of ideas and new beliefs that had been developing for some time. Within the university this would help erode the dominant position of the ideal of character with its emphasis on responsibilities, obligations and individual sacrifice and instead help posit an alternative vision of development focused on self-realization and individual rights.

Conclusion

American historians and social critics from the 1960s on have identified the growing popularity of psychology and shift to personality in the early twentieth century as the rise of a therapeutic culture, part of a reorientation from a producer to consumer society. Their interpretation of this development has been overwhelmingly negative.[66] Warren Susman, for example, argues that the development of personality led to a focus on "the realization of the self's own abilities," drawing attention away from the inner self towards the outer self, with a concomitant shift from self-sacrifice to self-realization.[67] In other words, in concentrating on personality, experts emphasized individual skills and development and individual distinctiveness. Attention fell on the self, on self-realization. And in focusing on the individual, on the personal, the self became shorn of any communal context or obligations to the community and nation.

More recently, scholars have begun to question older interpretations that equate the focus on self only with a negative turn to a therapeutic culture or that perceive a shearing of the self from a communal context. In his examination of Alcoholics Anonymous, Jeffrey Brown argues that character – in terms of "accountability and personal integrity" remains central to the therapeutic culture. He admits that the concept of self-realization and living in the moment can lead to an emphasis on "immediate gratification."[68] Yet he argues that "central components of the therapeutic culture are precisely about making character, and that this endeavor has proceeded through modes of thought and action which, though ungrounded in the sort of religious conviction and institutional authority that may once have served to calibrate the internal gyroscopes of moral agents, can foster ethical rigor, social responsibility, and civic engagement nonetheless."[69] In her analysis of the rise of therapeutic culture in Australia, Katie Wright notes that while it has sometimes led to an emphasis on self-indulgence, it has also "facilitated the assertion of individual rights to bodily autonomy, emotional well-being and personal safety."[70] Indeed, she argues that "in the opening up of private life the therapeutic has been profoundly political."[71] For his part, Mathew Thomson argues that the new emphasis on psychological development "continued to draw on existing models of citizenship and character" and "emphasized the importance of service" while at the same time providing "a new alternative: a less public, less political vision of ideal personal development." Still, he also argues that psychology provided "a model for the reconstruction and potential liberation of forms of behavior." Thomson cites, for example, the consciousness-raising projects of second-wave feminists as well as the belief in the 1960s and 1970s in individuals' right to sexual expression.[72] In his examination of the new left, Doug Rossinow puts forward a strong case for the idea that the "therapeutic quest for authenticity" encouraged a thorough engagement with politics and encouragement of collective action.[73] Paul Leinberger and Bruce Tucker have argued that what has been called "the self ethic" was not rooted in narcissism but rather "based on a genuine moral imperative – the *duty* to express the authentic self."[74]

Nikolas Rose sees the emphasis placed by critics on the rise of therapeutics as missing the impact and significance of the rise of psychology. He argues that the general adoption of psychological techniques and modes of thinking has become the prime means by which liberal democracies have attempted to make "it possible to reconcile the requirement that human beings conduct themselves simultaneously as subjects of freedom and subjects of society."[75] Put another way, "The individualizing techniques embodied in the psychology of development and personality are not linked to a repressive project. On the contrary, they enable us to construe a form of family life, education, or production that simultaneously maximizes the capacities of individuals, their personal contentment, *and* the efficiency of the institution."[76] For Rose, that rethinking involved a shift away from the ideals of character, emphasizing such traits as "sobriety, diligence, thrift" or "cleanliness, healthy diet, and hygiene," and towards greater attention to the subjective, to "anxieties, attitudes, relationships, conflicts."[77] This was not just the replacing of one term with another, a case of old wine in new bottles. Rather, he argues, "To master one's will in the service of character through the inculcation of habits and rituals of self-denial, prudence, and foresight, for example, is different from mastering one's desires through bringing its roots to awareness through a reflexive hermeneutics in order to free oneself from the self-destructive consequences of repression, projection, and identification."[78] It has resulted in new social authorities – psychologists, psychiatrists, counsellors – and has "come to infuse the practices of other social actors such as doctors, social workers, managers, nurses, even accountants."[79] It is about a new mode of thinking in which freedom is understood as "maximizing self-fulfillment of the active and autonomous individual."[80] "These new practices of thinking, judging, and acting are not simply 'private' matters," he argues. "They are linked to the ways in which persons figure in the political vocabulary of advanced liberal democracies – no longer as subjects with duties and obligations, but as individuals with rights and freedoms."[81]

The intellectual and political shifts that Rose tracks from the vantage point of the late twentieth and early twenty-first centuries were only still emerging on the mid-twentieth century Canadian campus. The focus on inner adjustment and the gradual disappearance of the broader Christian context had the effect of rendering the links between individual and community less visible and comprehensible. Yet if that connection had become vague, this does not mean that it had disappeared in favour of a cult of the individual. Rather, it simply became more difficult to articulate, as there was no longer one path to service or citizenship. For some, citizenship would continue to occur in traditional ways. For others, it might lead instead to opposing the state or building alternative communities. Equally, it might mean developing one's own sense of masculinity, femininity, and sexuality – of having the freedom to become who one really was.

In adopting the discourse of personality, educators and health experts were doing more than simply updating the aims and purposes of character formation. Rather, both consciously and unconsciously, they helped introduce a new means of thinking about the self and of the relationship between the individual and his or her community. The gradual shift in discourse occurred at the same time as physical educators reformulated the types of activities in which students should engage, as health experts began to articulate the need for resources to be put into hiring psychologists and psychiatrists within health services, and as administrators accepted and encouraged the development of guidance and vocational counselling. The structural and curricular changes occurring within physical education and health services corresponded with an ideological shift in the aims and purposes of student health services on campus. In the early part of the century, the notion of tending to the student body had been integrated into a conception of the university as contributing to the moral, spiritual, intellectual, and physical development of the country's future citizens. This vision did not disappear, but by mid-century it was receding as the field of health, much like other disciplines, became specialized and fragmented. University administrators and health experts would continue to create institutions that provided the services necessary for individual development and to articulate the important role that their institutions played in creating an educated citizenry. However, for both better and worse, students would increasingly be left on their own to determine how to integrate the various aspects of their education and to consider how those aspects might inform their role as citizens.

Conclusion

In November 1931, Dr Edna Guest was optimistic about both the contribution a centre of health education could make to the lives of Victoria College's female students and her own role in supervising the living quarters and physical and moral health of these women. While Guest's call for the creation of a mandatory health course within the academic curriculum did not materialize at Victoria or elsewhere, her hope for an "educational health centre" was realized on many campuses. By the 1960s, most institutions provided a health service offering medical advice and treatment as well as counselling. The end product – in terms of its function, purpose, and place on campus – was, however, something quite different from what Guest had imagined.

While many educators, health experts and administrators in the early-twentieth century envisioned physical training and health care as entwined, by the 1960s and early 1970s most universities had terminated their physical training programs.[1] It would be easy to assume that physical culture met its demise at the hands of the cultural shifts of the late 1960s. In some cases this is true. The women's program at the University of Toronto lingered until 1969, when female students protested their continuing obligations, particularly in light of the termination of the men's program the previous year.[2] Yet at other institutions, compulsory physical training had already begun to disappear in the 1950s and early 1960s.[3] Others significantly reduced their requirements through the period.[4] In most cases, administrators terminated these programs without much fanfare or explanation. The drastic rise in student enrolments and resulting lack of facilities was likely a very real factor in their disappearance. Indeed, at the same time that universities ended their programs, some began to shift the burden of physical examinations onto students, requiring them to undergo a physical examination by their family physician prior to university entrance.[5] Yet if on the surface the causes of the termination of such programs appear to have been financial, the ease with which they vanished can be attributed to the seismic shifts in university culture that had occurred over the course of the first three-quarters of the century.

While programs in physical training began to disappear, student counselling and student services more generally took on a bureaucratic life of their own. This formed part of a broader societal development. Personnel departments, employing the expertise of a variety of experts, including psychologists, began to appear within larger corporations in the early twentieth century in order to test and screen potential workers.[6] "Employment Management" first appeared as a course in the department of social services at the University of Toronto in 1919.[7] During the Second World War, as the federal department of labour attempted to manage labour shortages, it drew on these corporate methods, employing the techniques and expertise of industrial psychologists and management consultants, and the methods of intelligence and aptitude testing.[8] Such methods had also begun to filter into institutions of higher education. In the United States, theories regarding personnel, drawn from the field of industrial psychology, began to take root in a handful of institutions as early as the 1920s and 1930s, becoming a dominant feature in the late 1940s and 1950s. The aim was to provide academic, vocational, and personal counselling in order to increase the social efficiency of higher education.[9] In Canada in the 1950s and 1960s, university administrators began to gradually recognize the need for some of these processes, particularly in relation to students. Psychological and psychiatric services, guidance counselling, and in some cases aptitude testing, came to be perceived as one means of dealing with the issue of student alienation. While faculty could be found emphasizing integrative courses, tutorials, and small class sizes, administrators turned to other venues such as student counselling and academic advising. In the late-1960s, these services appeared in piecemeal form. Only much later would the clear burgeoning of a whole range of student services be evident. Yet in retrospect, the development of this area within the university had already begun to appear in the 1950s and 1960s. Health services formed an early part of that process.

The growth of health care on campus, along with the implementation, and later, disappearance of physical training programs, reveals much about the changing nature of the university in the twentieth century, about shifting beliefs regarding student formation, and about the role of ideals of health in this process. In the first half of the twentieth century, physical training and student health were embedded within a particular vision of the purpose of the university – one which encompassed the nurturing of the intellectual, moral, physical, and spiritual development of students in order to create citizens and leaders who could contribute towards the broader goals of community and national development. Providing health care had, of course, the very practical aim of identifying individual illness and preventing contagion, both of which could affect the functioning of residential institutions and the university at large. Yet that endeavour does not seem to have been the only, or even the primary, reason for providing health care. Rather, those in charge of student life perceived the physical health of the students and the students' environment as key to furthering intellectual success and a healthy citizenry.

Physical training, and physical education more generally, was rooted in nineteenth-century biological ideas about femininity and masculinity. Physical educators and physicians differed over the impact of biology. A.S. Lamb and Ethel Cartwright at McGill University believed women's physical activity should be significantly curtailed while others were more supportive of expanding women's sporting opportunities. Most physical educators worked to increase women's access to physical activity, departing from Victorian restrictions on female movement and encouraging women to experience greater bodily freedom. Yet all physical educators accepted the need for more medical and personal surveillance of women than of men and created programs that reinforced existing ideals of femininity and masculinity. In the case of both men and women, however, the aim of physical educators was to create healthy and moral citizens, and they drew on the latest science – from anthropological measurements to a tested regimen of exercises – to explain and reinforce the need for their programs.

The concerns and beliefs of a small and elite group of physical educators was never the only reason such programs gained a foothold in Canadian universities. Their ideas meshed with a host of contemporary anxieties regarding female frailty, the health of athletes, the need to create productive citizens, and the spread of disease. They intersected, too, with administrators' need to present Canadian universities as modern and up to date. And they reflected new intellectual currents in social and applied sciences in which researchers focused on identifying general laws and principles of society and determining normalcy and its deviations. Moreover, the programs were supported by a whole range of actors: university presidents, deans of men and women, physicians, nurses, as well as some faculty and students.

To separate physical culture from medical diagnoses is largely artificial, particularly at institutions that combined compulsory physical training with compulsory medical examinations. Indeed, doctors, physical instructors, and in the case of female students, deans of women, worked together to ensure the pure environment and moral setting they believed necessary for the development of healthy bodies. Examining medical soundness and gathering anthropological measurements were often the first steps towards sorting students into physical training programs. This formed part of a broader program in the early-twentieth century in which, as Cynthia Comacchio comments, "young people increasingly became objects of study, both in medicine and in the emerging social sciences," as experts attempted to define and delimit "the idea of 'the normal' in individual and social groups."[10] It also illuminates the ways in which both medical experts' and educators' assessments of health involved not only evaluations of body parts, but also social and cultural judgments. Diagnoses of drooping shoulders or poor posture were not just medical issues but reflective of individual character. Health talks by doctors and deans of women complemented the work of physical educators. Neither doctors nor physical instructors nor deans hesitated to make pronouncements in any of these spheres but rather saw it as their role to connect the medical and moral, the physical and spiritual.

Yet even as educators advocated a holistic interpretation of student life and used new scientific ideas to bolster moral beliefs, the general turn towards expertise would aid the fragmentation of that vision. One of the things that this study illustrates is the very gradual way in which expectations about access to health facilities and services gained headway. In 1900, few students would have had contact with a physician for the purpose of preventative health. Through the twentieth century, increasing numbers of students were exposed to not only physical examinations, but also to the belief that visits to a physician should become incorporated into their regular health routine.

Physicians, health experts, and educators concerned about health were central to increasing the social and cultural authority of medical experts. Examining the American context, Paul Starr contends that physicians developed social and institutional authority as they gained the power of action and command, such as the ability to authorize medical examinations or to exercise power over other health professionals such as nurses. Undergirding that social authority was a growing sense of cultural authority.[11] As Starr argues, "The authority to interpret signs and symptoms, to diagnose health or illness, to name disease, and to alter prognoses is the foundation of any social authority the physician can assume. By shaping the patients' understanding of their own experience, physicians create the conditions under which their advice seems appropriate."[12] In many circumstances a patient may either accept or reject the authority of a physician. But in other cases that authority is compulsory. Starr notes, "For purposes of certification, patients often have no choice but to submit to professional examination. In their capacity as cultural authorities, doctors make authoritative judgments of what constitutes illness or insanity, evaluate the fitness of persons for jobs, assess the disability of the injured."[13]

These forms of authority existed within the university. Physicians and physical educators asserted their medical knowledge through lectures and information regarding proper exercise, or by identifying and diagnosing illness. Their use of a growing set of medical instruments and tools for diagnostics reinforced their cultural authority.[14] They quickly added new procedures such as vaccination, Wasserman tests, tuberculin tests and chest X-rays, to health service practices. They also presented themselves as experts by providing solutions, in the form of various exercises, to ailments from flat feet to poor posture. Their authority was reinforced by the compulsory nature and institutionalization of physical training and health exams.

On the one hand, physicians' and health experts' growing authority enabled them to carve out a new space for themselves within the university. On the other hand, in doing so, they also helped compartmentalize medical expertise and knowledge. Physicians turned away from a broad sanitarianism towards the treatment of specific diseases, as seen in the focus on immunization or the eradication of tuberculosis. Equally, whereas earlier in the century administrators, deans, and physical educators had all made pronouncements on public health, the diagnosis and treatment of both tuberculosis and mental health fell primarily within the purview of medical experts, and more specifically, physicians within student health services.

As health care became compartmentalized and fragmented, with physicians focused on a specific disease, or body part, access to such care broadened through the growth of the collectivist, or welfare, state. By mid-century, a growing number of Canadians viewed access to affordable health care as an entitlement and expressed this view through a rights-based discourse. Thus, ironically, as collectivist notions of the state gained ground, ideas about overall health, and particularly mental health, came to focus on individual self-development. The self-realized individual would be achieved through the provisions of the collectivist welfare state.

Neither administrators nor medical staff nor students linked the creation of health services on campus to the gradual emergence of the welfare state. Yet in many respects, in supporting health services, university staff and students both consciously or unconsciously participated in the creation of a new conception of the state, one that emphasized social citizenship. Historians have illuminated the ways in which a variety of players from the 1930s to the 1950s began to articulate a sense of entitlement, and demand access, to state welfare provisions.[15] On the one hand, administrators early on developed health programs as part of the responsibilities and duties of the university to stand *in loco parentis*. Yet as universities provided such services, students began to assume their provision, indeed, even demanded better facilities. In some cases, as for example with students belonging to Toronto's Co-op residences, such demands were articulated as part of their rights as students. Others did so in terms of personal needs that they felt the university could meet. In either case, in providing such services and in seeking them out, administrators and students respectively participated in supporting the idea of social citizenship.

The changing justifications for the need for physical culture and health services on university campuses helps to illuminate the way in which the nineteenth-century underpinnings of citizenship were reconfigured for a new age. By the 1950s, the belief in creating character had been replaced with a focus on personality development. The shift in language highlights the increasing influence of psychology well beyond its academic field. But it also denotes more than just the rise of one discipline or the adoption of a more modern terminology. The concept of personality both reflected, and contributed to, new understandings of the self as well as the relationship between one's self and one's community.

I have argued elsewhere that for much of the first three-quarters of the twentieth century, English-Canadian universities remained institutions in transition. On the one hand, they began to experience the forces of modernization and secularization – the rise of the social sciences, of an ideal of research, and by the 1940s and 1950s, the expansion in facilities – that allowed for the growth of the multiversity. On the other hand, many remained small, rooted in the liberal arts and shaped by a vision of a moral community. Nancy Christie and Michael Gauvreau have illustrated the way in which religious ideals and beliefs remained central to the thought of social scientists in the 1930s and 1940s.[16] In the post-war years, as the work of Mona Gleason and Mary-Louise Adams has shown, experts reinforced traditional moral beliefs.[17] While many did so without the explicit language of Christianity, Christian assumptions and a broadly Christian society gave credence to experts' rhetoric.

Yet although, between the 1920s and 1950s, religious and scientific views were held together in new ways, they also began to break apart. Indeed they were doing so even as they remained seemingly entwined. Physical educators began searching for new means of developing their own field and bringing credibility to that field. They embraced the scientific study of physical education at the expense of training in physical activity, research at the expense of an emphasis on physical movement. The ideals inherent in physical culture became increasingly distant from the realities of the university. The growth of the university meant that it was difficult to create a unified program in physical culture, while physical culture itself began to move away from the Christian-based influences of nineteenth-century gymnastics and towards sport, skills, and achievement.

The increasing turn towards personality reflected the new research culture of the university, new ideas about citizenship, and changing social and cultural mores. The consequence was a shift away from an emphasis on self-denial, service, and sacrifice to nation, and towards a focus on self-fulfilment, self-realization, and the idea of citizenship rights. This turn has allowed greater room for individual expression and diversity. Self-realization did not have to come through a particular religion, commitment to family and community, or national service. Rather, it could occur through any number of philosophies of life and ways of being. At the same time, the path that one should take has become more vaguely defined. Commentators on a rights-based citizenship have argued that the notion of responsibility has always been an integral part of the equation.[18] In the heyday of 1960s student radicalism, the moral duties of citizenship may have been clear for some. Subsequently, however, just how one should execute one's responsibility has become murkier. In the context of university health, it is clear that the aims of physical training became much more amorphous. In focusing on self-realization, physical educators dropped the outdated nineteenth-century moral language, but in doing so they also lost the broader force that that language had imparted to the aims and purpose of physical training. While opening up options has increased individual freedom, it has also in some ways made it more difficult for individuals to perceive both how they might usefully contribute to civil society and how to turn the activities of a proliferation of social groups into forceful collective action.

The university, of course, was never the only site or source for shifting ideas regarding the self. Educators were affected by new intellectual developments, forces of secularization, changing notions of citizenship, modern social mores, emerging forms of youth culture, among many other things. Yet through their employment on university campuses and their highly regarded position within society, they also played an influential role in the transformations occurring within society. Despite the increasing intellectual and economic prominence of universities since the 1950s, their historical and cultural influence remains overlooked. Yet university personnel have played a significant role in shaping and reshaping the moral values, beliefs, and ideals held by individuals and contributing to their notions of citizenship.

This is not a story of linear progression, with, for example, one model of the university replacing another or of beliefs and practices informed by psychology usurping a Christian-based ideal of the self. The existence of the idea of the university as a moral community can be seen today. It reveals itself in the treatment of students as still immature youth, to be guided to full adulthood. There continues to be an emphasis on student experience – of the importance of involvement in activities well beyond the classroom. And there is an ideal – perhaps naive – that the university and its members serve local, national, and global communities. Indeed, while the idea of the university as a research centre is dominant, the notion of the university as a site that contributes to broad personal development endures.

Contemporary debates over the nature of the university continue to reflect the tensions between older ideals and newer realities. They include, among many others, academics' critique of the corporatization of the university versus the need for corporate-type skills in running a conglomerate; the tensions between teaching and research; the building of multiversities versus the attempt to maintain institutions providing intimacy and promoting individual growth; and the emphasis on technical training versus the belief in the need to produce students able to think critically. These debates are not new, but rather have their roots in the gradual transformations occurring since at least the turn of the twentieth century.

The rise of university health services and the implementation and dismantling of physical training provide one means of examining and understanding that transformation. The university of the early twentieth century was never simply a site of intellectual development. Rather, administrators and educators conceived of their institutions as places conducive to moral and spiritual formation. And that moral formation was inextricably connected with physical health. For a variety of reasons, and in a number of ways, educators' understanding of student development underwent change during the twentieth century, with self-realization becoming the dominant language through which they expressed their ideas about formation. Newer interpretations about the development of the self never fully eclipsed older ones. The particular historical configuration of the university within which Edna Guest worked in the 1920s and 1930s has disappeared. Yet Guest's notion that the university should embody something more than development of intellect remains at the centre of some of the current tensions surrounding the idea of the university – and of its aims and purposes. Moreover, while universities today may have a more fragmented method of caring for students' bodies and minds than in the past, administrators continue to attempt to find new ways to tend to the student body.

Appendix
Physical Training at the University of Toronto

	Unrestricted Physical Activity		Corrective Exercises/ Restrictions on Physical Activity		Unable to Undertake Physical Training		Military Pulhems
	Men	Women	Men	Women	Men	Women	Men
1921–2	93	83.3	5	15.5	2	4.2	
1923–4	92.2	90.58	6	7.6	1.8	1.82	
1924–5	93.8	88.6	4.7	10.8	1.5	6	
1925–6	95.27	84.9	2.26	13.1	2.13	2	
1926–7	92	83.66	6	14.68	2	1.66	
1927–8	94.3	88	3.3	9	2.4	3	
1928–9	93	83.9	4.2	12.2	2.8	3.9	
1929–30	93	87	5	10	2	3	
1930–1	92	88.3	5	11.9	3	7.8	
1931–2	95	83	3	8	2	9	
1932–3	95	86.8	3	5.7	2	7.5	
1933–4	96	77	2.5	7	1.5	16	
1934–5	95	84.5	3	8.2	2	7.2	
1935–6	94	91	4	6	2	3	
1936–7	96	86.2	2.5	7.4	1.5	6.4	
1937–8	96	83.2	2.5	11.2	1.5	5.6	
1938–9	94	86	4.5	10	1.5	4	
**1939–40	94.5	60	4	35	1.5	5.2	
1940–1	94	55	4	39	2	6	
1941–2	79.8	N/A	18.6	N/A	1.6	N/A	78.4
1942–3	68.4	N/A	25	N/A	6.6	N/A	70
1943–4	66.8	N/A	25	N/A	8.2	N/A	67
1944–5	79.6	N/A	10.2	N/A	6.6	N/A	74
1945–6	89	96	8	3	3	1	75.5
1946–7	94	95.9	4.5	3.8	1.5	.3	77
1947–8	93	95	6	4	1	1	75.7
1948–9	94.1	93.7	2.7	5.6	3.2	.7	

	University Classification – Activity Unrestricted		Military Pulhems Grading – Service Unrestricted
	Men	Women	Men
1952–3	93	93.9	79.6
1953–4	93.1	93.8	78.7
1954–5	94.7	93.9	76.1
1955–6	95.7	96.3	75.0
1956–7	95.4	96.2	72.2
1957–8	96.7	96	72.3
1958–9	97.1	97.3	67.6
1959–60	97.1	97.7	68.1
1960–1	97	97.8	63.6
1961–2	97.6	97.7	61.5
1962–3	97.2	97.9	61.1
1963–4	97.9	97.6	63.2
1964–5	97.8	98.04	61
1965–6	97.8	97.9	N/A
1966–7	98.3	97.4	N/A

**New medical adviser hired for female students.

Note: All numbers are percentages.

Sources: Reports of the University Health Service and Medical Adviser of Women in University of Toronto, *President's Reports*, 1921–67.

Abbreviations

AUM	Archives de l'Université de Montréal
ECWA	Esther Clark Wright Archives, Acadia University
DUA	Dalhousie University Archives
McMUA	McMaster University Archives
MtAUA	Mount Allison University Archives
MUA	McGill University Archives
UAA	University of Alberta Archives
UBCA	University of British Columbia Archives
UCC/VUA	United Church of Canada/Victoria University Archives (now Victoria University Archives)
UMA	University of Manitoba Archives
USA	University of Saskatchewan Archives
UTA	University of Toronto Archives
UWOA	University of Western Ontario Archives (now Western Archives)

Notes

Introduction

1 UCC/VUA, Dean of Women Fonds, Box 1-12, "Report of the Examining Physician," 12 November 1931.

2 For reference to this motto see, for example, "Report of the Principal," McGill University, *Annual Report*, 1946–7, 15.

3 My thanks to Carey Watt for bringing my attention to the motto and to David Mawhinney, Mount Allison University Archivist, for providing information on the erection of the building.

4 Howell, *Blood, Sweat, and Cheers*; Kidd, *The Struggle for Canadian Sport*; Metcalfe, *Canada Learns To Play*.

5 Mangan, "Discipline in the Dominion," 149–50; McKillop, "Marching As to War," 75–93.

6 Mangan, "Discipline in the Dominion," 146–67. See also Mangan, *Athleticism in the Victorian and Edwardian Public School*, 16–18. For the United States see, for example, Smith, *Sports and Freedom*, chap. 7, and for Canada see Howell, *Blood, Sweat, and Cheers*, 32.

7 Howell, *Blood, Sweat, and Cheers*, 32–3.

8 Bederman, *Manliness and Civilization*, chap. 5.

9 For youth groups see Howell, *Northern Sandlots*, 104–12, and *Blood, Sweat, and Cheers*, 33; Howell and Lindsay, "Social Gospel and the Young Boy Problem, 1895–1925," 75–87; Macleod, *Building Character in the American Boy*, xiv, 44–8; Kidd, *The Struggle for Canadian Sport*, 44. For the concern about keeping young men within the folds of Christianity, see Marks, "A Fragment of Heaven on Earth," 258–9. By the late nineteenth century, physical culture and bodybuilding had gained significant popular attention in the

Anglo-American world. See, for example, Churchill, "Making Broad Shoulders," 341–70; Daley, *Leisure and Pleasure*, 4.

10 Scraton, *Shaping Up to Womanhood*, chap. 2; McCrone, *Playing the Game*, 101; Fletcher, *Women First*, 3–4, 17–40. On the influence and spread of physical culture, see also Keys, *Globalizing Sport*, 19–24.

11 See, for example, Cahn, *Coming on Strong*, 12; Todd, *Physical Culture and the Body Beautiful*, 79–81; Horowitz, *Alma Mater*, 26–39.

12 Smith, "Graceful Athleticism," 123–6; Hall, *The Girl and the Game*, 27–33; Morrow, "The Strathcona Trust in Ontario, 1911–1939," 72–90; Moss, *Manliness and Militarism*.

13 Starr, *The Social Transformation of American Medicine*, 7. See also Whorton, *Crusaders for Fitness*.

14 See, for example, MacDougall, *Activists and Advocates*; Duffy, *The Sanitarians*; Tomes, *The Gospel of Germs*.

15 Meckel, "Going to School, Getting Sick," 188; Smith, "Dampness, Darkness, Dirt, Disease," 196, 204–5.

16 See, for example, Axelrod, *The Promise of Schooling*, 104–14, 111–21; Dehli, "'Health Scouts' for the State?" 247–9; Smith, "Dampness, Darkness, Dirt, Disease," 196, 211; Comacchio, "'The Rising Generation,'"150–2; Gleason, "Race, Class, and Health," 95–112, and *Small Matters*, chap. 4; Poutanen, "Containing and Preventing Contagious Disease," 401–28; Lewis, "Physical Perfection for Spiritual Welfare," 144–6; Sutherland, *Children in English-Canadian Society*, 191–2. For the medicalization of education in the United States, see Petrina, "The Medicalization of Education," 503–31, and Cohen, "The Mental Hygiene Movement, the Development of Personality and the School," 123–49. For Britain, see Welshman, "Physical Education and the School Medical Services in England and Wales," 31–48, and, Scraton, *Shaping Up to Womanhood*, 22–5. For Australia see Kirk, *Schooling Bodies*.

17 Comacchio, *Dominion of Youth*, 18–21.

18 Howell, *Blood, Sweat, and Cheers*, 33. For the international context, see, for example, Reiss, "Sport and the Redefinition of Middle-Class Masculinity," 173–97; Vernon, "The Health and Welfare of University Students in Britain, 1920–1939," 232; Zweiniger-Bargielowska, "Building a British Superman," 601.

19 Mott, "Confronting 'Modern' Problems through Play," 59–63; Mackinnon, *Love and Freedom*, chap. 2.

20 Such concerns fuelled a growing enthusiasm for wilderness vacations, camping, and cottage life. See, for example, Cameron, "Tom Thompson, Antimodernism, and the Ideal of Manhood" 185–208, and Wall, *The Nurture of Nature*.

21 See, for example, McKillop, *Matters of Mind*; Christie and Gauvreau, *A Full-Orbed Christianity*; Owram, *The Government Generation*.
22 See, for example, Starr, *The Social Transformation of American Medicine*; Gidney and Millar, *Professional Gentlemen*; Comacchio, *"Nations are Built of Babies"*; Arnup, *Education for Motherhood*; Gleason, *Normalizing the Ideal*; Bailey, "Scientific Truth … And Love," 711–32.
23 See most recently, Campbell, *Respectful Citizens*; Fahrni, *Household Politics*; Tillotson, *Contributing Citizens*.
24 See, for example, Axelrod, *Making a Middle Class*; Gidney, *A Long Eclipse*.
25 On the importance of understanding disease as both a biological issue and a social and cultural construct, see, for example, Rosenberg, "Introduction," xiii–xxvi; Harley, "Rhetoric and the Social Construction of Sickness and Healing," 407–35; Duffin, *Lovers and Livers*.
26 For a good summary of this literature see Wright, "Theorizing Therapeutic Culture," 321–36.
27 For aspects of the increasing societal influence of psychology – its infiltration into the military, schools, popular imagination, and in the later part of the century the culture of human resources – see, for example, Gleason, *Normalizing the Ideal*; M.L. Adams, *The Trouble With Normal*; Wright and Myers, *History of Academic Psychology*; Stephen, *Pick One Intelligent Girl*; Jasen, "Student Activism, Mental Health, and English-Canadian Universities in the 1960s," 455–80; Dowbiggin, *Keeping America Sane*; Moran and Wright, *Mental Health and Canadian Society*. For a powerful argument regarding the growth in influence of psychology see Rose, *Inventing Our Selves*.
28 See, for example, Frager and Patrias, *Discounted Labour*, 93–113; Iacovetta, *Gatekeepers*; Sangster, *Regulating Girls and Women*; Strange and Loo, *Making Good*, 9.
29 Axelrod, *Making a Middle Class*, 21–9; Porter, *Vertical Mosaic*, 178. In the first part of the century in Ontario, some 10 to 15 per cent came from working-class backgrounds. Female students were more likely than male students to originate from families with a father who held a professional or managerial position. After the Second World War, the student body witnessed slightly greater diversification in background. See Gaffield, Marks, and Laskin, "Student Populations and Graduate Careers: Queen's University, 1895–1900," 12; Millar and Gidney, "'Medettes': Thriving or Just Surviving?" 218, 227; Gidney, *A Long Eclipse*, 90–1.
30 For example, Helen Kemp and Northrup Frye faced uncertainty over their futures. Kemp's father, chief graphic designer for a Toronto cork and seal company had little work in the early 1930s, while Frye's father, a hardware and building supplies salesman based in Moncton, could barely pay

the bills. See Denham, *The Correspondence of Northrup Frye and Helen Kemp,* 5, 94.

31 For examples of the treatment of university students as youth, see Gidney, *A Long Eclipse,* chap. 2; Hébert, "Between the Future and the Present," 163–200. For the United States, see Prescott, "The White Plague Goes to College," 744.

32 See, for example, David Whitson, "The Embodiment of Gender: Discipline, Domination, and Empowerment," 353–71; Verbrugge, "Recreating the Body," 275; Hall, *Feminism and Sporting Bodies.*

33 There is a fairly extensive literature on girls' and women's physical education. See, for example, Hall, *The Girl and the Game;* Lathrop, "Elegance and Expression,"; Kidd, *The Struggle for Canadian Sport,* chap. 3; Smith, "Graceful Athleticism or Robust Womanhood," 120–37; Lenskyj, *Out of Bounds,* "The Role of Physical Education in the Socialization of Girls in Ontario, 1890–1930," and "Femininity First: Sport and Physical Education for Ontario Girls, 1890–1930," 4–17; Gurney, *Girls' Sports;* Bryans, "Secondary School Curriculum for Girls," 124–39. The literature in relation to boys and young men is much smaller. See, for example, Mangan, "Discipline in the Dominion," 142–67; Barman, *Growing Up British in British Columbia,* chaps. 4 and 5; Moss, *Manliness and Militarism,* chap. 5.

34 The institutions examined in detail include: Dalhousie University, Acadia University, St. Francis Xavier University, Mount Allison University, McGill University, the University of Montreal, Laval University, Victoria College, the University of Toronto, the University of Manitoba, the University of Alberta, and the University of British Columbia. This has been supplemented with material from other institutions such as Queen's University, Western University, and the University of Saskatchewan. While I have attempted to provide a pan-Canadian story and include two francophone universities in Quebec, these institutions did not provide physical training and students had access to some form of medical service only as of the 1940s. As a result, this is substantially an English-Canadian study.

1. Institutional Development of Student Health Programs

1 For example, in the 1840s, the Coburg Female Academy advertised its healthy environment. As early as the 1850s, some universities had begun to set aside a basement room or small separate building as a gymnasium. By the 1890s, larger institutions such as McGill and Toronto provided well-equipped facilities and maintained fields adjacent to classroom space. In 1897, administrators at St. Francis Xavier University asked the Sisters of

St. Martha to establish a mission near the institution in order to provide
a variety of services to priests and students, including nursing. See Selles,
Methodists and Women's Education in Ontario, 1836–1925, 44; Moriarty, "The
Organizational History of the Canadian Intercollegiate Athletic Union Central," 51–63; Cameron, *For the People*, 102.

2 See, for example, Cahn, *Coming on Strong*, 12; Vertinsky, *The Eternally
Wounded Woman*, 144; Prescott, *Student Bodies*, chap. 1. For the debates of the
1870s and 1880s in Canada, see Burke, "Women of Newfangle," 111–33, and
"'Being unlike Man,'" 11–31.

3 UCC/VUA, Annesley Hall Committee of Management, 90.064v, Box 2-6,
Dean's Reports, 10 March 1910.

4 Mitchinson, "'All Matter Peculiar to Women and Womanhood,'" 158–69.

5 For some of the extensive literature on this topic see Gidney, *A Long Eclipse*,
168n1. More recently, see Burke, "Women of Newfangle," 111–33 and
"'Being unlike Man,'" 11–31.

6 The founder of Royal Victoria College, the women's college at McGill
University, initially paid for medical attendance for students as well as the
academic and domestic staff. By the first decades of the twentieth century, administrators had replaced the college physical exam with a medical certificate, filled out by a family physician on a form provided by the
College. This continued until at least 1940. Through this period, students
had access to a physician free of charge. Administrators also instituted
compulsory physical training for two periods a week for first-year students
in 1905–6. This was extended to students in second year in 1908–9 and to
those in third year, though only for one period a week, in 1909–10. When
Annesley Hall, the women's residence at Victoria College, University of Toronto, opened in 1903, administrators hired a doctor, instructor in physical
training, and nurse. Prior to the First World War administrators at Victoria
College expected residents to take gym during their first three years unless
exempted by the examining physician. In the 1920s, the program fell by
the wayside but was revived for several years in the mid-1930s. As of 1942,
students fell under the University of Toronto's requirements for physical
training. Administrators required women at University College and in the
University of Toronto's professional faculties to participate in physical education in the early years of the twentieth century, with times set aside in the
course schedule for this activity. Mount Allison provided an infirmary from
at least 1904. See MUA, RG 42, 3-177, RVC Residence Physician 1939–42,
"Extract from the letter of August 4th 1939 from Mrs. Walter Vaughan to
Mrs. W.L. Grant," 2-137, Physical Education – General, 1869-37, "Evolution of the Department of Physical Education," January 1936, and 2-135,

"Physical Education – Program for Women, 1905–1915"; "Royal Victoria College," McGill University *Calendar*, 1910–11 and 1940–1; UCC/VUA, Fonds 2045, 92.010v, Box 6-4, Medical Report, May 1904, 90.064v, Box 1-1, Minutes of the Committee of Management, 22 March 1905 and 10 April 1907, and 90.065v, Box 1-9, Annual Meeting of Women's Council, 28 May 1942; Gurney, *A Century to Remember*, 20; MTAA, Raymond Clare Archibald Fonds, 5501/6/1/8, p. 28, Saint John *Daily Sun*, 2 April 1904, n.p.

7 In 1905, at the height of the progressive reform movement, a series of journalistic exposés highlighted these problems. President Theodore Roosevelt, along with leading university administrators, seized on the opportunity to attempt to implement reform. See Smith, *Sports and Freedom*, chap. 14.

8 See, for example, "Athletics," *Acta Victoriana*, 1905, 251–3.

9 Reed, *Blue and White*, xi, 31–33; UTA, Office of the President, A67-0007, Box 22, File: Barton, letter, President Falconer to Dr James W. Barton, 3 December 1912.

10 F.H. Harvey, Medical Director of Physical Education, "Gymnasium Report," McGill University, *Principal's Report*, 1911–12; Walton, "The Life and Professional Contributions of Ethel Mary Cartwright," 34–5.

11 Queen's University, *Principal's Report*, 1914–15, 21.

12 UTA, Office of the President, A67-0007, Box 68, File: Athletic Association, letter: T.A. Reed to Falconer, 28 April, 1920, and Faculty of Medicine Council Minutes, A86-0027, Reel 21, Minutes, Committee on Students' Health, 3 March 1921 and 21 March 1921. James Pitsula notes that at the University of Saskatchewan men could choose between military drill and physical training, though most enrolled in the former. See "Manly Heroes," 132.

13 University of Toronto, *Calendar*, 1917–18; "Physical Education," UBC, *Calendar*, 1915–16; Walton, "The Life and Professional Contributions of Ethel Mary Cartwright," 41.

14 McGill required all female students to engage in two classes of physical culture a week. In 1918, physical education became compulsory for first- and second-year women at the University of Alberta, although the program was limited to folk dancing and basketball. See "Royal Victoria College," McGill University, *Calendar*, 1915; UAA, Office of the President, RG3, Tory, 68-9-280, Cecil E. Race, Registrar, to Dean Kerr, Acting President and Chairman, Committee on Physical Education, 11 April 1918.

15 This was, however, not universal. UBC had compulsory military training for men from 1915 to 1919. McGill's program for men became defunct in 1926 due to lack of facilities. See University of Toronto, *Calendar*, 1919–20; "Department of Physical and Military Training," UWO, *Announcement*, 1920–1; UAA, Office of the President, RG3, 68-9-280, "Regulations of Corporation

Regarding Physical Education," McGill University, attached to letter: A.S. Lamb, Department of Physical Education, McGill to Dr Tory, 15 March 1920; "Health," Acadia University, *Calendar*, 1920–21. For UBC see Vertinsky, "Memory and Monument," 23.

16 Vernon, "Health and Welfare of University Students," 232–4, and "A Healthy Society for Future Intellectuals," 195–6.

17 Stewart, "John Ryle, the Institute of Social Medicine and the Health of Oxford Students," 63.

18 As of 1923, students at Mount Allison had to register for two hours a week of physical education in their first and second years. By 1936–7, St. Francis Xavier required students to undergo an annual physical examination and had instituted three hours a week of physical education for first- and second-year students. The University of Western Ontario established a student health service in 1935. In 1937–8, the University of Manitoba established a medical service for students in the faculty of medicine and for those living in residence that consisted of access to an infirmary and a daily visiting physician for student consultations. A year later, gymnastics and swimming classes became compulsory for diploma students in agriculture. See "Physical Training," University of Saskatchewan, *Calendar*, 1920–1, "Report of the President," University of Saskatchewan, *President's Report*, 1928–9, 7–8, and "Health Report" in University of Saskatchewan, *Annual Report of the President*, 1938–9; MtAUA, *President's Report*, 1923–4; "Gymnasium," *The McMaster University Monthly* (November 1922), 77; "Physical Education," McMaster University, *Calendar*, 1930–1; "Health," Dalhousie University, *Calendar*, 1924–5 and 1932–3; DUA, President's Office, UA3, Box 39, File 9, Remarks by President Stanley, 8 April 1938; "Physical Education," *Calendar of St. Francis Xavier University*, 1936–7; University of Manitoba, *President's Report*, 1937–40; UMA, UPC PROP 94, Hilary Findlay, "Physical Education at the University of Manitoba: An Historical Overview," unpublished paper, 1978; Schwarz, "Report on Health and Psychiatric Services on Canadian Campuses," 27.

19 By 1941, 43 per cent of men "called up for military training ... had been rejected on the grounds of poor health." See McCuaig, *The Weariness and the Fever*, 181.

20 McKillop, *Matters of Mind*, 524.

21 In 1942–3, the University of Alberta made women's war service compulsory, with drill and physical education for first-year students. Women at UBC were required to engage in war work, including one hour a week of physical training. The University of Toronto instituted compulsory war work. This did not consist of physical training, though many students at that institution

were already engaged in physical exercise. See UAA, "President's Report," in *Report of the Board of Governors of the University of Alberta*, 1942–3; "Report of the Instructor in Physical Education for Women," in UBC, *President's Report*, 1942–3; Kiefer and Pierson, "The War Effort and Women Students at Toronto," 175–6.

22 UAA, University of Alberta, *Calendar*, 1915–16, and 1940–1, 1967–8.

23 "Health Services," McGill University, *Calendar*, 1945.

24 The program does not seem to have continued after that year. "University Health Service," UBC, *Calendar*, 1929–30; "Report of the Director of Physical Education for Men" and "Report of the Director of Physical Education for Women," in *Report of the President of the University of British Columbia*, 1945–6; *UBC Handbook*, 1932–3, 1935–6; "University Health Service," *The Tillicum*, 1942–3, 86.

25 UMA, UPC PROP 94, Hilary Findlay, "Physical Education at the University of Manitoba: An Historical Overview," unpublished paper, 1978.

26 Gleason, *Normalizing the Ideal*; Stephen, *Pick One Intelligent Girl*, 52, 211, 218; Poutanen, "Containing and Preventing Contagious Disease," 410; Bender, "Inspecting Workers," 51–75.

27 Porter, "Preserving the Health of the Student Body," 289.

28 UMA, UA20, Box 99-28, pamphlet: "McGill University, General Information, 1948–9." See also UBCA, UBC Subject File Collection, Box 22, pamphlet: *This is YOUR Health Service*, n.d.

29 UCC/VUA, 90.065v, Box 1-2, Medical Report, 1935; Grant, "Students' Health Service of Dalhousie University," 485–90; MUA, RG 30, Faculty of Education, 64–169, Minutes of Committees on Health Service, 1931.

30 UTA, Office of the President, A67-0007, Box 77, File: Gordon, letter: E. Gordon to R. Falconer, 17 January 1923. For the reference to men, see "Report of the University Health Service, Men Students," in University of Toronto, *President's Report*, 1921–2.

31 UCC/VUA, 90.064v, Box 3-20, Report by Guest, n.d.

32 Lowe, *Looking Good*, 23.

33 MUA, RG 42, 2-137, Physical Education – General, 1869–1937, Evolution of Department of Physical Education for Women, January 1936.

34 UCC/VUA, 90.064v, Committee of Management, Box 4-3, Correspondence, 1904–13, n.d. For the 1930s, see page 1 of the introduction. Similar data was collected at American women's colleges. See Lowe, *Looking Good*, 23–4.

35 Starr, *The Social Transformation of American Medicine*, 136–7.

36 Carr and Beamish, *Manitoba Medicine*, 86.

37 "Health," Dalhousie University, *Calendar*, 1931–2, 17–18. In the same period, the examination at McGill University included urinalysis and at the

University of Toronto both urinalysis and a haemoglobin count. See "Department of Physical Education," in McGill University, *Annual Report,* 1934–5 and 1935–6; UTA, A68-0028, Box 15, File: University Health Services, "General Information for Students: University Health Service," ca 1938.

38 Prescott, *Student Bodies,* 3, 64–5, and "The White Plague," 743. A 1935 survey of health programs in small northeastern colleges found that 50 per cent required physical exams prior to registration, while at most of the rest the exam occurred after registration. See Way, "A Survey of Small College Health Service Programs," 18–19.

39 MUA, RG 46, 14-33, Minutes, Sub-Committee on Student Health, 3 November 1936.

40 UCC/VUA, 90.064v, Box 3-20, Report of Dr Guest, November 1929.

41 MUA, RG 46, 14-33, Minutes, Sub-Committee on Student Health, 1 May 1936.

42 Professor Simpson, speaking at "Sixth Session," Congress of the Universities of the Empire, *Report of Proceedings,* 1926, 182.

43 Report of the Physical Director, in University of Toronto, *President's Report,* 1908–9.

44 Barton, "What Physical Examination of Students Shows," 51–2.

45 See UAA, Office of the President, RG3, 68-9-280, letter, A.S. Lamb to Dr. Tory, 15 March 1920; UTA, School of Physical and Health Education, A83-0046, Box 3, File: Presidential Committee on Required Physical Education, Minutes, 21 September 1955.

46 UCC/VUA, 90.065v, Box 1-10, Report of Physician, ca 1934.

47 UCC/VUA, Dean of Women Fonds, 90.141v, Box 2-20, Dean's Council Minutes, 20 September 1928.

48 MUA, RG 30, Faculty of Education, 64-169, Minutes of Committees on Health Service, 1931.

49 MUA, RG 30, 67-191, Frank G. Pedley, University Medical Officer, "Memorandum on Proposed Health Service," 1940.

50 UAA, Student Medical Services, 75-144-1119, pamphlet, "Medical Services, 1935–6."

51 "Report of the Medical Examiner," in *Report of the President of UBC,* 1936–7; Grant, "Students' Health Service of Dalhousie University," 485–90; University of Toronto, *Calendar,* 1941–2.

52 McGill University, *Calendar,* 1920.

53 "Report of the Medical Examiner," in *Report of the President of the University of British Columbia,* 1936–7.

54 Prescott, *Student Bodies,* 66–7.

55 "Student Health Insurance," UWO, *President's Report,* 1930–1.

56 UCC/VUA, 90.065v, Women's Council, Box 1-2, "Report of the Acting Dean of Women," 29 May 1934.
57 UTA, Office of the President, A67-0007, Box 77, File: Gordon, letter: E. Gordon to R. Falconer, 17 January 1923. This situation continued to exist at least into the 1940s. See University of Toronto, *Calendar*, 1941–2.
58 Similarly, the University College Women's Union had an infirmary with two beds. See UCC/VUA, Dean of Women Fonds, 90.141v, Box 2-17, letter Edna Guest to Miss Addison, n.d.; UTA, B74-0011, Box 1-20, Report of the Work of the Women's Union by the Acting Dean, University College, 3 March 1931.
59 UCC/VUA, Dean of Women Fonds, 90.141v, Box 2-17, Dean of Women's Correspondence Re Women's Health 1910–32, letter, Edna Guest to Miss Addison, n.d.
60 MtAUA, Raymond Clare Archibald Fonds, 5501/6/1/8, p.28, Saint John *Daily Sun*, 2 April 1904.
61 UTA, B79-0011, University College, Dean of Women, Box 3, File 1, pamphlet: "Shirreff Hall, Dalhousie University," 1927.
62 This was true, for example, of the men's infirmary at Victoria College. See UCC/VUA, Fonds 2000, Board of Regents, 87.195v, Burwash Hall and Men's Residence Committee, Box 1-1, Victoria University Men's Residences, c. 1948.
63 UTA, A76-0044, Box 96, University Health Service, "A Report for the Medical Advisory Committee," c. 1946; UCC/VUA, Fonds 2021, President's Office, 89.130v, Box 77-11, "University of Toronto Health Service," c. 1942.
64 UTA, B74-0011, Box 3-3, "House Regulations 1942–3."
65 UAA, Student Medical Services, 75-144-1119, pamphlet: "Medical Services, 1935–6."
66 "Report of the President" in University of Saskatchewan, *President's Report*, 1928–9, 7–8, and "Report of the Accident and Sick Benefit Fund," University of Saskatchewan, *President's Report*, 1928–9, 61.
67 UAA, University of Alberta, *Calendar*, 1915–16; UAA, Student Medical Services, 75-144-1119, pamphlet: "Medical Services, 1935–6."
68 MUA, RG 46, 14-33, meeting, Sub-Committee on Student Health, 16 December 1935.
69 MUA, RG 30, 67-191, University Medical Officer, "Memorandum on Proposed Health Service," 1940;
70 "Department of Physical Education," UWO, *Announcement*, 1930–1.
71 UCC/VUA, Fonds 2021, President's Office, 89.130v, Box 77-11, "University of Toronto Health Service," ca 1942.

72 DUA, UA 12, Faculty of Medicine, Dean of Medicine, 60-1, Students'
Health Service, Notice from W. Holland, Director, 7 March 1947. Dalhousie
University did not offer hospitalization coverage when it started its service:
"Students' Health Service," Dalhousie University, *Calendar*, 1932–3, 11–12

73 UAA, Student Medical Services, 75-144-1119, pamphlet: "Medical Services,
1935–6." Dalhousie had a similar policy, although did not list what it meant
by "misconduct." See "Students' Health Service," Dalhousie University, *Calendar*, 1932–3, 11–12.

74 UAA, Student Medical Services, 75-144-1119, pamphlet: "Medical Services,
1947–8."

75 UAA, University of Alberta, *Calendar*, 1915–16, 1919–20, 1925–6, 1950–1,
and Student Medical Services, 75-144-1119, pamphlet: "Medical Services,"
1935–6; "Health," Dalhousie University, *Calendar*, 1931–2, 17–18, and DUA,
President's Office, 234-7, Business Manager to President Kerr, 31 October 1951; University of Toronto, *Calendar*, 1922–3, 1939–40; UCC/VUA,
Women's Council, 90.065v, Box 1-2, Report of Acting Dean of Women, 29
May 1934, and Dean of Women Fonds, 87.071v, Box 1-12, E.W. Wallace
to N. Ford, 2 June 1932, and Fonds 2021, President's Office, 89.130v, Box
77-11, Brown to Dr. Macdonald, 9 April 1941; MUA, RG 46, 14-33, Minutes,
subcommittee on student health, 16 December 1935; St. Francis Xavier
University, *Calendar*, 1930–1 and 1951–2; UMA, UA20, Box 51-12, Report of
Health Inquiry Committee, 11 March 1941, and Box 148-19, "Welcome to
the Residence," 4 December 1952; UBCA, UBC Subject File Collection, Box
22, pamphlet: *This is YOUR Health Service*, n.d. For the limited implementation of some of these types of schemes in Britain, see Vernon, "The Health
and Welfare of University Students in Britain, 1920–39," 243–45.

76 UCC/VUA, 90.064v, Box 3-19, Report by Scott Raff, January 1913; "Suspension of Drill a Temporary Measure," *The Varsity*, 22 January 1919; University
of Toronto, *Calendar* 1923–4 to 1939–40.

77 UCC/VUA, Fonds 2021, President's Office, 89.130v, Box 77-11, "University
of Toronto Health Service," ca 1942; "Campus Co-op Leads in Health Service Plan," *The Varsity*, 14 March 1941.

78 University of Toronto, *Calendar*, 1942–3. Same rate 1950–1.

79 University of Toronto, *Calendar*, 1938–9.

80 University of Toronto, *Calendar*, 1926–7.

81 UCC/VUA, Dean of Women Fonds, 97.071v, Box 1-12, letter: Guest to Ford,
2 May 1932.

82 UCC/VUA, 90.064v, Box 4-5, letter: Guest to Addison, 11 November 1926.

83 UCC/VUA, Dean of Women Fonds, 97.071v, Box 1-12, letter: Guest to Ford,
2 May 1932.

84 UAA, Provost's Office, Student Affairs, RG 17, 74-70, Minutes of the Committee on Student Affairs, October 1916–January 1917, and, Report of the Students' Medical Service, 22 January 1916, and, Student Medical Services, 75-144-1119, Minutes, Medical Service Committee, 28 February 1918.

85 UAA, Office of the President, 68-1, 3/4/8/10-1, Letter: President R. Newton to J.M. MacEachran, Chairman, Committee on Medical Services, 5 October 1944. In response, the board of governors felt the honorarium might be increased. See UAA, Office of the President, 68-1, 3/4/8/10-1, letter: MacEachran to Newton, 28 September 1944.

86 MUA, RG 30, 67-191, University Medical Officer, "Memorandum on Proposed Health Service," 1940.

87 "Report of Medical Adviser of Women," in University of Toronto, *President's Report*, 1922–3 and 1936–7.

88 In 1934–5 they treated 275 students. By 1934–5 this number had increased to 741. See Report of the Director of the Connaught Laboratories, in University of Toronto, *President's Report*, 1935–6.

89 "New Department Doing Good Work," *McGill News* 4/1 (December 1922): 9.

90 Grant, "Students' Health Service of Dalhousie University," 485–90.

91 UCC/VUA, Fonds 2045, 92.010v, Box 6-4, 1904–6, Report of Annesley Hall Gymnasium, May 1904.

92 UAA, Student Medical Services, 75-144-1119, pamphlet: "Medical Services, 1935–6." For McGill University, see MUA, RG 30, 67-191, University Medical Officer, "Memorandum on Proposed Health Service," 1940.

93 "Hospital and Health Service," Acadia University, *Bulletin*, 1951–2.

94 "Department of Physical Education," in McGill University, *Annual Report*, 1934–5; "Report of the Medical Adviser for Women," in University of Toronto, *President's Report*, 1940–1.

95 "Report of the Medical Examiner of Students," in *Report of the President of UBC*, 1929–30.

96 UAA, Student Medical Services, 75-144-1119, Meeting, Medical Service Committee, 27 September 1944; UAA, Office of the President, 68-1, 3/4/8/10-1, J.M. MacEachran, Chairman Committee on Medical Services, to President R. Newton, 28 September 1944, and Newton to J.M. MacEachran, 5 October 1944.

97 "Health of Students," McGill University, *Principal's Report*, 1931–2.

98 "Report of the University Health Service (Men)," in University of Toronto, *President's Report*, 1931–2.

99 "Report of Medical Adviser of Women," in University of Toronto, *President's Report*, 1933–4.

100 "Report of Medical Adviser of Women," in University of Toronto, *President's Report*, 1937–8.
101 "Report of the Director of the University Health Service," in University of Toronto, *President's Report*, 1947–8.
102 "Report of Medical Adviser of Women," in University of Toronto, *President's Report*, 1933–4.
103 "Report of Medical Adviser of Women," in University of Toronto, *President's Report*, 1937–8.
104 "Report of the Director of the University Health Service," in University of Toronto, *President's Report*, 1947–8.
105 "Report of the University Health Service (Men)," in University of Toronto, *President's Report*, 1921–2.
106 "Faculty of Dentistry," in University of Manitoba, *President's Report*, 1960–1.
107 "Report of Medical Adviser of Women," in University of Toronto, *President's Report*, 1936–7.
108 "Report of the Director of the University Health Service," in University of Toronto, *President's Report*, 1948–9.
109 McHenry, Crawford, and Barber, "The Heights and Weights of a Canadian Group," 37–41.
110 Hawgood, "Go East Young Woman," 91.
111 Prescott, "Using the Student Body," 16–20.

2. Ailments and Epidemics

1 See MUA, RG 42, 1-69, Health Service 1934–47, "A Survey of the Absences among RVC Students, October 1934–7." The physicians' and nurses' reports for 1900 to 1940 at Victoria College document similar trends. These records can be found within larger holdings of the Women's Council (90.065v), Dean of Women Fonds (90.141v), and the Annesley Hall Committee of Management Records (90.064v) at UCC/VUA.
2 Doctors recorded individual cases of measles in 1906–7, 1915, 1916, 1917, 1923, 1925, 1935–6, 1941–2, and mumps in 1916, 1921, 1928, 1935–6, 1939–40. See UCC/VUA, Fonds 2069, 90.064v, Boxes 2 and 3, Dean's Reports and Nurses' Reports for the period 1903 to 1940. Unfortunately, the rich records on student health at Victoria College exist only for the period from 1900 to the Second World War.
3 Similarly, in 1930–1, the nurse reported one case each of measles and scarlet fever while in 1937–8 she listed one case of typhoid fever, nine cases of scarlet fever, and one case of mumps. In 1941–2, two students contracted chickenpox; six, the mumps; twelve, rubella; and three,

scarlet fever. See UAA, Office of the President, RG3, 68-1, 3/2/8/8-2, Infirmary Report, 1928–9, 1930–1; 3/3/5/4-2, Report of the Director of Medical Services, 1937–8; 3/4/8/10-1, Annual Report of the Students' Medical Service from the University Infirmary, 1941–2; and Student Medical Services, 75-144-1119, Annual Report from the Infirmary, 1947–8.

4 MUA, RG 42, 1-69, Health Service 1934–47, "A Survey of the Absences Among RVC Students, October 1934–7; "Report of the Public Health Supervisor," in *Report of the President of UBC*, 1935–6; UAA, "Report of the Provost," in *Report of the Board of Governors of the University of Alberta*, 1920–1, 1935–6, 1940–1.

5 Carr and Beamish, *Manitoba Medicine*, 87, 92.

6 Scientists discovered a diphtheria antitoxoid in the 1890s; an antityphoid vaccine, which would be used widely by the First World War, in 1897; and Salvarsan, for the treatment of syphilis, in 1910. See Tomes, *The Gospel of Germs*, 5–6; Weindling, "The Immunological Tradition," 197; Weatherall, "Drug Treatment and the Rise of Pharmacology," 264.

7 Weindling, "The Immunological Tradition," 197–200; Mark Harrison, *Disease and the Modern World*, 149.

8 UCC/VUA, 90.065v, Box 1-4, Women's Council Annual Meeting, Report of the Physician, 20 May 1937.

9 UCC/VUA, 90.065v, Box 1-2, Medical Report, Fall 1935; 90.141v, Box 2-17, Dean of Women's Correspondence, 1910–32, Report of Nurse Maitland, 30 November 1932.

10 UTA, Office of the President, A67-0007, Box 81, File: Health Services, letter, J.J.R. Macleod to R. Falconer, 1 March 1923.

11 Professor Tait Mackenzie [*sic*], speaking at "Sixth Session," Congress of the Universities of the Empire, 1926, *Report of Proceedings*, 168–9.

12 H.J. Cody, speaking at session, "Physical Education in the Universities," Fifth Quinquennial Congress of the Universities of the British Empire, 1936, *Report of Proceedings*, 218.

13 "Report of the Physical Director," in University of Toronto, *President's Report*, 1908–9.

14 Indeed, there was at least one case in each of January 1915, 1916–17, 1918–19, 1919–20, fall 1921, fall 1929, and fall 1931, all of which required removal of the appendix in a hospital. See UCC/VUA, Physicians' and Nurses' Reports, 1900–40, in holdings of the Dean of Women Fonds, and Committee of Management Records. Similarly, cases of hernia and appendicitis frequently recurred at Queen's University. See Queen's University, *Principal's Report*, 1927–8, 66.

15 Of the 476 exams performed at McGill University in 1912–13, 87 turned up "defects of the eyes." In 1930 at Victoria College, 31 of 179 female residents needed their eyes re-examined. Eyesight was a problem at other institutions as well. The dean of the faculty of medicine at Dalhousie University listed vision as the chief defect in 1933. Studies of male students at Oxford in the 1940s and 1950s revealed that undergraduates' sight was four times worse than that of the male population in general. See "Report of the Department of Physical Education," McGill University, *Annual Report*, 1912–13; UCC/ VUA, 90.064v, Box 3-20, Report of the Examining Physician, November 1930; H.G. Grant, "Students' Health Service of Dalhousie University," 485; Stewart, "John Ryle," 67. See also Macleod, *A Bridge Built Halfway*, 42.

16 "Report of the Medical Examiner of Students," in *Report of the President of the UBC*, 1934–5.

17 "Report of the University Health Service (Men)," in University of Toronto, *President's Report*, 1934–5.

18 "Medical Advisor Says Co-Eds Here of Splendid Type," *Varsity*, 15 December 1924.

19 UCC/VUA, 90.064v, Box 3-20, "Physician's Report," n.d.

20 UCC/VUA, 90.065v, Box 1-2, "Medical Report," Fall 1935.

21 UCC/VUA, Margaret Burwash, Fonds 2045, 92.010v, Box 6-4, Report of Annesley Hall Gymnasium, May 1904. In the 1950s, the University of Toronto sent students with poor posture to the Physiotherapy Department. See UTA, School of Physical Health and Education, A83-0046, Box 3, File: Presidential Committee, Minutes of the Presidential Committee on Required Physical Education, 21 September 1955.

22 "Report of the Medical Adviser of Women," in University of Toronto, *President's Report*, 1923–4.

23 UTA, Faculty of Medicine Council Minutes, A86-0027, Reel 21, Committee on Students' Health, 3 March 1921 and 21 March 1921. For similar concerns about lack of medical inspection in the public school system, see Gordon, "The Need of Physical Training in Schools," 131.

24 The full implementation of school medical inspections differed by province and level of urbanization. By 1914, Nova Scotia had a system of school medical inspection in place, though primarily in urban centres such as Halifax, Sydney, Amherst, and Truro. Gleason notes that in 1914 one-quarter of students in British Columbia did not receive medical examinations. Comacchio argues that by 1940, "most Canadian cities still did not carry out any health inspection or instruction in their high schools." See respectively Michael Smith, "Dampness, Darkness, Dirt, Disease," 210; Gleason, "Race, Class, and Health," 101; Comacchio, "'The Rising Generation,'" 155.

25 "University Smallpox Epidemic is Checked," *Toronto Daily Star*, 19 October 1927. The fact that officials considered the outbreak to be limited to Victoria College suggests that these students must have attended classes only at Victoria on that Monday morning. Students registered at Victoria attended science courses at the University of Toronto but took all of their arts courses at the College.

26 "Report of the Dean of Women," in University of Manitoba, *President's Report*, 1937–8.

27 Belmont was a small town just north of Toronto. See UCC/VUA, 90.064v, Box 3-2, Report or the Nurse, 9 March 1916.

28 UCC/VUA, 90.064v, Box 2-8, Dean's Report, 14 March 1912, and, Box 1-4, Nurse's Report, 20 May 1937.

29 UCC/VUA, Fonds 2069, 90.064v, Box 1-4, Annesley Hall Committee of Management Minutes, 14 February 1918.

30 Influenza likely originated in the Midwest of the United States. See Patterson and Pyle, "The Geography and Mortality of the 1918 Influenza Pandemic," 4. For a detailed history of the epidemic in the United States see Barry, *The Great Influenza*. For the spread of the pandemic in Canada, see Humphries, "The Horror at Home," 235–60.

31 Johnson and Mueller, "Updating the Accounts," 106–7, 115; McGinnis, "The Impact of Epidemic Influenza: Canada 1918–1919," 122–3.

32 "Spanish Influenza Visits Victoria," *Varsity*, 9 October 1918; UCC/VUA, Fonds 2069, 90.064v, Box 3-2, Dean's Report, 13 March 1919.

33 Andrews, "Epidemic and Public Health," 24.

34 "Report of the University Health Service (Men)," in University of Toronto, *President's Report*, 1934–5.

35 UAA, Office of the President, 68-1, 3/3/5/4-2, Report of the Director of Medical Services, 1935–6.

36 "Report of the Director of the University Health Service," in *Report of the President of UBC*, 1941–2.

37 "Report of the Director of the University Health Service," in University of Toronto, *President's Report*, 1957–8.

38 "Flu Stews U's In Canada," *Xaverian Weekly*, 11 October 1957, 1; H.M. Simms, "Report of the University Physician," in Acadia University, *Report of the President*, 1957–8.

39 UCC/VUA, 90.064v, Box 3-20, Report by Dr Guest, 1 November 1921. By the late 1920s, tuberculin testing was common at American universities.

40 "Report of the Acting-Head of the University Health Service," in *Report of the President of UBC*, 1929–30, and, "Report of the Director of the University Health Service," in *Report of the President of UBC*, 1941–2.

41 Gleason, "Race, Class, and Health," 98–9; Norah Lewis, "Physical Perfection for Spiritual Welfare," 147; Sutherland, *Children in English-Canadian Society*, 41.

42 UCC/VUA, 90.064v, Box 3-2, Nurse's Report, 10 December 1914. For mumps, see UCC/VUA, 90.064v, Box 2-1, Annesley Hall Committee of Management Minutes, 10 February 1928.

43 UCC/VUA, 90.064v, Box 2-4, Dean's Report, 1906–7, and Box 3-21, Nurse's Report, 9 May 1917, and Box 2-1, Minutes, 8 November 1923.

44 UCC/VUA, 90.064v, Box 3-2, Report by Marion Clark, Nurse, 9 December 1915.

45 UCC/VUA, 90.065v, Women's Council, Box 1-3, Report of the Physician, 14 May 1936.

46 University of Guelph, Archival and Special Collections, McLaughlin Library, RE1 MAC ADD 14, Correspondence Box 5, Macdonald Institute, Director Watson to Miss C. Weaver, 24 March 1905. My thanks to Mary Wilson for this information.

47 UCC/VUA, 90.064v, Box 2-8, Dean's Report, 14 March 1912.

48 UCC/VUA, 90.064v, Box 2-8, Dean's Report, 14 March 1912.

49 UAA, Office of the President, 68-1, 3/3/5/4-2, Report of the Director of Medical Services, 1935–6.

50 UAA, Office of the President, 68-1, 3/3/5/4-2, Report of the Director of Medical Services, 1935–6.

51 UAA, Student Medical Services, 75-144-1119, Report of the Acting Provost, 9 May 1919.

52 "Victoria College Lit Holds Opening Meeting," *The Varsity*, 11 October 1918.

53 "Spanish Influenza Visits Victoria," *The Varsity*, 9 October 1918.

54 The University of Alberta, for example, closed its doors from 16 October to 6 December, the University of Toronto from 18 October until the 5th of November, and UBC closed its door for three weeks, starting October 20th 1918. See UAA, Student Medical Services, 75-144-1119, Meeting, Medical Service Committee, Report of the Acting Provost, 9 May 1919; "University Buildings Closed," *Varsity*, 18 October 1918; Miller, *Our Glory and Our Grief*, 185; Logan, *Tuum Est*, 73.

55 UCC/VUA, 90.064v, Box 3-1, Dean's Report, 14 November 1918.

56 UCC/VUA, 90.141v, Box 2-16, Dean Addison to Registrar, University of Toronto, 2 May 1912.

57 UCC/VUA, 90.064v, Box 3-2, Dean's Report, 12 June 1919.

58 UCC/VUA, 90.064v, Box 3-2, Nurse's Report, 12 April 1916.

59 For rheumatic fever, see UCC/VUA, 90.141v, Box 1-12, Correspondence, 18 March 1912; Report of the Dean of Women, in University of Manitoba,

President's Report, 1937–8. For tuberculosis, see for example, MUA, RG 46, 14-33, Sub-committee on Student Health, 16 December 1935; "Report of Medical Adviser of Women," in University of Toronto, *President's Report,* 1937–8; Report of the Director of the University Health Service, in *Report of the President of the UBC,* 1938–9; Archives de l'Université de Montréal, Fonds du Secrétariat général, D35/1400, letter, Gaetan Jarry, M.D., La Ligue Antituberculeuse de Montréal, to the Rector, Monseigneur Olivier-Maurault, 31 October 1947.

60 While the cause of death is unknown, one St. Francis Xavier student died in each of the years 1894, 1896, 1899, and 1904. During the 1918 influenza outbreak, the Victoria College student journal recorded three student deaths in October alone. In that year, one residence student died at the University of Alberta and at least three at UBC. Students did not die only from contagious diseases. C. Stuart Houston notes that in 1926, eight students at Regina College died from drinking unpasteurized milk. See James D. Cameron, *For the People,* 102; *Acta Victoriana* (October 1918): 68; UAA, Student Medical Services, 75-144-1119, Meeting, Medical Services Committee, Report of the Acting Provost, 9 May 1919; Logan, *Tuum Est,* 73; Houston, *Steps on the Road to Medicare,* 24–5.

61 McPherson, *Bedside Matters,* 141.

62 UCC/VUA, 90.064v, Box 3-1, Dean's Reports, 14 November 1918.

63 UCC/VUA, 90.064v, Box 2-4, Dean's Reports, October 1907.

64 UCC/VUA, 90.064v, Box 3-3, Dean's Reports, 15 April 1920.

65 UCC/VUA, 90.064v, Box 2-1, Annesley Hall Committee of Management Minutes, 10 May 1928.

66 "Report of the Dean of Women," in University of Manitoba, *President's Report,* 1936–7.

67 "Quarantine Raised," *The Varsity,* 19 December 1911.

68 Andrews, "Epidemic and Public Health," 27–8; Pettigrew, *The Silent Enemy,* 15, 33, 48–9; Quiney, "'Filling the Gaps'," 361–2.

69 UAA, Student Medical Services, 75-144-1119, Report of the Acting Provost, 9 May 1919.

70 UCC/VUA, 90.064v, Box 3-1, Dean's Report, 14 November 1918 and 13 March 1919.

71 Logan, *Tuum Est,* 73.

72 "Report of the Director of the University Health Service," in University of Toronto, *President's Report,* 1957–8.

73 Fahrni, "'Elles sont partout ...'," 68, 73; Jones, "Contact Across a Diseased Boundary," 121; Miller, *Our Glory and Our Grief,* 187.

74 "Report of the Dean of Women," in University of Manitoba, *President's Report*, 1939–40.
75 UAA, Student Medical Services, 75-144-1119, Meeting, Medical Service Committee, Report of the Acting Provost, 9 May 1919.
76 "The Flu," *The Argosy* 15, 5 (March 1919): 163–4.
77 Quoted in Cleveland and Conrad, "Mary Dulhanty (1909–1999)," in *The Small Details of Life*, 347–8.
78 Fahrni, "'Elles sont partout …,'" 84–5.
79 Prescott, "Sending Their Sons into Danger," 298–9.
80 "Hospital," *Acadia Bulletin*, 1925–6.
81 "Ban Is Not Lifted," *Varsity*, 20 February 1920.
82 UAA, "President's Report," in *Report of the Board of Governors of the University of Alberta*, 1928–9.
83 "The Smallpox Scare," *Acta Victoriana* 52, 2 (November 1927): 34. See also "University Smallpox Epidemic is Checked," *Toronto Daily Star*, 19 October 1927; "Smallpox Checked," *Varsity*, 20 October 1927; O'Grady, *Margaret Addison*, 201–2.
84 University of Guelph, Archival and Special Collections, McLaughlin Library, RE1 MAC A0014, Box 5, Correspondence, Miss Weaver to Director Watson, 23 March 1905 and Director Watson to Miss Weaver, 24 March 1905.
85 McGill University, *Principal's Report*, 1885.
86 "The Smallpox Scare," *Acta Victoriana*, 52, 2 (November 1927): 34; "Smallpox Epidemic Regulations," *Varsity*, 20 October 1927; "Immediate Vaccination Advised," *Varsity*, 20 October 1927; "Smallpox Checked," *Varsity*, 20 October 1927; Editorial, "Vaccination Edict Earns Silent Approbation," *Varsity*, 17 November 1927. By 1914, the Ontario *Vaccination Act* had made vaccination mandatory in the case of an outbreak. See Arnup, "'Victims of Vaccination?'"165.
87 In 1928–9, the Medical Examiner noted that 77.7 per cent of students had been vaccinated. Still, during a 1932 outbreak of smallpox in the city, university officials urged some 250 students (or about 7.5 per cent of the student population) who had not been vaccinated, to do so. See "Report of the Medical Examiner of Students," in *Report of the President of UBC*, 1928–9; "Epidemic Hits City Warning Issued to U.B.C.," *The Ubyssey*, 5 February 1932, 1.
88 Alberta seems to be one of the few places that did not require smallpox immunization. By at least 1934, students at Toronto had access to Schick, Dick, and TB tests through Connaught Laboratories. UMA, UA20, Box 51-12, Report of Health Inquiry Committee, 11 March 1941; UTA, A68-0028,

Box 15, File: University Health Services, "General Information for Students: University Health Service," ca 1938; MUA, RG 46, 14-33, Minutes, Committee on Student Health, 1 March 1939; "University Health Service," UBC, *Calendar*, 1940–1; AUM, Fonds du Secrétariat général, D35/1405, letter, Association générale des étudiants to Mr. Eugene Poirier, secrétaire de la Société d'Administration de l'Université de Montréal, 30 June 1945.

89 "Report of the Director of the University Health Service," in *Report of the President of UBC*, 1941–2.

90 The women's residence at Victoria College took in students from other faculties and professional programs when they could not fill residence rooms with their own arts students. See UCC/VUA, 90.064v, Box 3-2, Nurse's Report, 9 March 1916.

91 For the United States, see Leavitt, "Gendered Expectations," 159–60; Kraut, *Silent Travelers*; Prescott, "The White Plague Goes to College," 738. For Canada, see Gleason, "Race, Class, and Health," 97; Helen Harrison, "In the Picture of Health," 53, 267–70.

92 MtAUA, *President's Report*, 18 May 1938, 3.

93 UCC/VUA, 87.071v, Box 1-12, Women's Council Resolution, June 1933.

94 UCC/VUA, 90.065v, Women's Council, Executive Committee Minutes, 1932–5, Box 1-10, Report of Physician to Women Students, ca 1934.

95 ECWA, "University Physician," in Acadia University, *Report of the President*, 1944–5, 34–5.

96 Jane Lewis, "The Prevention of Diphtheria," 163; Norah Lewis, "Physical Perfection for Spiritual Welfare," 148.

3. Physical Culture and Character Formation

1 No explanation was ever provided for this gender difference. In general, the few statistics available at other universities seem to suggest a similar pattern of students' good health. For example, in 1922 at McGill University, 93.7 per cent of male and female students who had a medical examination fell into Category A; in 1931–2, 83 per cent did so; in 1935–6, 95.6 per cent did so; and in 1941–2, 72.7 per cent of men and 69 per cent of women did so. Similarly, at Victoria College, 81 per cent of female students fell into Category A in 1923–4; 94 per cent in 1930; and 95 per cent in 1935–6. At the University of Alberta, 92 per cent of first-year students were approved for physical training in 1948–9. This seems also to have been the case at Queen's University. However, these high results did not always hold. In 1941–2, at Macdonald College, students rated significantly lower, with only 51.6 per cent

of men and 57.8 per cent of women in Category A. Class certainly played a factor in health. Macleod notes that physical examinations for the student body at Memorial University in 1943–4 indicated that outport students were less healthy than students from St. John's. See "New Department Doing Good Work," *The McGill News* 4, 1 (December 1922): 9–11; "Department of Physical Education," in McGill University, *Annual Report*, 1931–2; MUA, RG 42, C.2, 130, Physical Education Survey, 1935–6 and RG 30, Faculty of Education, C.6S, 175, Minutes of the Senate Committee on Physical Education, 26 January 1943; UCC/VUA, 90.064v, Box 3-20, "Report of the Examining Physician," 7 November 1923 and November 1930 and 90.065v, Women's Council, Box 1-2, Medical Report, Fall 1935; UAA, Student Medical Services, 75-144-119, "Committee on Medical Services Meeting, 6 October 1948"; Queen's University, *Principal's Report*, 1926–7; Macleod, *A Bridge Built Halfway*, 42.

2 McCrone, *Playing the Game*, 101.
3 Ainsworth, *History of Physical Education in Colleges for Women*, 8, 41; Fletcher, *Women First*, 17, 31.
4 Lathrop, "Contested Terrain," 167. See also Ainsworth, *History of Physical Education in Colleges for Women*, 8.
5 Fletcher, *Women First*, 4, 17; Scraton, *Shaping Up to Womanhood*, 28.
6 McCrone, *Playing the Game*, 101.
7 Ainsworth, *History of Physical Education in Colleges for Women*, 8–9, 18–22; Fletcher, *Women First*, 4, 31; McCrone, *Playing the Game*, chap. 4.
8 Cosentino and Howell, *A History of Physical Education in Canada*, 26–9.
9 Welch, *History of American Physical Education and Sport*, 119–37.
10 Ainsworth, *History of Physical Education in Colleges for Women*, 8, 25, 40–1.
11 Bennett, "Dr. Dudley A. Sargent and the Harvard Summer School of Physical Education," 131.
12 Lathrop, "Elegance and Expression," 38; Welch, *History of American Physical Education and Sport*, 115; Michael Smith, "Graceful Athleticism," 125. See also Ruyter, "American Delsatism," 2015–30, and Vertinsky, "Transatlantic Traffic in Expressive Movement," 2031–51.
13 Ainsworth, *History of Physical Education in Colleges for Women*, 8–9, 18–22; Welch, *History of American Physical Education and Sport*, 119–137.
14 Ainsworth, *History of Physical Education in Colleges for Women*, 11. For more on Bukh, see Bonde, "Globalization Before Globalization," 2000–14.
15 Cosentino and Howell, *History of Physical Education in Canada*, 35; Walton, "The Life and Professional Contributions of Ethel Mary Cartwright," 16, 35, 114–15.
16 McCrone, *Playing the Game*, 110.

17 Lathrop, "Elegance and Expression," 34–37, 86. For the importance of Scott
   Raff and the School to the cultural milieu of Toronto see Murray, "Making
   the Modern."
18 For example, in 1900 Royal Victoria College hired Vendla M. Holstrom,
   a graduate of the Posse Gymnasium in Boston and the Harvard Summer
   School program. The first directress of athletics and physical education for
   women at the University of Toronto, Ivy Coventry, was equally a graduate of
   the Sargent School. The women hired by Victoria College, Toronto, to assist
   Scott Raff in the years prior to the First World War had all studied at the Sargent School, while one was a graduate of both the Sargent School and Hemenway Gymnasium. Florence Somers, one of the first faculty members of the
   University of Toronto's School of Physical Education, created in 1940, was
   not only director of the Margaret Eaton School in the 1930s, but prior to
   that, had been associate director of the Sargent School. E. Winnifred Briggs,
   appointed in 1916 as the first head of the department of physical training
   and physiology at Mount Allison Ladies' College was also a graduate of
   the Sargent School, as was Margaret Dobbs, who worked at Mount Alison
   University in the 1930s. See "RVC Gymnasium," in McGill University, *Calendar*, 1900–1; Parkes, *Development of Women's Athletics*, 2; Byl, "The Margaret
   Eaton School," 84 and Appendix E1; Lathrop, "Elegance and Expression,"
   127, 218; Gurney, *A Century to Remember*, 17; MtAUA, "Three Cheers for Old
   Mount A! Curriculum Expands" at http://www.mta.ca/threecheers/sports-
   gymnasticswomens05.html, accessed 11 December 2008, and "Meeting of
   Regents," in *President's Report*, 31 October 1934.
19 Dorothy Jackson, who provided instruction at Victoria College for several
   years in the 1930s, graduated from the Margaret Eaton School and worked
   full time at the School between 1934 and 1941. Instructors at Mount Allison
   University in the 1930s and 1940s included: Lois Fahs, who had obtained an
   MA from Columbia University, as well as Della MacFarlane and Rosamund
   Crocker, both graduates of the Margaret Eaton School. Jessie Herriott, Ethel
   Cartwright's successor at McGill University, received her training at Colum-
   bia University. In the early 1930s, Dalhousie University hired Florence R.
   Harris, a graduate of McGill, as its physical instructor for women students.
   Iveagh Munro, a graduate of McGill's School of Physical Education became
   director of physical education for women at that institution from 1939 to
   1966. Zerada Slack, who taught at McGill University between 1928 and 1939,
   Mount Allison from 1939 to 1942, and then at the University of Toronto
   from 1945 to 1965, obtained her credentials from McGill University. In
   1942–3, Acadia University hired Miss Norma Burgess, a graduate of McGill
   University. See MtAUA, "Three Cheers for Old Mount A! Curriculum

Expands" at http://www.mta.ca/threecheers/sportsgymnasticswomens05.
html, accessed 11 December 2008, and "Report of the President," in *President's Report*, October 1939 and 19 November 1946; ECWA, "Department
of Physical Education" in Acadia University, *Report of the President*, 1942–3;
"Physical Instructor for Women," Dalhousie University, *President's Report*,
1930–1, 26; Kidd, *The Struggle for Canadian Sport*, 122; Gillett, *We Walked Very
Warily*, 227.

20 Bennett, "Dr. Dudley A. Sargent," 132; Walton, "The Life and Professional
Contributions of Ethel Mary Cartwright," 35.

21 Similarly, in 1941 the department of athletics and physical training at the
University of Toronto added to its staff M.G. Griffiths, who had received his
BSA at Toronto and MPE from Springfield. Keith King, co-director of
physical education at Dalhousie University in the 1950s, had taken some
graduate coursework at Springfield College. There were, however, also
notable exceptions to this pattern. A number of male physical directors
gained their appointments at least partly as a result of their earlier success
as athletes. This seems to have been the case for Maurice Van Vliet, physical director at UBC from 1935 to 1945 and for thirty years thereafter at the
University of Alberta; for Robert Osborne, director of the School of Physical
Education at UBC from 1945 to the late 1970s; and for Warren Stephens,
director of athletics at the University of Toronto beginning in the 1930s.
See Markham, "The Indelible Mark of Springfield College," 16; Kirkconnell, *The Fifth Quarter-Century*, 47; "Report on Athletics and Physical Training
(Men)," in University of Toronto, *President's Report*, 1941–2; "Report of the
Physical Education Department of Men, 1950–4," in Dalhousie University,
President's Report, 1950–4; "John Howard Crocker (1870–1959)" at http://
www.uwo.ca/olympic/lectures/crocker_about.html, accessed 27 February
2011; "Maury Van Vliet" at http://www.ubcsportshalloffame.com/cgi-bin/
search.cgi?person_id=67, accessed 27 February 2011; "Biographical Sketch,"
Robert Osborne Fonds at http://www.library.ubc.ca/archives/u_arch/
osborne.pdf, accessed 27 February 2011; UTA, A73-0026, Box 443 (80),
Varsity, 17 March 1933.

22 "Report on Athletics and Physical Training," in University of Toronto, *President's Report*, 1932–3, 89–90.

23 Parkes, *Development of Women's Athletics*, 2.

24 MUA, RG 42, 2-135, "Report of the Work in the RVC Gymnasium, 1906–7,"
and 2-135, Physical Education – Programme for Women, 1905–15,
"Demonstration of Gymnastics and Dancing," n.d.

25 For these types of exercises see Ainsworth, *History of Physical Education in
Colleges for Women*, 8, 41.

26 UCC/VUA, 90.064v, Box 3-19, "Report of the Director of Physical Education," 1905, 14 October 1908, October 1909, January 1912.

27 UCC/VUA, 90.064v, Box 3-19, "Report of the Director of Physical Education," 1905. For similar comments see UCC/VUA, 90.064v, Box 1-1, Minutes of Committee of Management, 8 April 1909.

28 UCC/VUA, 90.064v, Box 3-19, "Report of the Director of Physical Education," 1905, and 14 October 1908; Hall, *The Girl and the Game*, 33.

29 Scraton, *Shaping Up to Womanhood*, 28.

30 UCC/VUA, 90.064v, Box 3-19, "Report of the Director of Physical Education," 1905, and January 1908, and Box 2-7, Dean's Report, 9 March 1911; Hall, *The Girl and the Game*, 33.

31 UCC/VUA, 90.064v, Box 3-19, "Report of the Director of Physical Education," 14 October 1908, and January 1912; F.H. Harvey, Medical Director, "Report of the Department of Physical Education," in McGill University, *Principal's Report*, 1912–13. Same emphasis 1925.

32 UCC/VUA, 90.064v, Box 3-20, "Report of Medical Examiner," 10 May 1905.

33 Although some American women's colleges such as Smith and Bryn Mawr instituted drills and marching, this does not seem to have been the case in Canada. Yet, as Helen Lenskyj argues, the concern over fitness for both soldiers and civilians made it easier during the war to promote physical education for girls. See Ainsworth, *History of Physical Education in Colleges for Women*, 31; Lenskyj, "The Role of Physical Education in the Socialization of Girls in Ontario," 215.

34 University of Saskatchewan, *Calendar* 1920–1, 1930–1, 1940–1; "Department of Physical and Military Training," UWO, *Announcement*, 1920–1; "Physical Education," *Calendar of Mount St. Bernard*, with *Calendar of St. Francis Xavier University*, 1936–7. For the continuation of these elements at Victoria College, the University of Toronto, and for women at McGill University, see UCC/VUA, 90.065v, Box 1-2, "Report of Dean of Women," 10 November 1934; UTA, Office of the President, A67-0007, Box 77, File: Gordon, "University of Toronto Women's Athletic Association, 5 February 1923; "Department of Physical Education," McGill University, *Calendar*, 1935. Posture and folk dancing formed part of the voluntary program at UBC. See "Report of the Instructor in Physical Education for Women," in *Report of the President of the University of British Columbia*, 1935–6.

35 MUA, RG 42, 2-137, "Evolution of Department of Physical Education for Women," January 1936. This was also the case at Queen's University. See "Report on Women's Classes in Physical Training," in Queen's University, *Principal's Report*, 1937–8.

36 "Department of Physical Education," McGill University, *Calendar*, 1935; "Department of Physical and Military Training," UWO, *Announcement*, 1920–1.

37 ECWA, "Department of Physical Education," in Acadia University, *Report of the President*, 1939–40, 21–22. UWO offered a similar broad introduction to different physical activities. See "Department of Physical and Military Training," UWO, *Announcement*, 1920–1.

38 Smith, "Graceful Athleticism," 121.

39 "The Gym Exhibition," *Argosy* (6 March 1894): xxiii, cited in partial research notes on the history of sports at Mt. Allison University, MtAUA.

40 "Report of the Medical Director of Physical Training," in McGill University, *Principal's Report*, 1905–6. See also the same source for 1913–14.

41 "Gymnasium Report," in McGill University, *Principal's Report*, 1908–9.

42 "Gymnasium Report," in McGill University, *Principal's Report*, 1908–9.

43 "Compulsory Physical Training A Fact," *Varsity*, 22 October 1917.

44 "Department of Physical and Military Training," UWO, *Announcement*, 1920–1.

45 UTA, Office of the President, A67-0007, Box 75, File: Health Services, "Regulations," ca 1921–2; "Report on Athletics and Physical Training," University of Toronto, *President's Report*, 1929–30.

46 ECWA, "Department of Physical Education," Acadia University, *Report of the President*, 1939–40.

47 Kiefer and Pierson, "The War Effort and Women Students," 162–3.

48 See chap. 1, note 18.

49 Griswold, "The 'Flabby American,' the Body, and the Cold War," 323–48.

50 See, for example, "Report of the Director of Physical Education for Women," University of Toronto, *President's Report*, 1949–50; "Department of Physical Education," UWO *Announcement*, 1945–6; "Physical Training," University of Saskatchewan, *Calendar*, 1950–1 and 1955–6. One hour of the two-hour requirement for female students at Dalhousie consisted of instruction in a variety of activities including tumbling, apparatus, square dancing, and social dancing. See "Report of the Physical Director for Women," Dalhousie University, *President's Report*, 1949–50.

51 "Report of the Physical Director," University of Toronto, *President's Report*, 1912–13.

52 McGill University, *Annual Report*, 1914–15.

53 Kirk Wipper, "A Record of the School of Physical and Health Education, University of Toronto, 1940–65," quoted in Cosentino and Howell, *History of Physical Education in Canada*, 45.

54 DUA, President's Office, UA3, 39-9, S.A. Korning, "Communication from the Physical Education Department about Physical Activities at Dalhousie," 1938–9.

55 ECWA, "Department of Physical Education," Acadia University, *Report of the President*, 1939–40.

56 Howell, *Blood, Sweat, and Cheers*, 31. See also Metcalfe, *Canada Learns to Play*, 120–1. For the United States, see Dyreson, "Regulating the Body," 122, 126, 137; Reiss, "Sport and the Redefinition of Middle-Class Masculinity," 179–80, 185; Mrozek, "Sport in American Life," 18-19; Szasz, "The Stress on 'Character and Service' in Progressive America," 145; Susman, "'Personality' and the Making of Twentieth-Century Culture," 214.

57 Nicolson, *Inventing Personality*, 15; Szasz, "The Stress on 'Character and Service' in Progressive America," 147; McKillop, "Marching as to War," 80–4.

58 Atkinson, "Fitness, Feminism and Schooling," 116; Scraton, *Shaping Up to Womanhood*, 33. On the gendered nature of "character," see also White and Hunt, "Citizenship: Care of the Self, Character and Personality," 103–4.

59 "Report of the Physical Director," in University of Toronto, *President's Report*, 1912–13.

60 See Pitsula, "Manly Heroes," 121–22, and Kuhlberg, "An Acute Yet Brief Bout of 'Returned-soldier-itis,'" 57.

61 Lamb, "Physical Education," 163.

62 Cartwright, "Athletics and Physical Education for Girls," 278.

63 UTA, Department of Graduate Records, A73-0026, Box 121/91, "Sports for Girls Develop Citizenship," *Mail*, 6 September 1928.

64 UCC/VUA, Fonds 2045, 92.010v, Box 6-4, Report on Gymnasium, 1905–6.

65 F.H. Harvey, "Gymnasium Report," in McGill University, *Principal's Report*, 1909–10.

66 UAA, Office of the President, RG3, 68-9-280, "Regulations of Corporation Regarding Physical Education," McGill University, attached to letter, A.S. Lamb, Department of Physical Education, McGill, to Dr Tory, 15 March 1920; UTA, A86-0028, Box 15, University Health Services, Proposal Regarding the University Health Service, Faculty of Medicine, 7 October 1938.

67 McCrone, *Playing the Game*, 101.

68 Ainsworth, *History of Physical Education in Colleges for Women*, 8.

69 Lathrop, "Elegance and Expression," 39.

70 Gordon, "The Need of Physical Training in Schools," 131.

71 Porter, "Exercise and Health," 223.

72 Macdonald, "The Relation of Play to the Education of the Child," 343.

73 Allen, *The Social Passion*; Baltutis, "'To Enlarge Our Hearts and To Widen Our Horizon'"; Dennis, "Beginning to Restructure the Institutional Church"; McGowan, "The Maritimes' Region and the Building of a Canadian Church."

74 Gidney, *A Long Eclipse*, chap. 1.

75 UCC/VUA, 90.064v, Box 3-19, "Report of Physical Training," February 1907; "Report of the Dean of Women," in *Report of the President of UBC*, 1936–7; Tait McKenzie, speaking at "Sixth Session," Congress of the Universities of the Empire, 1926, 168–73. See also "Report of the President," in University of Saskatchewan, *Annual Report of the President*, 1957–8, 15.

76 UTA, "Report of the Physical Director," in University of Toronto, *President's Report*, 1908–9. For similar comments see McGill University, *Annual Report*, 1914–15.

77 McGill University, *Principal's Report*, 1913–14.

78 McGill University, *Principal's Report*, 1914–15.

79 MUA, RG42, 2-135, "Report of the Work in the RVC Gymnasium, 1906–7." See also, UCC/VUA, 90.064v, Box 2-6, Dean's Reports, 10 March 1910; "Health of its Women Interests University," *Varsity*, 14 June 1922.

80 John Hughes, speaking at session on "Physical Education in the Universities," Congress of the Universities of the British Empire, 1936, 217. For similar comments earlier in the century in the United States, see Lowe, *Looking Good*, 16.

81 UCC/VUA, 90.064v, Box 3-19, "Director of Physical Education, Reports," 1909, quoted in Lathrop, "Elegance and Expression," 53.

82 "Health of its Women Interests University," *Varsity*, 14 June 1922. See also "Report of the Physical Director," in University of Toronto, *President's Report*, 1908–9.

83 UAA, Office of the President, RG3, 68-9-280, "Regulations of Corporation Regarding Physical Education," McGill University, attached to letter, A.S. Lamb, Department of Physical Education, McGill University, to Dr Tory, 15 March 1920.

84 J. Howard Crocker, "Physical Education and the University," *Occidentalia*, 1931, quoted in Keyes, "John Howard Crocker, LL.D., 1870–1959," 113.

85 Warren Stevens, "Why Athletics?" *Health*.

86 Zweiniger-Bargielowska, "Building a British Superman," 596.

87 MUA, RG 42, 2-133, Physical Education Reorganization, "Memorandum Re Required Program of Physical Activity for Meeting of Senate, 21 February 1940.

88 MUA, RG 42, 1-69, Health Service, Department of Physical Education, "Circular for Men Students, 1945–6."

89 Strong-Boag, *New Day Recalled*, 13. For similar attitudes of American female students in the 1920s, see Fass, *The Damned and the Beautiful*, 82.

90 For the strongest articulation of this position, see Lenskyj, *Out of Bounds*, chaps. 1–3; "The Role of Physical Education in the Socialization of Girls in Ontario," 245; and "Femininity First," 4–17. See also Scraton, *Shaping Up to Womanhood*, 35.

91 Kidd, *The Struggle for Canadian Sport*, 114–15, 121–4, 127–8; Hall, *The Girl and the Game*, 74–9. On the conservative nature of women's athletics at UBC in the 1940s, see Vertinsky, "'Power Geometries,'" 59–60.

92 Cartwright, "Athletics and Physical Education for Girls," 281.

93 Cartwright, "Athletics and Physical Education for Girls," 279–81.

94 Cartwright, "Athletics and Physical Education for Girls," 281. For the late nineteenth century, see Vertinsky, *The Eternally Wounded Woman*, chap. 1.

95 Cartwright, "Athletics and Physical Education for Girls," 281.

96 On the division among Canadian sportswomen, see Kidd, *The Struggle for Canadian Sport*, 119–30.

97 UTA, A83-0045, Box 1-3, Women's Athletic Directorate Minutes, 1920–5.

98 UTA, Department of Graduate Records, A73-0026, Box 121/91, "Sports for Girls Develop Citizenship," *Mail*, 6 September 1928.

99 Kidd, *The Struggle for Canadian Sport*, 116–19.

100 UTA, Department of Graduate Records, 356/52, "Doctor Lauds Women Discarding Dress," *Star*, 20 April 1929.

101 Hall, *The Girl and the Game*, 51, chap. 3; Harrigan, "Women's Agency and the Development of Women's Intercollegiate Athletics," 39.

102 Kiefer and Pierson, "The War Effort and Women Students at Toronto," 177.

103 ECWA, "Department of Physical Education," in Acadia University, *Report of the President*, 1942–3.

104 Verbrugge, "Recreating the Body," 280.

105 Verbrugge, "Recreating the Body," 302. See also Verbrugge, *Active Bodies*, 8.

106 McCrone, *Playing the Game*, 286.

107 Lathrop, "Elegance and Expression," 54.

108 MUA, RG 42, 2-135, "Physical Education – Programme for Women, 1905–1915."

109 Gillett notes this of McGill, but it is equally true of other institutions. See *We Walked Very Warily*, 200.

110 UCC/VUA, Fonds 2045, 92.010v, Box 6-2, Notes, 1903.

111 UCC/VUA, Fonds 2045, 92.010v, Box 6-4, 1904–6, "Report of the Annesley Hall Gymnasium, 1905–6."

112 UCC/VUA, 90.064v, Box 1-1, Minutes of the Committee of Management, 8 April 1909, and Box 3-19, Report by Scott Raff, January 1910 and 14 November 1912.

113 Letter to Editor, *Varsity*, 21 October 1921.

114 Cited in Gillett, *We Walked Very Warily*, 264.

115 UWOA, Office of the President Fonds, AFC 40, 28/2, University Physician to the Principal, University College, UWO, 22 April 1955.

116 "Obituary: Archie Campbell, Teacher, Lawyer, and Judge, 1942–2007," *Globe and Mail*, 19 April 2007, R5.

117 UCC/VUA, 90.064v, Box 1-1, Committee of Management Minutes, 13 February 1907, and 90.064v, Committee of Management, Director of Physical Education's Reports, 1905–13, Box 3-19, Report of Gymnasium, 1905.

118 For similar comments about male students prior to compulsory training see "Report of the Physical Director," in University of Toronto, *President's Report*, 1908–9.

119 F.W. Harvey, "Report of the Department of Physical Education," in McGill University, *Principal's Report*, 1915–16.

120 UCC/VUA, 90.064v, Box 3-19, "Report of Physical Training," 14 March 1907.

121 UAA, "Report of the Chairman of the Committee on Physical Education," in *Report of the Board of Governors*, 1947–8.

122 See, for example, UTA, A83-0046, Box 3, File: Program – Required, "Report on Compulsory Physical Education for 1st Year Women, 1969"; "Health Services," McGill University, *Calendar*, 1945.

123 "Report of the Physical Director for Women 1949–50," Dalhousie University, *President's Report*, 1945–50. Same comments made for 1951–4 report.

124 UCC/VUA, 90.064v, Box 3-19, Emma Scott Raff, "Report to the Victoria Women's Residence Association," 14 April 1910.

125 Axelrod, *Making a Middle Class*, 112.

126 UTA, Office of the President, A67-0007, Box 22, File: Barton, letter Dr Barton to President Falconer, 10 April 1913.

127 That program began in 1946. "Report of the Instructor in Physical Education for Women," in *Report of the President of the UBC*, 1942–3; Logan, *Tuum Est*, 132, 143, 158–9; Stewart, *"It's Up to You,"* 119–120.

4. Health in Home and Body

1 Gidney, *A Long Eclipse*, 33.
2 For examinations of residences as a physical environment, see King, "Centres of 'Home-Like Influence,'" 39–59; Adams, "Rooms of Their Own," 29–41; Horowitz, *Alma Mater*.
3 UCC/VUA, 90.141v, Box 1-12, Report of the Examining Physician, 13 November 1930 and 12 November 1931.
4 UTA, B74-0011, University College, Box 3-2, Submission from Alumnae Association, University College, n.d.
5 Tomes, *The Gospel of Germs*, 8–9, 27, 96. See also Meckel, "Going to School, Getting Sick," 196–7; Hoy, *Chasing Dirt*, 61.
6 Tomes, *The Gospel of Germs*, 57.
7 Hoy, *Chasing Dirt*, 69–70.
8 Quoted in McLaren, *Our Own Master Race*, 36. See also Dowbiggin, *Keeping America Sane*, 165.
9 "Report of the University Health Service, Women Students," in University of Toronto, *President's Report*, 1921–2.
10 "Report of the University Health Service, Women Students," in University of Toronto, *President's Report*, 1921–2.
11 UCC/VUA, 90.141v, Box 1-5, letter: H.M. Griffin to the Dean of Women, 19 April 1904. See also UCC/VUA, 90.064v, Box 3-2, Nurse's Report, 14 October 1915.
12 UCC/VUA, 90.141v, Box 2-17, letter: Edna Guest to Dr Ford, 3 December 1932, and Box 1-12, "Report of Examining Physician, 12 November 1931, and 90.064v, Box 3-20, "Dr. Guest's Report," 1927.
13 UCC/VUA, 90.141v, Box 2-17, letter: Edna Guest to Dr Ford, 3 December 1932.
14 UTA, B74-0011, University College, Box 3-2, Submission from Alumnae Association, University College, n.d.
15 UCC/VUA, 90.064v, Box 3-20, "Dr. Guest's Report," 1927. See also UCC/VUA, 90.141v, Box 1-12, Report of Examining Physician, 13 November 1930, and Box 2-17, letter: Edna Guest to Dr Ford, 3 December 1932.
16 UCC/VUA, 90.064v, Box 2-3, Dean's Reports, May 1905.
17 UCC/VUA, 90.064v, Box 3-2, Nurse's Report, 9 March 1916.
18 "Report of the Department of Physical Education," in McGill University, *Annual Report*, 1924–5.
19 Cited in King, "The Experience of the Second Generation of Women Students," 159.

20 UTA, B74-0011, University College, Box 3-2, Submission from Alumnae Association, University College, n.d.
21 UCC/VUA, 90.065v, Box 1-2, Report of the Acting Dean of Women, 29 May 1934.
22 UTA, B74-0011, University College, Box 3-2, Submission from Alumnae Association, University College, n.d.
23 Hoy, *Chasing Dirt*, 87.
24 Ibid.
25 UTA, B74-0011, University College, Box 3-2, Submission from Alumnae Association, University College, n.d.
26 Forty-six per cent of students surveyed lived in houses containing both sexes. See UTA, B74-0011, University College, Box 3-2, Submission from Alumnae Association, University College, n.d.
27 "Report of the University Health Service, Women Students," in University of Toronto, *President's Report*, 1921–2.
28 Drawing on school board medical records in the 1920s, Sutherland notes that three-quarters of school children in Vancouver shared a room and argues that significant numbers of these would have shared a bed. See Sutherland, *Growing Up*, 38.
29 Fifty-one per cent of those surveyed shared a double bed. See UTA, B74-0011, University College, Box 3-2, Submission from Alumnae Association, University College, n.d.
30 Bliss, "'Pure Books on Avoided Subjects,'" 258.
31 UTA, B74-0011, University College, Box 3-2, Submission from Alumnae Association, University College, n.d.
32 Gidney, "'Less Inefficiency, More Milk': The Politics of Food and the Culture of the English-Canadian University, 1900–1950," 298.
33 For the history of anthropometry on campus see, for example, Urla and Swedlund, "The Anthropometry of Barbie," 288; Park, "Muscles, Symmetry and Action" 378–80, and "'Taking their Measure,'" 193–217; Vertinsky, "Embodying Normalcy," 95–113; Lowe, *Looking Good*, 22–3.
34 Urla and Swedlund, "The Anthropometry of Barbie," 286–7. For the rise of statistical analysis in the nineteenth century, see for example, Porter, *The Rise of Statistical Thinking*. For Canada, see Curtis, *The Politics of Population*; Emery, *Facts of Life: The Social Construction of Vital Statistics*.
35 Tanner, *A History of the Study of Human Growth*, 142.
36 Urla and Swedlund, "The Anthropometry of Barbie," 287.
37 Porter, *The Rise of Statistical Thinking, 1820–1900*, 6. Anthropometric measurements came to form the basis of early actuarial assessments

and continue to provide graphs and charts to determine health in modern medical practice. See Urla and Swedlund, "The Anthropometry of Barbie," 289.

38 Park, "Muscles, Symmetry and Action," 379–80.

39 Prescott, *Student Bodies*, 40–1; Tanner, *A History of the Study of Human Growth*, 185–9, 196; Urla and Swedlund, "The Anthropometry of Barbie," 288.

40 Urla and Swedlund, "The Anthropometry of Barbie," 290. For the problematic role of anthropometry in the creation of a "normal" body type, see also Vertinsky, "Embodying Normalcy," 95–113.

41 Kline, *Building a Better Race*, 39.

42 Urla and Swedlund, "The Anthropometry of Barbie," 289–91.

43 Yosifon and Stearns, "The Rise and Fall of American Posture," 1084.

44 Vertinsky, *The Eternally Wounded Woman*, 145; Lowe, *Looking Good*, 22.

45 "Department of Physical Education," in McGill University, *Annual Report*, 1923–4.

46 "Sophs Wax Fat, Freshmen Lean," *Varsity*, 26 October 1923; "Report of the Director of the University Health Service," in University of Toronto, *President's Report*, 1940–1.

47 It may also have occurred earlier. Records for the University of Toronto indicate one study completed in 1923–4. Physicians at Victoria College recorded female students' posture and chest expansion measurements in the early 1930s. In the first two decades of the twentieth century, the University of Toronto offered a diploma course in gymnastics and physical drill which included instruction in anthropometry. See "Report of the Medical Adviser of Women," in University of Toronto, *President's Report*, 1923–4; UCC/VUA, 90.141v, Box 1-12, "Report of the Examining Physician," 1931–2; UTA, A83-0046, Box 1, pamphlet: "Department of Athletics and Physical Education for Women, 1947–8," and "Department of Athletics and Physical Education, Women, 1961–62"; O'Bryan, "Physical Education – A Study of Professional Education in Ontario Universities," 129–31.

48 "Medical Advisor Says Co-Eds Here of Splendid Type," *Varsity*, 15 December 1924; "Department of Physical Education," in McGill University, *Annual Report*, 1930–1, and "Report of Principal," in McGill University, *Annual Report*, 1937–8.

49 "Department of Physical and Military Training," UWO, *Announcement*, 1920–1; "Report of the Instructor in Physical Education," in *Report of the President of UBC*, 1935–6.

50 UCC/VUA, 90.064v, Report of Lelia A. Davis, 9 April 1909; "Report of the Physical Director," in University of Toronto, *President's Report*, 1920–1; "Macdonald College," in McGill University, *Principal's Report*, 1909–10; "Report of

the Medical Examiner of Students," in *Report of the President of UBC*, 1930–1; "Report of the University Health Service (Men)," in University of Toronto, *President's Report*, 1934–5.

51 UCC/VUA, 90.064v, Box 3-19, "Report to the Victoria Women's Residence Association," 14 April 1910.

52 At the University of Toronto, male students on average gained in both height and weight over the course of the 1920s and 1930s. In 1923, the average freshman was 5 feet 8 inches and weighed 137 lbs. By 1932–3, this had increased to 5 feet 8½ inches and 141 lbs. And in 1940–1, the average male student measured 5 feet 9¼ inches and weighed 145½ lbs. Such increases accord with a general North American pattern of weight and height increases over the course of the first half of the twentieth century. See "Sophs Wax Fat, Freshmen Lean," *Varsity*, 26 October 1923; "Report of the University Health Service (Men)," in University of Toronto, *President's Report*, 1932–3; "Report of the Director of the University Health Service," in University of Toronto, *President's Report*, 1940–1. For references to this North American Pattern, see Levenstein, *Revolution at the Table*, 194.

53 "Report of the University Health Services (Men)," in University of Toronto, *President's Report*, 1937–8.

54 Lowe, *Looking Good*, 30.

55 Ibid., 31.

56 UCC/VUA, 90.064v, Box 3-2, Nurse's Report, 12 November 1914. See also her comments, 12 March 1914. Clark did note in November 1914 the benefit to one student of a weight loss of two pounds. This was the only mention of concern about an overweight student.

57 UCC/VUA, 90.064v, Box 2-1, Minutes, 13 January 1921.

58 "Health of its Women Interests University," *Varsity*, 14 June 1922.

59 Graham, "Health Work in a Junior College," 288–9.

60 "Report of the Medical Examiner of Students," in *Report of the President of UBC*, 1934–5.

61 UCC/VUA, 90.064v, Box 3-20, Dr Guest's Report, 1927.

62 "Report of the Medical Examiner of Students," in *Report of the President of UBC*, 1934–5.

63 Lowe, *Looking Good*, 147.

64 Ibid., 148.

65 UCC/VUA, 90.065v, Box 1-2, Nurse's Report, 29 May 1934

66 DUA, UA12, Faculty of Medicine, Dean of Medicine (personal Files), 60-1, Student Health Service 1934–54, W.A. Murray, Director of Student Health to Dean Grant, 30 November 1953.

67 For Canada, see for example, Gleason, "'Lost Voices, Lost Bodies'?" 145. For the United States see Todd, *Physical Culture and the Body Beautiful*, 176–82, 265; Lowe, *Looking Good*, 29; Park, "Muscles, Symmetry and Action," 365–95.

68 "New Department Doing Good Work," *McGill News*, 4, 1 (December 1922): 9. For similar comments regarding male athletes, see Memorandum by Director of the Department of Physical Education, McGill University, in "Sixth Session," Congress of the Universities of the Empire, 1926, 198.

69 Gordon, "The Need of Physical Training in Schools," 132–3.

70 Capt. Kennedy, "Posture, and How To Correct It," *ATA Magazine*, 4, 8 (January 1924): 24. My thanks to R.D. Gidney and Wyn Millar for this reference.

71 Ellis, "'Backward and Brilliant Children,'" 256.

72 See respectively, UCC/VUA, 90.064v, Box 3-20, Report of Lelia A. Davis, 9 April 1909; "Medical Advisor Says Co-Eds Here of Splendid Type," *Varsity*, 15 December 1924; UCC/VUA, 90.064v, Box 3-20, Report by Guest, n.d. For other, similar, comments on uneven development, see also UCC/VUA, Fonds 2045, 92.010v, Box 6-4, "Report of Annesley Hall Gymnasium," May 1904, and 90.064v, Box 3-19, "Report of Gymnasium," 1905, and Box 1-1, Committee of Management, 12 May 1910. At Vassar in the 1930s, approximately one-third of students received special exercises for posture problems. See Yosifon and Stearns, "The Rise and Fall of American Posture," 1078.

73 "Health of its Women Interests University," *Varsity*, 14 June 1922.

74 UCC/VUA, 90.141v, Box 2-17, letter: Edna Guest to Miss Addison, n.d.

75 UCC/VUA, 90.064v, Box 3-2, Nurse's Report, 14 October 1915.

76 UCC/VUA, 90.064v, Box 3-20, Dr Guest's Report, 1927.

77 UCC/VUA, 90.141v, Box 1-12, "Report of Examining Physician," 12 November 1931. For the attack on high heels by American university administrators see Lowe, *Looking Good*, 107.

78 Tanner, *A History of the Study of Human Growth*, 196.

79 Dudley Allen Sargent, "The Physical Proportions of the Typical Man," *Scribner's Magazine* 2 (1887): 17, cited in Vertinsky, "Embodying Normalcy," 104.

80 C. Lamb, in "Sixth Session," Congress of the Universities of the Empire, 1926, 176; "Report of the Instructor in Physical Education for Women," in *Report of the President of UBC*, 1935–6.

81 "Sophs Wax Fat, Freshmen Lean," *Varsity*, 26 October 1923.

82 UCC/VUA, 90.065v, Box 1-2, "Report of the Acting Dean of Women," 29 May 1934.

83 UCC/VUA, 90.064v, Box 3-20, Report of Edna Guest, November 1929.

84 UCC/VUA, 90.064v, Box 3-20, Report of Edna Guest, 7 November 1923.

85 Robinson, *Give My Heart*, 182.

86 McLaren, *Our Own Master Race*, 30–1, 37; Sangster, *Regulating Girls and Women*, 88, 135. For a personal account of the devastating effects of such beliefs, see Demerson, *Incorrigible*, 10–11, 72–82. Read against the information in this chapter, that account also illuminates the very different treatment by Dr Edna Guest of women who attended Victoria College as opposed to those incarcerated in the Mercer Reformatory.

87 Churchill, "Making Broad Shoulders," 350. Promoters of physical culture in interwar Britain took a similar approach. See Ina Zweiniger-Bargielowska, "Building a British Superman," 596, 599. So too did Canadian government programs during this period. See Macdonald, *Strong, Beautiful and Modern*, 13.

88 "Report of the Director of the University Health Services," in University of Toronto, *President's Report*, 1940–1.

89 UCC/VUA, 90.064v, Box 3-19, Report by Scott Raff, March 1911. See also in the same source, Report by Scott Raff, 1905.

90 UTA, Department of Graduate Records, A73-0026, Box 151/33, "Upholds Eugenics to College Girls," *Telegram*, 14 February 1929.

91 Guest, "Problems of Girlhood and Motherhood," 193–4.

92 DUA, UA 12, Faculty of Medicine, Dean of Medicine (personal files), Box 72-7, Report of the Director of the Students' Health Service, ca 1932; H.G. Grant, "Students' Health Service of Dalhousie University," *Canadian Public Health Journal* (October 1933), 485–90; George D. Porter, "Preserving the Health of the Student Body," *University of Toronto Monthly*, 22, 7 (April 1922): 289; UCC/VUA, 90.064v, Box 1-1, Minutes of the Committee of Management, 9 February 1911; MUA, RG 30, 67-191, Memorandum on Proposed Health Service, 1940, by Frank G. Pedley, University Medical Officer; ECWA, "University Physician," in Acadia University, *Report of the President*, 1944–5. As late as 1959–60 the University of Western Ontario provided nine weeks of health lectures to first-year students. See UWOA, Office of the President, AFC 40, 41/36, Report of the University Physician, 1959–60.

93 "Dr. Porter Gives U.C. Men Useful Rules for Health," *Varsity*, 23 January 1922; "Report of the University Health Service (Men)," University of Toronto, *President's Report*, 1935–6; "Hospital and Health Service," Acadia University, *Calendar*, 1951–2.

94 UCC/VUA, 90.064v, Box 1-2, "Report of Dean of Women," 4 June 1935; "Department of Physical Education," in McGill University, *Annual Report*, 1934–5.

95 MUA, RG 42, 1-69, Health Services 1934–47, College Hygiene Course to Women Students, 1938–9.

96 Lowe, *Looking Good*, 26.

97 "Dr. Porter Gives U.C. Men Useful Rules for Health," *Varsity*, 23 January 1922.

98 MUA, RG42, 1-69, Health Service, 1934-47, Department of Physical Education, Announcement for Women Students, 1940–1.

99 Fraser, "What Can the University Contribute to Public Health Education?" 426.

100 Ibid., 427.

101 Axelrod, *Making a Middle Class*, 115.

102 Cassel, *The Secret Plague*, 214.

103 O'Grady, *Margaret Addison*, 174–5.

104 Ibid., 174–5; Robinson, *Give My Heart*, 181.

105 Jeanne Bell, cited in "A Whispering Campaign," in Light and Roach Pierson, eds., *No Easy Road*, 110–11.

106 Ruth (Manning) Alexander, quoted in "Home Away From Home," *Vic Report* (Winter 2002–3): 6.

107 UCC/VUA, Dean of Women Fonds, B1-12, Report of the Examining Physician of the Women Students in Residence, Victoria University, 1931–2, by Guest, 12 November 1931.

108 Axelrod, *Making a Middle Class*, 116.

109 MUA, RG 42, 1-69, Health Service 1934–47, College Hygiene Course to Women Students, 1938–9.

110 Bailey, "Scientific Truth ... And Love," 711–32; Hébert, "Carabines, poutchinettes co-eds, ou freschettes sont-elles des étudiantes?" 599. For a general introduction to the topic in Quebec, see Gauvreau, "The Emergence of Personalist Feminism," 319–47.

111 Strange, *Toronto's Girl Problem*, 205.

112 Fass, *The Damned and the Beautiful*, 75.

113 Quoted in Moody, "Esther Clark Goes to College," 47.

114 See McLaren, *The Bedroom and the State*, 67.

115 Quoted in McLaren, *Our Own Master Race*, 79.

116 McLaren, *Our Own Master Race*, 79.

117 For comments by a professor of psychology at McGill, published in the *Dalhousie Review*, see McLaren, *Our Own Master Race*, 79.

118 Cited in Strange, *Toronto's Girl Problem*, 169.

119 Kirkwood, *For College Women ... and Men*, 28–9.

120 Moran, *Teaching Sex*, 27.

121 McLaren, *Our Own Master Race*, 72; Moran, *Teaching Sex*, 27–8.

122 Cassel, *The Secret Plague*, 123.

123 McLaren, *Our Own Master Race*, 73.

124 Cassel, *The Secret Plague*, 4, 171.

125 Prescott, *Student Bodies*, 93.
126 UMA, UA 20, Box 51-12, Report of Health Inquiry Committee, 11 March 1941.
127 UTA, Office of the President, A67-0007, Box 73, File: Porter, "University Health Service," 1921–2. In the early twentieth century, doctors at Toronto General Hospital performed Wasserman tests on 1,674 women at the time of delivery, discovering a 4.3 per cent positive reaction. See Mitchinson, *Giving Birth*, 149.
128 UAA, Student Medical Services, 75-144-1119, Meeting, Medical Service Committee, 3 September 1947.
129 Such tests in New York City "exposed only 1.34 per cent positive for syphilis." See Brandt, *No Magic Bullet*, 149.
130 Brandt, *No Magic Bullet*, 154.
131 "Report of the University Health Service (Men)," University of Toronto, *President's Report*, 1921–2. See also, MUA, RG 46, 14-33, Minutes, Sub-committee on Student Health, 14 April 1937.
132 "Dr. Porter Gives U.C. Men Useful Rules for Health," *Varsity*, 23 January 1922. See also UCC/VUA, 90.064v, Box 3-11, Dean's Reports to the Committee of Management, 13 February 1930, and Box 1-2, Report of Dean of Women, 4 June 1935, and President's Office, 89.130v, B55-1, Report of the Dean of Women to the Women's Council of Victoria University, 30 May 1938.
133 MUA, RG 42, 1-69, Health Service 1934–47, College Hygiene Course to Women Students, 1938–9.
134 "Report of the Director of the University Health Service," in *Report of the President of the UBC*, 1944–5.
135 MUA, RG 42, 1-69, Health Service, 1934-47, Department of Physical Education, Circular for Men Students, 1945–6.
136 Archives de l'Université de Montréal, Fonds du Secrétariat général, D35/1523, letter: Jacques Saucier, President, Anti-Venereal Disease Campaign, to Monseigneur Olivier Maurault, 4 March 1944, and response from Chef du Secrétariat général, 18 March 1944.
137 MUA, RG 42, 1-69, Health Service, 1934–47, Department of Physical Education, Circular for Men Students, 1945–46.
138 MUA, RG 42, 1-69, Health Service, 1934–47, Department of Physical Education, Circular for Men Students, 1945–6.
139 Kirkwood, *For College Women ... and Men*, 9.
140 Dorothy Ainsworth notes that by the 1920s, the examinations at many elite American women's colleges had come to focus more extensively on orthopaedic examination, especially of the feet and back, with reduced

emphasis on collecting anthropometric measurements. See Ainsworth, *The History of Physical Education in Colleges for Women*, 66–8.

141 Brandt, *No Magic Bullet*, 154.

5. Female Students' Health and the Creation of New Occupational Opportunities for Women

1 Kinnear, *In Subordination*; Prentice, "Bluestockings, Feminists, or Women Workers?" 231–61; Fingard, "Gender and Inequality at Dalhousie," 687–703; Smyth, et al., *Challenging Professions*. For the United States, see for example, Glazer and Slater, *Unequal Colleagues*; Clifford, *Lone Voyagers*.

2 There are brief references to these groups in Prentice, "Bluestockings, Feminists, or Women Workers?" 242–3; Ford, *A Path Not Strewn With Roses*, 61–4; Gillett, *We Walked Very Warily*, Appendix D, 428–31. University-educated women also found employment in university and hospital laboratories. See Twohig, "'Local Girls' and 'Lab Boys,'" 55–75.

3 Victoria College provides a useful case because of its rich sources on women's residential life in the early part of the twentieth century and the secondary material now available on the women employed at the institution.

4 Margaret Addison was dean of residence from 1903 until 1920, when she became dean of women and took on responsibility for both residents and commuters. O'Grady, *Margaret Addison*, 3. To avoid confusion, I refer to her throughout the text as dean of women.

5 O'Grady, *Margaret Addison*, 34–55. Deans of women often held postgraduate degrees. For example, Mary Bollert, adviser to women at UBC, obtained an MA from the University of Toronto in 1902 and from Columbia University in 1906. See King, "The Experience of the Second Generation of Women Students at Ontario Universities," 106.

6 O'Grady, *Margaret Addison*, 158.

7 Ford, *A Path Not Strewn With Roses*, 48.

8 Gidney, *A Long Eclipse*, 40; McCarthy, *A Fool in Paradise*, 84.

9 Ford, *A Path Not Strewn With Roses*, 58.

10 Byl, "Margaret Eaton School," Appendix E1; O'Grady, *Margaret Addison*, 88.

11 On MacMurchy's life and beliefs, see Prentice, "Bluestockings, Feminists, or Women Workers?" 237; Hacker, *Indomitable Lady Doctors*, 141, 224; Dodd, "Helen MacMurchy"; Kendrick and Slade, *Spirit of Life*, 85; McLaren, *Our Own Master Race*, 30–1.

12 Mann and Inglis, "The Early Years," 10.

13 UCC/VUA, 90.141, Box 1-12, Report of the Examining Physician, 1931–2; Hacker, *Indomitable Lady Doctors*, 188–9; Kendrick and Slade, *Spirit of Life*, 84.

14 Hacker, *Indomitable Lady Doctors*, 232; Kendrick and Slade, *Spirit of Life*, 97–8; Mitchinson, "Marion Hilliard," 227.

15 Byl, "Margaret Eaton School," Appendix E1, 297–8.

16 UCC/VUA, 90.064v, Box 4-3, letter from Elliott to Addison, 18 May 1913, and from Clark to the Ladies' Board of Annesley Hall, 30 May 1913, and Box 4-5, letter from Phelps to Addison, 18 February 1925, and Minutes of the Committee of Management, 14 May 1925.

17 UCC/VUA, 90.064v, Box 4-3, Correspondence Re Appointments: 1904–13, letter Mina Richardson to Addison, 23 January 1904.

18 UCC/VUA, 90.064v, Box 2-1, Committee of Management Minutes, 1920 to 1926; Box 2-4, Dean's Reports, October 1907; Box 1-4, Committee of Management Minutes, 6 September 1917 and 29 June 1920; and, 90.065v, Box 1-8, Report of the Dean of Women, 29 May 1941.

19 O'Grady, *Margaret Addison*, 124.

20 UCC/VUA, 90.064v, Box 3-24, Reports of the Committee Re Dieticians, 10 April 1913.

21 After receiving her training at the Drexel Institute in Philadelphia, in 1902 Laird became senior instructor at the Lillian Massey School of Household Science in Toronto, established by Lillian Massey-Treble. In 1903 she became principal of the school. Nathaniel Burwash, who supported Massey-Treble's work, was instrumental in having household science incorporated into the University of Toronto curriculum. See Heap, "From the Science of Housekeeping to the Science of Nutrition," 145.

22 UCC/VUA, 90.064v, Box 4-3, letter from Mina Richardson to Addison, 23 January 1904.

23 Byl, "The Margaret Eaton School," 90, 99, 228; Lathrop, "Elegance and Expression," 37, 58–9, 64.

24 O'Grady, *Margaret Addison*, 61, 81–2.

25 Ibid., 124.

26 Robinson, *Give My Heart*, 281.

27 UCC/VUA, 90.064v, Box 4-3, letter from Fife to Addison, 25 January 1904, and letter from Clark to Addison, 30 May 1913, and letter from Elliott to Addison, 18 May 1913, and, Box 4-5, letter from Phelps to Addison, 18 February 1925.

28 The ability to reconstruct salaries is partial at best. Victoria did not employ medical advisers on a full-time basis, providing instead a fee per student until the 1930s when the per capita payment was changed to an equivalent salary of $1,000. In contrast, a full-time female medical adviser at the University of Toronto received approximately $2,500. Similarly, physical instructors worked at Victoria for only a couple of hours each week, earning several hundred dollars from this work. Because most worked full-time at

the Margaret Eaton School, their income can be gleaned from research into
that school. See UCC/VUA, 90.141v, Box 2-3, Correspondence, 5 May 1920,
and 90.064v, Box 1-4, Committee of Management Minutes, 13 November
1919, and 90.065v, Women's Council, Box 1-2, Minutes, 10 November 1934,
and 90.064v, Box 4-4, letter from Henderson to Addison, 20 February 1921,
and letter from Addison to Schreiber, 23 March 1921, and Box 2-2, Minutes
of the Committee of Management, 14 November 1929, and Box 2-1, Minutes of the Committee of Management, 12 June 1924, 12 Jan. 1926,
15 September 1927, and Box 1-3, Committee of Management Minutes,
14 May 1914, and Box 1-4, Minutes of the Committee of Management,
13 November 1919, and Box 4-2, letter from Committee of Management to
Chancellor Wallace, 22 May 1930; UTA, A83-0046, Box 1, File: Estimates,
Coventry to Bursar's Office, 8 July 1922; Byl, "The Margaret Eaton School,"
Appendix E1.

29 The dean's salary at Victoria was higher than that of the Superintendent of
University Hall at the University of Saskatchewan, who earned $1,380 plus
room and board in 1920. Still, it was somewhat lower than at other places.
At the University of British Columbia, Mary Bollert received $3,000 in 1921.
At the University of Manitoba, Ursilla Macdonnell received $2,800 in 1920,
$3,100 in 1921, and $4,000 in 1926. Their slightly higher salaries may reflect
the fact that they also taught at their institutions. Nurses at Victoria received
approximately the same wages as those elsewhere. Their income was slightly
higher than that of private-duty nurses, who at the top end might receive
$70 a month in the early 1920s, but slightly lower than the first public
health nurses in Ontario, who received $1,500 a year, or $125 a month.
Their income was also slightly lower than at the University of Alberta, which
hired a nurse in 1921–2 at $100, a rate increased to $150 a month by 1928
and then reduced to $120 in 1933. Nurses at Canadian universities such as
Victoria College and the University of Alberta received salaries comparable
to those at some elite American universities, and considerably less than
those at others. For example, at Vassar College nurses received $80 to $90 a
month and at Smith College, $800 for the academic year, whereas a nurse at
Radcliffe College received $1,800 with room and board (estimated at $2,300
for the college year) and at Columbia University anywhere from $1,200 to
$2,900. In 1946, University College hired a dietician at $110 a month with
board. McGill University hired one in 1942–3 at $1,350 a year with free
board. As with those for nurses, the salaries for dieticians were close to,
but slightly lower than those at leading American institutions. Vassar, for
example, paid $1,500-$2,000 a year; Smith, $1,300; Radcliffe, $3,100; and
Columbia, anywhere from $1,800 to $3,000. See UCC/VUA, 90.141v, Box

2-3, Correspondence, 5 May 1920, and 90.064v, Box 1-4, Committee of Management Minutes, 13 November 1919, and Committee of Management, Box 4-5, Summary of Nurses and Dieticians' Pay at other Colleges, ca 1929; UTA, A83-0046, Box 1, File: Estimates, 1930–1, and, B74-0011, Box 3-7, Dean of Women to Principal Taylor, 24 August 1946; UAA, Student Medical Services, 75-144-1119, Meeting, Medical Service Committee, 6 October 1921, 10 December 1928, and 4 January 1933; MUA, RG 42, 1-35, letter from Cyril James, Principal, to Prof. R.D. Maclennan, Douglas Hall, 17 June 1942; Kinnear, *In Subordination*, 34; Drover, "A Place for Everyone," 60; Stuart, "War and Peace," 179–80; McPherson, *Bedside Matters*, 39, 48, 52, 135–7.

30 UTA, A86-0028, Box 15, File: University Health Services, Budget 1938-39, and, A68-0006, Box 52, File: Health Services, Salary Estimates for the Year 1942–3.

31 Byl, "The Margaret Eaton School," 378–401; Lathrop, "Elegance and Expression," 248–58.

32 At the University of Saskatchewan, the 1915 pay scale for non-academic staff saw clerical staff receiving $60 a month, janitors anywhere from $35 to $70, with some inclusion of board and meals. In 1945, an infirmary maid at the University of Alberta earned approximately $50, less meals. See Drover, "A Place for Everyone," 59; UAA, Student Medical Services, 75-144-1119, Meeting, Medical Service Committee, 11 April 1945.

33 For example, Lulu Gaiser earned $2,000 as a lecturer in botany at McMaster and $2,800 in 1930 as associate professor. Winnifred Hughes earned $2,500 in 1929 as assistant professor in zoology at the University of Alberta and $2,600 by 1941. Dixie Pelluet was hired in the department of zoology at Dalhousie University in 1931 at a salary of $2,600. Germaine Lafeuille became assistant professor of French at Dalhousie University in 1942 at a salary of $2,800. See Ainley, "Last in the Field?" 37, 44, 50-51; Fingard, "Gender and Inequality at Dalhousie," 688.

34 Marsh, *Canadians In and Out of Work*, 166–7, 180. For a comparison to teachers' salaries, see Gidney and Millar, "The Salaries of Teachers in English Canada," 9–11.

35 UTA, Office of the President, A67-0007, Box 109, File: Reed, letter from Reed to Falconer, 9 September 1927.

36 UTA, A86-0028, Box 15, File: University Health Services, Budget 1938–9; UTA, A68-0006, Box 52, File: Health Services, Salary Estimates for the Year 1942–3.

37 Gidney and Millar, "The Salaries of Teachers in English Canada," 13–14.

38 UTA, A83-0046, Box 1, File: Appointments, Ivy Coventry to Falconer, 5 February 1925.

39 UTA, A73-002, Board of Governors, Box 61-3, "Staff – Sessional Appointments," 20 August 1948.

40 Prentice, "Bluestockings, Feminists, or Women Workers?" 259.

41 Baskerville, *A Silent Revolution?* 245.

42 UCC/VUA, 90.064v, Box 4-3, letter from Committee of Management to Marion L. Clark, 25 June 1913.

43 UCC/VUA, 89.130v, Box 37-1, Duties of Dean of Women and Duties of Head of Residences, 1931.

44 Hacker, *Indomitable Lady Doctors,* 188–9.

45 UTA, Department of Graduate Records, A73-0026, Box 151/33, *Torontonensis* 1927.

46 Lathrop, "Elegance and Expression," 114.

47 UTA, B74-0011, Box 3-7, University College Women's Residences, Application for Position of Dietitian, August 1952.

48 McPherson, *Bedside Matters,* 23, 17–18, 32–40, 165, 271n49. See also Dehli, "'Health Scouts' for the State?" 248.

49 UCC/VUA, 90.064v, Box 2-23, Report from Infirmary Committee, October 1913.

50 UCC/VUA, 90.064v, Box 4-3, letter from the Committee of Management to Marion L. Clark, 25 June 1913, and, 89.130v, Box 55-1, Report of the Dean of Women to the Women's Council of Victoria University, 30 May 1938.

51 UCC/VUA, 90.064v, Box 4-3, letter from Elliott to Addison, 18 May 1913, and, letter from Clark to Addison, 30 May 1913.

52 UCC/VUA, 90.064v, Box 1-1, Committee of Management Minutes, 13 February 1907.

53 UCC/VUA, 90.064v, Box 1-1, Committee of Management Minutes, 12 February 1908 and 15 April 1908.

54 UCC/VUA, Dean of Women Fonds, 87.071v, Box 1-12, Minutes of the Advisory Committee to the Dean, 12 September 1932.

55 UCC/VUA, Dean of Women Fonds, 90.141v, Box 2-17, letter from Guest to Ford, 3 December 1932.

56 UCC/VUA, 90.065v, Women's Council, Box 1-16, Minutes of the Committee on Medical Service, 1934–5, 1 November 1934.

57 "Report of the Residence Nurse," in University of Manitoba, *President's Report,* 1945–6.

58 See note 18. This was also the case at the University of Saskatchewan. Similarly, Phyllis Wray, physical-training instructor at Dalhousie University departed after her marriage in 1943. See Drover, "A Place for Everyone," 54; DUA, President's Office, UA3, 39-9, Physical Instructors for Women Students.

59 Cited in Prentice, "Bluestockings, Feminists, or Women Workers?" 256.

60 For Canada, see for example, Kinnear, *In Subordination*, 48–50; Ford, *A Path Not Strewn With Roses*. For the British world, see Pickles, "Colonial Counterparts"; Mackinnon, *Love and Freedom*.

61 UCC/VUA, 90.064v, Box 2-1, Committee of Management Minutes, 14 October 1920.

62 For this incident, see Gidney, "'Less Inefficiency, More Milk,'" 288–9.

63 O'Grady, *Margaret Addison*, 167, 179.

64 UCC/VUA, Fonds 2069, 90.064v, Box 3-1, Dean's Report, 14 November 1918, and Box 1-4, Annesley Hall Committee of Management Minutes, 13 November 1919.

65 In the late nineteenth century, administrators at Royal Victoria College hired a number of resident and non-resident tutors and instructors in a variety of fields, several holding an MA or PhD. See Gillett, *We Walked Very Warily*, 167.

66 UCC/VUA, 90.064v, Box 2-9, Dean's Report, 13 March 1913, and Box 2-10, Dean of Women's Annual Report for the Senate of Victoria College, 1914, and Box 2-1, Committee of Management Minutes, 11 June 1923; O'Grady, *Margaret Addison*, 142, 161,179.

67 UCC/VUA, 90.064v, Box 3-8, Dean's Report, 14 October 1926, and 90.065v, Women's Council, Box 1-1, Report of Dean, ca 1932.

68 UCC/VUA, 90.065v, Women's Council, Box 1-1, Report of Dean, ca 1932.

69 Gurney, *A Century to Remember*, 19.

70 Ford, *A Path Not Strewn With Roses*, 62, 72–4.

71 Gurney, *A Century to Remember*, 26–7. For similar activities on the part of American deans of women in Southern colleges, see Bashaw, *"Stalwart Women,"* 79.

72 James, "A Passion for Service," 111.

73 O'Grady, *Margaret Addison*, 113. See also Ford, *A Path Not Strewn With Roses*, 33. Marion Ferguson, dean of women at University College from 1931 to 1955, was a member, as was Mossie May (Waddington) Kirkwood, dean of women at University College, 1921–9, and principal of St. Hilda's, Trinity College, as of 1936. See *Who's Who in Canada* 1947–8, 350, 1142.

74 James, "A Passion for Service," 111, 113, 116.

75 O'Grady, *Margaret Addison*, 116. For the circumstances around this issue, see Burke, "'Being Unlike Man.'"

76 Gillett, *We Walked Very Warily*, 378–82.

77 O'Grady, *Margaret Addison*, 180. On the NADW, see Bashaw, "Reassessment and Redefinition," 163.

78 Gillett, "The Heart of the Matter," 191.

79 Mitchinson, "Marion Hilliard," 231.
80 Heap, "From the Science of Housekeeping to the Science of Nutrition," 151, 154.
81 Gillett, *We Walked Very Warily*, 227.
82 Clara Benson was a member of the national executive of the YWCA. Marion Ferguson, dean of women at University College, 1931–55, had been a YWCA secretary posted overseas and in Canada in the 1920s and remained active thereafter. See Heap, "From the Science of Housekeeping to the Science of Nutrition," 155; *Who's Who in Canada* 1947–8, 350.
83 McCarthy, *A Fool in Paradise*, 84.
84 UCC/VUA, 90.064v, Box 3-20, Report by Guest, n.d.
85 "Report of the Dean of Junior Women," in University of Manitoba, *President's Report*, 1940–1.
86 Griffiths, *The Splendid Vision*, 29–30. Addison was also a member of the Toronto local. O'Grady, *Margaret Addison*, 253n46.
87 *Who's Who in Canada*, 1947–8, 944.
88 Gillett, *We Walked Very Warily*, 304–6.
89 Scott, *Natural Allies*; Rupp, *Worlds of Women*; Griffiths, *The Splendid Vision*, 20.
90 O'Grady, *Margaret Addison*, 137.
91 "The Position of Women in Universities," Congress of the Universities of the Empire, 1912, *Report of Proceedings*, 346, 352–3.
92 O'Grady, *Margaret Addison*, 181.
93 Susan Cameron Vaughan, who became warden of Royal Victoria College in the 1930s, was president from 1923 to 1926. See Pickles, "Colonial Counterparts," 280–8, 296n83.
94 Prentice, "Three Women in Physics," 131.
95 Rupp, *Worlds of Women*, 37–40.
96 Hallman and Lathrop, "Sustaining the Fire of 'Scholarly Passion,'" 50–1.
97 Heap, "From the Science of Housekeeping to the Science of Nutrition," 150.
98 Coburn, *In Pursuit of Coleridge*, 64–5.
99 See Prentice, "Three Women in Physics," 128, and Mitchinson, "Marion Hilliard," 229. Cameron Duder has documented the explicit romantic relationship between Frieda Fraser, a faculty member in the school of hygiene at the University of Toronto, and her long-term companion, Bud Williams. See "Two Middle-Aged and Very Good-Looking Females," 344–5.
100 Gidney, *A Long Eclipse*, chap. 2.
101 Margaret Addison invited a host of other speakers such as various travelling secretaries of the YWCA, the World Student Christian Federation, and

the women's missionary societies, as well as speakers able to discuss the new careers opening up for women. O'Grady, *Margaret Addison*, 123–4, 183.

102 Mrs. Ramsay-Wright offered a trophy in 1905 for women's intercollege tennis championships, Margaret Addison in 1908 for hockey, and Scott Raff in 1912 for interyear basketball. See Parkes, *Development of Women's Athletics*, 6; UTA, A83-0045, Box 1, Women's Athletic League, Minutes, 14 October 1908, *Acta Victoriana*, January 1912, 192.

103 Mann and Inglis, "The Early Years," 10.

104 UTA, A83-0045, Box 1-3, Women's Athletic Directorate Minutes, 1920–5. Clara Benson was president of the University of Toronto Athletic Club from 1922 to 1945. See Heap, "From the Science of Housekeeping to the Science of Nutrition," 155.

105 Gurney, *A Century to Remember*, 21.

106 UTA, A83-0045, Box 1-3, Women's Athletic Directorate Minutes, 1920–5.

107 UTA, Department of Graduate Records, A73-0026, Box 121/91, "Dr. E.H. Gordon Dies Suddenly," *Globe and Mail*, 18 December 1939.

108 Pickles, "Colonial Counterparts," 289–90.

109 Ibid., 286.

110 Hébert, "Carabines, poutchinettes co-eds ou freshettes sont-elles des étudiantes?" 593–625.

111 O'Grady, *Margaret Addison*, 7, 100–2.

112 Strong-Boag, "Canada's Women Doctors: Feminism Constrained,"124; O'Grady, *Margaret Addison*, 5–8.

113 "Character Moulded by Capable Teacher," *Globe and Mail*, 20 October 1923.

114 Mitchinson, "Marion Hilliard," 228.

115 Axelrod, *Making a Middle Class*, 119.

116 Hébert, "Carabines, poutchinettes co-eds ou freshettes sont-elles des étudiantes?" 609.

117 Pickles, "Colonial Counterparts," 289.

118 Ibid., 279.

119 Ford, *A Path Not Strewn With Roses*, 58–9.

120 Kinnear, *In Subordination*, 157.

121 Prentice, "Scholarly Passion," 271–2.

122 Kirkwood, *For College Women ... and Men*, 66.

123 Mitchinson, "Marion Hilliard," 237.

124 See Kinnear, *In Subordination*, 148.

125 This was true of deans of women at other colleges. For the United States, see for example, Bashaw, *"Stalwart Women,"* 14.

126 UCC/VUA, 90.064v, Box 3-19, Report by Scott Raff, March 1911.

127 Cartwright, "Athletics and Physical Education for Girls," 278.

128 "Woman Doctors Cast Off Halo," *Globe and Mail*, 22 January 1931. The quote is by Hilliard. But other doctors made similar comments. See Mac-Murchy, "The Woman in the Medical Profession," 28.

129 Fingard, "Gender and Inequality at Dalhousie"; Prentice, "Bluestockings, Feminists, or Women Workers?"; Kinnear, *In Subordination*. For elsewhere, see Graham, "Expansion and Exclusion: A History of Women in American Higher Education," 759–73; Pickles, "Colonial Counterparts."

130 Rossiter, *Women Scientists in America*, 314.

131 See for example, Palmieri, *In Adamless Eden*; Glazer and Slater, *Unequal Colleagues*.

132 Mitchinson, *Giving Birth*, 40.

133 Heap, "From the Science of Housekeeping to the Science of Nutrition," 142; James, "A Passion for Service," 105–30.

134 Prentice notes this in "Scholarly Passion," 273.

135 Ford, *A Path Not Strewn With Roses*; Gillett, *We Walked Very Warily*; LaPierre, "The First Generation," 20.

136 Kinnear, *In Subordination*, 47.

137 Prentice, "Three Women in Physics," 128. For evidence of the lack of kinship, see also Hallman and Lathrop, "Sustaining the Fire of 'Scholarly Passion,'" 58.

138 Pickles, "Colonial Counterparts," 281–2.

139 Quoted in O'Grady, *Margaret Addison*, 111.

140 UTA, Department of Graduate Records, A73-0026, Box 121/91, "Woman Doctors Cast Off Halo," *Globe and Mail*, 22 January 1931. See also MacMur-chy, "The Woman in the Medical Profession," 28.

141 Rupp, *Worlds of Women*. See also Scott, *Natural Allies*; Mackinnon, *Love and Freedom*, 213–18.

142 For specific arguments relating the creation of these health-related professions to the emergence of a professional women's feminism, see Gidney, "Feminist Ideals and Everyday Life," 96–117.

6. Changing Contexts and Programs, 1930s to 1960s

1 The information for the next few pages draws on Gidney, *A Long Eclipse*, 7, 91, chap. 5. For the continuing presence of Christianity within public institutions and as a shaping force within Canadian society well into the twentieth century, see also Miedema, *For Canada's Sake*; Gauvreau, *The Catholic Origins of Quebec's Quiet Revolution*; Gidney and Millar, "The Christian Recessional in Ontario's Public Schools," 275–93.

2 Christie and Gauvreau, *A Full-Orbed Christianity*.
3 McKillop, *Matters of Mind*; Owram, *The Government Generation*.
4 UTA, University Historian, A83-0036, Box 34, file: University Health Service, G.E. Wodehouse, "University Health Service, University of Toronto."
5 University of Toronto, *Calendar*, 1946–7.
6 The men's infirmary, with sixteen beds, was located in Hart House, while the women's infirmary, with ten beds, was located in University College's Women's Union. In 1950, there were approximately eight small infirmaries in the various colleges and residences. Four years later, only the women's infirmary at Victoria College and the male and female infirmaries at St. Michael's College remained. UTA, A76-0044, Box 96, University Health Service, "A Report to the Medical Advisory Committee," ca 1946, and, Faculty of Medicine, Box 96, File: University Health Service Advisory Committee, Minutes, 9 December 1954.
7 The university developed the service in stages, organizing a service to students in the faculty of medicine in 1942, a year later to students in the faculty of science, and then to all students. See Université de Laval, *Annuaire Général*, 1945–6, 39.
8 AUM, Fonds du Secrétariat général, D35/1405, letter: Association Générale des Etudiants to Mr. Eugene Poirier, Secrétaire de la Société d'Administration de l'Université de Montréal, 30 June 1945, and pamphlet, "L'A.G.E.U.M. en vingt-cinq points," ca 1948; "Notre Service Médical," *Quartier Latin*, 23 October 1945.
9 MtAUA, Norman A. Hesler Fonds, 7654/20, Report of the Campus House Committee, 23 September 1946.
10 "Report of Residence Nurse," in University of Manitoba, *President's Report*, 1945–6, and "Department of Student Health Service," in University of Manitoba, *President's Report*, 1953–4.
11 Schwarz, "Report on Health and Psychiatric Services on Canadian Campuses," 25–35.
12 UAA, Student Medical Services, 75-144-1119, Minutes, 20 January 1943; Schwartz, "Report on Health and Psychiatric Services on Canadian Campuses," 24.
13 "University Health Service," UBC, *Calendar*, 1955–6.
14 Schwartz, "Report on Health and Psychiatric Services on Canadian Campuses," 23.
15 Letter to editor, *The Varsity*, 13 November 1922. For a similar complaint regarding lack of university services, see "Student Health Services," *Acta Victoriana* (March 1941): 8–12.
16 Report of the Director of the University Health Service, in *Report of the President of the UBC*, 1938–9.

17 "Report of the Dean of the Men's Residence," in University of Manitoba, *President's Report*, 1936–7. This was similarly a problem at American universities. See Prescott, *Student Bodies*, 91.

18 UMA, UA20, Box 51-12, Report of Health Inquiry Committee, 11 March 1941.

19 UAA, Provost's Office, Student Affairs, RG17, 69-123, 2052, letter: R.C.W. Hooper, Adviser to Men Students, to Professor McLachlin, School of Physical Education, 23 March 1964.

20 UAA, Provost's Office, Student Affairs, RG17, 69-123, 2052, Medical Services 1959–64, letter: J.D. Wallace, Executive Director, University of Alberta Hospital to Major R.C.W. Hooper, Advisor to Men Students, 25 March 1964.

21 UAA, Office of the President, 68-1, 3/3/5/4-2, Report of the Director of Medical Services, 1935–6.

22 UMA, UA20, Box 51-12, Report of Health Inquiry Committee, 11 March 1941.

23 Ibid.

24 Ibid.

25 "Student Health Services," *Acta Victoriana* (March 1941): 8–12.

26 Starr, *The Social Transformation of American Medicine*, 237.

27 Ibid., 258.

28 Ibid., 259.

29 "Student Health Insurance," UWO, *President's Report*, 1930–1 and 1932–3.

30 AUM, Fonds du Secrétariat général, D35/283, letter: Association Générale des Etudiants to M. Parizeau, Courtier d'assurances, 2 December 1941, and, D35/282, letter: Association Générale des Etudiants to Secrétaire, Université de Montréal, 21 December 1950. A similar situation existed at Laval where, in 1944, university officials turned down a hospitalization plan put forward by the Quebec Hospital Service Association. In the early 1950s, the university would pay some hospitalization costs, up to thirty dollars, an amount increased to fifty dollars in 1955. See Université Laval, Division des Archives, U525/20/1/1, letter from Directeur Général, Quebec Hospital Service Association to A. Labrie, 7 June 1944, and reply 10 June 1944, and Laval, *Annuaire Général*, 1950–1 and 1955–6.

31 Report of the University Physician, Helen M. Rossiter, "University Health Service," UWO, *President's Report*, 1950–1.

32 These began to develop in the late 1930s, usually as a prepayment plan run by physicians, with subscribers receiving direct services. See Bothwell and English, "Pragmatic Physicians," 485.

33 "Fees," University of Saskatchewan, *Calendar*, 1950–1. In addition to providing services by the university health services, by the early 1960s UBC had

arranged a voluntary program for extended health coverage with Medical Services Incorporated at a rate of eight dollars a year, covering in-hospital expenses not provided by the university health services, immediate home care for accidents and injuries, and specialist consultation after referral from a university health service physician. See "University Health Service," UBC, *Calendar*, 1965–6.

34 Report of the University Physician, Helen M. Rossiter, "University Health Service," UWO, *President's Report*, 1950–1.

35 "Blue Cross Plan Unsuitable – French," *Xaverian Weekly*, 12 October 1956, 3.

36 "Report of the Director of the University Health Service," Acadia University, *Report of the President*, 1967–8.

37 For example, Saskatchewan established a hospitalization plan in 1946, British Columbia in 1947, and Alberta in 1950. The federal government's Hospital Insurance and Diagnostic Services Act came into effect on 1 July 1958, which, by providing federal funds to provinces that instituted a hospital insurance plan, created a system that insured every Canadian for hospital and diagnostic services costs. The 1966 Medical Care Act was implemented in 1968 and had come into effect across Canada by 1971. See Naylor, *Private Practice, Public Payment*, 167, 239–40; Kealey, "Historical Perspectives on Health Care," 141.

38 Naylor, *Private Practice, Public Payment*, 167. In 1969–70, 25 per cent of Acadia students had no medical insurance coverage. See "Report of the Director of the University Health Service," Acadia University, *Report of the President*, 1970–1.

39 The other category of students who remained uninsured were those who were no longer covered by their parents due to their adult status but who had not applied for their own coverage. A survey of University of Toronto students in the early 1960s indicated that 90 per cent of students "have adequate hospital insurance," thus leaving 10 per cent with inadequate or no coverage. See Report of the Director of the University Health Service, in University of Toronto, *President's Report*, 1961–2, and "Report of the Director of the University Health Service," Acadia University, *Report of the President*, 1969–70. The same was true of medical plans. See "University Health Service," UBC, *Calendar*, 1968–9.

40 Wipper, *Retrospect and Prospect*, 13.

41 MUA, RG 42, 3-177, RVC Residence Physician 1939–42, letter: Cyril James to Doctor Hardisty, 27 November 1941; "Health Service," McGill University, *Calendar*, 1950.

42 For a list of degree programs see Meagher, "Professional Preparation," 69. As these programs were created, some were placed under the wing

of faculties or institutes of education, with the implication, according to Cosentino and Howell, that the main function in the latter was to train physical education teachers, while in the former physical education became a stand-alone program, an acknowledgment of the area as a field of study in its own right. See, *A History of Physical Education in Canada*, 62.

43 Ainsworth, "A History of Physical Education in College for Women (USA)," 170–2. For more on these individuals see Gerber, *Innovators and Institutions in Physical Education*.

44 Reese, "The Origins of Progressive Education," 1–24.

45 Gidney and Gidney, "Branding the Classroom," 352; Patterson, "Society and Education during the Wars and Their Interlude, 1914–1945," 373–4, and, "Progressive Education: Impetus to Educational Change in Alberta and Saskatchewan," 169–192. See also, Axelrod, *Promise of Schooling*, 110–15; von Heyking, *Creating Citizens*, 33–4; Christou, *Progressive Education*.

46 Ainsworth, "A History of Physical Education in Colleges for Women (USA)," 176.

47 See Bouchier and Cruikshank, "Abandoning Nature," 318. In New Zealand, governments began to subsidize school swimming and life-saving programs as early as the 1890s, with both becoming identified with good citizenship. See Daley, *Leisure and Pleasure*, 120.

48 "PT Situation Explained," *Varsity*, 26 October 1921.

49 ECWA, "Department of Physical Education," in Acadia University, *Report of the President*, 1939–40, 21–2.

50 UTA, School of Physical and Health Education, A83-0046, Box 3, File: Presidential Committee, Minutes, Presidential Committee on Required Physical Education, 21 September1955. See also University of Toronto, *Calendar*, 1945–6.

51 "Report of the Director of Physical Education for Women," in University of Toronto, *President's Report*, 1949–50.

52 "Department of Physical Education," UWO, *Announcement*, 1945–6.

53 "Physical Education," University of Saskatchewan, *Calendar*, 1955–6; MtAUA, *University Handbook*, 1965–6, 46, 64–6.

54 By the mid-1950s, female students at the University of Toronto had to pass the swim test but no longer had to take gymnastics. See UTA, School of Physical and Health Education, A83-0046, Box 1, pamphlet: Department of Athletics and Physical Education – women, 1956–7.

55 "Report of the Director of Physical Education for Women," in UBC, *President's Report*, 1945–6.

56 Ibid.

57 "Report of the Director of Athletics and Physical Education for Men," in University of Toronto, *President's Report*, 1947–8.
58 "Physical Training," University of Saskatchewan, *Calendar*, 1940–1. Same 1950–1.
59 "Physical Education," University of Saskatchewan, *Calendar*, 1955–6.
60 Ibid.
61 "Report of the Physical Director for Women," Dalhousie University, *President's Report*, 1945–50. Same comments made for 1951–4 report.
62 "Department of Physical Education," in Acadia University, *Report of the President*, 1955–6.
63 Gilbert W. Chapman, "Department of Physical Education and Athletics," in Acadia University, *Report of the President*, 1968–9.
64 Park, "'Taking their Measure,'" 209.
65 Yosifon and Stearns, "The Rise and Fall of American Posture," 1086, 1089.
66 von Heyking, *Creating Citizens*, 33–4.
67 Park, "'Taking their Measure,'" 210.
68 ECWHA, "Department of Physical Education," in *Report of the President*, 1939–40.
69 MUA, RG30, Faculty of Education, 65-175, Minutes of Senate Committee on Physical Education, 5 April 1944.
70 Howell, "Physical Education Research in Canada," 253.
71 "Physical, Health and Recreational Education," UWO, *Announcement*, 1960–1, 108.
72 Lathrop, "Elegance and Expression," 240.
73 When McGill University created a dean of students position in 1970, the effect was the subordination of an associate dean, responsible for female students, under the position of dean, responsible for male students. Eventually the associate dean position simply disappeared. See Gillett, *We Walked Very Warily*, 209–11, 397. Little research has been undertaken into the role of dean of women in Canada. In the United States, Robert Schwartz has demonstrated a clear pattern of the gradual disappearance of the position of dean of women after the Second World War or the subordination of that position to a dean of students or dean of student personnel, held by a man. See Schwartz, "How Deans of Women Became Men," 419–36.
74 This was a protracted and often difficult internal process. The renaming of "physical education" as "human kinetics" or "kinesiology" occurred between the late 1960s and 1990s and marked a departure from activity-based courses to a greater emphasis on science and theory-based courses. See for example,

Harrigan, *Finding their place*, 3–8, 18; O'Bryan, "Physical Education – A Study of Professional Education in Ontario Universities," 142–52.

75 Lathrop, "Elegance and Expression," 286.

76 This does not mean they had equal access to facilities. Women's athletic facilities often lagged significantly behind those provided for men. See, for example, Ford, *A Path Not Strewn With Roses*, 62, 72–4. At the University of Toronto, male students gained up-to-date social and athletic facilities with the opening in 1919 of Hart House, which remained closed to women until 1972. Women did not have a modern facility until 1959. Due to financial cutbacks, UBCs new War Memorial Gymnasium, completed in 1951, had no provisions for female students, who were left with the facilities of the old gymnasium, now vacated by the men. See Vertinsky, "Power Geometries," 48–73.

77 "Report of the Director of Physical Education for Women" in UBC, *President's Report*, 1945–6.

78 University of Alberta, *Calendar*, 1950–1, 82.

79 "Report of the Director of Physical Education for Women," in UBC, *President's Report*, 1945–6.

80 "Report of the Director of Physical Education for Women," in University of Toronto, *President's Report*, 1954–5.

81 "Physical, Health and Recreation Education," UWO, *Announcement*, 1960–1.

7. Shifting Health Priorities – Tuberculosis and Mental Health

1 Feldberg, *Disease and Class*, 35.

2 McCuaig, *The Weariness, the Fever, and the Fret*, 10, 12, 18; Feldberg, *Disease and Class*, 120; Prescott, "The White Plague," 752.

3 McCuaig, "Tuberculosis: The Changing Concepts of the Disease in Canada 1900–1950," 300.

4 McCuaig, *The Weariness, the Fever, and the Fret*, 248.

5 Ibid., 63.

6 Ibid., 106.

7 Prescott, "The White Plague," 735, 738, 757.

8 In 1921, the Saskatchewan Anti-tuberculosis Commission survey of 1,700 children found 44 per cent infected by age six, 60 per cent by age fourteen, and 76 per cent by age eighteen. See McCuaig, *The Weariness, the Fever and the Fret*, 61–4.

9 In 1920, McGill may have become one of the first universities to require all students to have an annual X-ray of their chest. If so, this was undertaken by students prior to entrance. Researchers at the university undertook an

early study from 1931 to 1934 consisting of chest surveys of first-year students. By the 1950s, medical staff examined all first- to third-year students. According to George Wherrett, Mount Allison began testing in 1925. In 1931–2 Dalhousie's examination included a chest fluoroscope and X-ray of all suspicious chest cases, though this was likely voluntary for students. The university expanded its testing from suspicious cases in new students to all students in the late 1940s. Women entering Toronto received a skin test in 1933. In 1935–6 this was extended to all women taking a physical and in 1938 to all men. Medical officers at UBC performed a skin test on a select number of students in 1937–8 and then expanded the scope of testing the next year to all students receiving a medical exam. Queen's University began compulsory testing of all first-year students in 1939–40. In 1941, the University of Alberta required chest plates only if tuberculosis was suspected, though the next year all students received a free tuberculin test courtesy of the provincial department of health. UWO required a chest X-ray of all new students as of 1942–3. Both the University of Manitoba and Acadia University had instituted a chest X-ray for incoming students as of 1944–5. The University of Montreal did so in 1945. See MUA, RG 30, 66-183, Correspondence, A.S. Lamb 1944–59, "Biographical Data"; "Department of Physical Education," in McGill University, *Annual Report*, 1932–3; MUA, RG 42, 2-137, Physical Education – General, 1869-1937, Evolution of Department of Physical Education for Women, Jan. 1936; "Health Service," McGill University, *Calendar*, 1950; "Health," Dalhousie University, *Calendar*, 1931–2, 17–18; DUA, UA 12, Faculty of Medicine, Dean of Medicine, 60-1, Students' Health Service, "Notice," 7 March 1947; "Report of the Medical Adviser of Women," University of Toronto, *President's Report*, 1933–4; UTA, A68-0028, Box 15, File: University Health Services, "General Information for Students: University Health Service," ca 1938; "Report of the Director of the University Health Service," in *Report of the President of the UBC*, 1938–9; "Report of the Medical Health Officer," in Queen's University, *Principal's Report*, 1938–9. UAA, "Report of the Provost," in *Report of the Board of Governors*, 1942–3; "Department of Physical Education," UWO, *President's Report*, 1942–3; UMA, UA20, Box 51-12, Report of Health Inquiry Committee, 11 March 1941, and Box 77-4, Board of Governors' Minutes, 11 October 1945; ECWA, "University Physician," in *Report of the President*, 1944–5, 34–5; AUM, Fonds du Secrétariat général, D35/1405, letter: Association Générale des Étudiants to Mr. Eugene Poirier, Secrétaire de la Société d'Administration de l'Université de Montréal, 30 June 1945; "Notre Service Médical," *Quartier Latin*, 23 October 1945; Wherrett, *The Miracle of the Empty Beds*, 1977.

10 The director of the university health services at UBC also noted that there were few variations according to sex, but that in terms of age, "39 per cent of students under twenty and 51 per cent of those over twenty years of age were positive" and "urban rates were higher than rural, 45 per cent of students from urban areas showing positive, while the rural figure was 33 per cent." See "Report of the Director of the University Health Service," in *Report of the President of the UBC*, 1938–9. See also, "Report of Medical Adviser of Women," University of Toronto, *President's Report*, 1937–8. For American statistics, see "Fifth Annual Report of the Tuberculosis Committee," American Student Health Association, Proceedings of the 16th Annual Meeting of the ASHA, *Bulletin*, 19 (1935), 63–6.

11 In 1932–3, at Dalhousie University, the number of active cases was 0.5 per cent. In 1934–5, at McGill, it was 0.5 per cent. In 1941–2, at the University of Toronto, it was 0.3 per cent. In 1944–5, at the University of Manitoba, it was 0.2 per cent. In 1946, at the University of Toronto, it was 0.4 per cent, and at the University of Alberta, it was 0.08 per cent. See Grant, "Students' Health Service of Dalhousie University," 485–90; MUA, RG 46, 14-33, Minutes, Subcommittee on Student Health, 16 December 1935; UTA, A68-0006, Box 52, File: Health Services, letter: R.W. Ian Urquhart to the President, 11 March 1942; UMA, UA20, 68-2, letter: E.L Ross, Medical Superintendent, Sanatorium Board of Manitoba, to President H.P. Armes, 29 November 1944; UTA, A76-0044, Faculty of Medicine, Box 96, University Health Service, Report of the Director of the University Health Service, 11 April 1946; UAA, Student Medical Services, 75-144-1119, Meeting, Medical Service Committee, 30 October 1946. For the United States, see Fifth Annual Report of the Tuberculosis Committee, American Student Health Association, Proceedings of the 16th Annual Meeting of the ASHA, *Bulletin*, 19 (1935), 63–6. This may have been the case in the public school system as well. In the 1921 survey of Saskatchewan children, for example, only 0.84 per cent of children tested had an active form of the disease. See McCuaig, *The Weariness, the Fever, and the Fret*, 64.

12 "Report of the Director of the University Health Service," in University of Toronto, *President's Report*, 1948–9.

13 "Report of the Medical Adviser of Women," in University of Toronto, *President's Report*, 1937–8, 1938–9, 1940–1, and, "Report of the Director of the University Health Service," in University of Toronto, *President's Report*, 1944–5.

14 Wherrett, *The Miracle of the Empty Beds*, appendix 6.

15 McCuaig, *The Weariness, the Fever, and the Fret*, 67.

16 Ibid., 62.

17 Ibid.
18 Prescott, "The White Plague," 766.
19 "Report of the Director of the University Health Service," in *Report of the President of UBC*, 1942–3.
20 "Report of the Director of the University Health Service," in University of Toronto, *President's Report*, 1947–8.
21 "Four TB Cases Discovered at UBC," *The Varsity*, 12 March 1948.
22 For the different approaches, see McCuaig, *The Weariness, the Fever, and the Fret*, 83–5, 191–3, 264–5, and Feldberg, *Disease and Class*, 8. Medical staff offered the BCG vaccine to these groups as of 1950 at the University of Alberta and by 1955 at UBC. See UAA, "Report of Director of Student Medical Services," in *Report of the Board of Governors*, 1950–1; "University Health Service," UBC, *Calendar*, 1955–6.
23 UAA, Student Medical Services, 75-144-1119, Medical Service Committee Minutes, 20 January 1943.
24 McCuaig, *The Weariness, the Fever and the Fret*, 189.
25 Ibid., 210.
26 ECWA, "The University Physician," in *Report of the President*, Acadia University, 1944–5, 1948–9, 1949–50, and 1954–55. See also "Artsmen – No Bones Says T.B. Mobile Unit," *Xaverian Weekly*, 23 October 1948, 1.
27 "University Physician," Acadia University, *Report of the President*, 1954–5.
28 "Report of the Director of the University Health Service," in *Report of the President of the UBC*, 1943–4; "University Student Health Service," UBC, *Calendar*, 1950–1; UAA, Student Medical Services, 75-144-1119, Meeting, Medical Service Committee, 18 April 1944; UMA, UA20, Box 77-4, Board of Governors' Minutes, 11 October 1945; "Department of Student Health Service," in University of Manitoba, *President's Report*, 1953–4; UTA, University Historian, A83-0036, Box 34, file: University Health Service, G.E. Wodehouse, "University Health Service, University of Toronto"; AUM, Fonds du Secrétariat général, D35/1405, letter: Association Générale des Étudiants to Mr. Eugene Poirier, Secrétaire de la Société d'Administration de l'Université de Montréal, 30 June 1945; "Department of Physical Education," UWO, *President's Report*, 1942–3.
29 McCuaig, "Tuberculosis: The Changing Concepts of the Disease in Canada 1900–1950," 304.
30 UTA, University Historian, A83-0036, Box 34, file University Health Service, G.E. Wodehouse, "University Health Service, University of Toronto."
31 Prescott, "The White Plague," 760.
32 Ibid., 738.

33 See, for example, McCuaig, *The Weariness, the Fever, and the Fret*, 247–8; Starr, *The Social Transformation of American Medicine*, 141.

34 McCuaig, *The Weariness, the Fever and the Fret*, 68–9.

35 Physicians recorded instances of nervous strain among Victoria College students in 1906–7, 1908–9, 1913–14, 1914–15, 1916–17, 1918–19, 1919–20. See UCC/VUA, 90.064v, Box 2-4, Report of Annesley Hall, 1906–7, and Box 2-5, Dean's Reports, 14 January 1909, and Box 3-2, Report by Marion Clark, 12 March 1914 and 9 May 1917, and Box 3-22, Report by Nurse Gregory, February 1919 and October 1919. It was also recorded elsewhere. See, for example, MUA, MG4014, c.2, Susan Vaughan Papers, Daybook, 1930–1.

36 Armstrong, *Political Anatomy of the Body*, 19–20.

37 Park, "Muscles, Symmetry and Action," 374.

38 Rotundo, *American Manhood*, 189.

39 UCC/VUA, 90.064v, Box 3-2, Report by Marion Clark, 10 December 1914, 12 March 1914, 13 January 1915, and Box 3-21, Report by Marion Clark, 9 May 1917, and, Box 3-22, Report by Nurse Gregory, February 1919, and Box 3-20, Report by Dr Guest, 1 November 1921, and Dean of Women Fonds, Box 1-12, Report of Examining Physician, 12 November 1931.

40 UCC/VUA, Annesley Hall Committee of Management, Box 2-5, Dean's Report, 11 February 1909.

41 UCC/VUA, 90.064v, Box 3-2, Report by Marion Clark, 10 December 1914.

42 UCC/VUA, 90.064v, Box 3-20, Report by Dr Guest, 1 November 1921.

43 UCC/VUA, Fonds 2000, Board of Regents, 87.195v, Box 1-2, Report of Burwash Hall and Men's Residences, n.d., ca 1933–4.

44 "Report of the Dean of the Men's Residence," in University of Manitoba, *President's Report*, 1936–7.

45 Lenskyj notes a similar timing in "The Role of Physical Education in the Socialization of Girls in Ontario, 1890–1930," 225.

46 Prescott, *Student Bodies*, 115–17; Gleason, *Normalizing the Ideal*, 20–2; Richardson, *The Century of the Child*, 1, 113; Wright and Myers, *History of Academic Psychology in Canada*, 17. For the history of mental hygiene in American schools and universities, see Cohen, "The Mental Hygiene Movement, the Development of Personality and the School," 123–49, and *Challenging Orthodoxies*.

47 Gleason, *Normalizing the Ideal*, 5, 38. For the spread of psychology into history and social studies curricula as well as the work of summer camps, see respectively, von Heyking, *Creating Citizens*, and Wall, *The Nurture of Nature*, chap. 4. For its influence in advertising, see Lears, "From Salvation to Self-Realization," 19. For its spread into mainline Protestant thought and particularly the field of pastoral counselling, see Warren, "The Shift from

Character to Personality," 537–55. More generally, see Rose, *Governing the Soul* and *Inventing Our Selves.*

48 Starr, *The Social Transformation of American Medicine*, 345.

49 Ibid. For the Canadian wartime context, see Copp, *Battle Exhaustion.*

50 Neary, "Canadian Universities and Canadian Veterans of World War II," 129–30.

51 Chenier, *Strangers in Our Midst*, 29. For the incursion of mental hygiene experts into wartime and post-war reconstruction, see also Stephen, *Pick One Intelligent Girl;* Wright and Myers, eds. *History of Academic Psychology in Canada*, 17; Fingard and Rutherford, "Social Disintegration, Problem Pregnancies, Civilian Disasters: Psychiatric Research in Nova Scotia in the 1950s," 195–6. On the incorporation of psychology into social work related to newcomers, see Iacovetta, *Gatekeepers*, 65–9.

52 Gleason, *Normalizing the Ideal*, 22–3; Richardson, *The Century of the Child*, 64. The CNCMH subsidized work in mental health undertaken by leading psychologists at the University of Toronto, such as Edward Bott, Wilhelm Blatz, William Line, J. Davidson Ketchum and S.N.F. Chant, later president of UBC. See Myers, "Psychology at Toronto," 84–7.

53 Danziger, *Naming the Mind*, 127; Cohen, "The Mental Hygiene Movement, the Development of Personality and the School," 126–7; Gleason, *Normalizing the Ideal*, 23–4; Dowbiggin, *Keeping America Sane*, 64–5, 86. While historians have linked the shift from hereditary to environmental explanations for mental development to a decline in eugenic thought, Wendy Kline powerfully argues that for the United States eugenic views remained strong into the 1950s as eugenicists adopted a positive eugenics or pronatalism that encouraged procreation by the fit and particularly the importance of the home environment in that process. See Klein, *Building a Better Race*, 123. More research is needed to understand this process in the Canadian context, but Kline's findings of the influence of positive eugenics from the 1930s to the 1950s seems to parallel findings in this study of the continued belief in the importance of general race betterment in the same period.

54 Armstrong, *Political Anatomy of the Body*, 22; Danziger, *Naming the Mind*, 110, 127.

55 Danziger, *Naming the Mind*, 110.

56 Blaine, "The Problems of Adolescence," 253.

57 Ibid., 254.

58 Ibid., 267.

59 Davies, "The Paradox of Progressive Education," 277; Ellis, "'Backward and Brilliant Children,'" 391–5. See also chap. 6, note 45.

60 Cohen, *Challenging Orthodoxies*, 210. Erik Erikson, one of the leading theorists of adolescence in the post-war period, helped popularize the belief that
   university life could contribute to an identity crisis through the very process
   of postponing adulthood. See Jasen, "Student Activism, Mental Health, and
   English-Canadian Universities in the 1960s," 461.

61 Prescott, *Student Bodies*, 118–19.

62 Ibid., 122.

63 Thompson, "Organization in a University for Instruction in Mental Hygiene
   and for Safeguarding the Mental Health of Students," 86.

64 Ibid., 89.

65 Legge, "The Relation of Mental Hygiene to a University Administrative
   Hygiene Program," 90–1.

66 R.W. Bradshaw, "New Values in Student Health," *The Lancet,* January 1935,
   quoted in Way, "A Survey of Small College Health Service Programs," 45–6.

67 Prescott, *Student Bodies*, 129.

68 Stewart, "John Ryle," 68.

69 Prescott, *Student Bodies*, 130.

70 As of 1920 students in Edmonton had access to a psychologist through the
   department of psychiatry at the University of Alberta Hospital. See Schwartz,
   "Report on Health and Psychiatric Services on Canadian Campuses," 29.
   As of 1939 the University Health Service at UBC had access to a psychiatric
   consultant for a half day a week through the Mental Hygiene Program of
   the Metropolitan Health Department. See UBCA, Annual Report, UBC
   Student Health Service – Psychiatric Service, 1962–3, 1.

71 H.J. Cody, Congress of the Universities of the British Empire, 1936, *Report of
   Proceedings*, 218.

72 "Department of Physical Education," McGill University, *Principal's Report*,
   1931–2.

73 UWO seems to have implemented such tests for first-year students for the
   year 1937. See Axelrod, *Making a Middle Class*, 57. On Laycock, see McMurray, "Psychology at Saskatchewan," 181.

74 "Freshmen Welcomed to Saskatchewan," *The Sheaf,* 25 September 1936, 1.

75 Laycock argued that the good grades but poor test results of some grade
   12 students revealed "their true capacity" as their grades were the result
   of "good fortune, [or] excessive drill" and implementation of tests as an
   entry requirement would thus correct "erroneous impressions which might
   be gained from Grade XII results." See "Report of Dean of the College of
   Arts and Science," in University of Saskatchewan, *President's Report*, 1938–9,
   16–19.

76 "Report of the University Health Service (Men)," in University of Toronto, *President's Report*, 1934–5; "Report of the Director of the University Health Service," in *Report of the President of UBC*, 1941–2; MUA, RG 30, 67-191, University Medical Officer, Memorandum on Proposed Health Service, 1940; UAA, Report of the Director of Medical Services, Dr J.W. Scott, in *Report of the Board of Governors*, 1945–6; "University Physician," in *Report of the President*, Acadia University, 1962–3; UTA, A76-0044, Faculty of Medicine, Box 96, University Health Service, Report of the Director of the University Health Service, 11 April 1946; St. F.X. Archives, RG 18/1/6631-6650, *President's Report*, 1969–70, p. 12; UMA, UA20, Box 99-28, Recommendations of the President's Committee for a Student Health and Counselling Service, 21 September 1948.

77 "University Health Service," UBC, *Calendar*, 1940–1.

78 "Report of the Dean of Junior Women," in University of Manitoba, *President's Report*, 1945–6.

79 MUA, RG 42, 1-69, Health Service 1934–47, Percy Vivian to Muriel Roscoe, 9 September 1947.

80 MUA, RG 42, 1-69, Health Service, 1934–47, Muriel Roscoe to Percy Vivian, 4 October 1947.

81 MUA, RG 42, 1-69, Health Service 1924–47, "C.S.I. - Form N2."

82 UTA, A76-0044, Faculty of Medicine, Box 96, University Health Service, Report of the Director of the University Health Service, 11 April 1946.

83 Psychologists included J. Davidson Ketchum and S.N.F. Chant of the University of Toronto and S.R. Laycock of the University of Saskatchewan. See UCA/VUA, SCM, Box 84-53, file: First Hazen Conference, 1941, "The influence of the University in Canada on the life of the Student," Account of First Canadian Hazen Conference, Chaffey's Lock, ON, June 23–29, 1941.

84 Prescott, *Student Bodies*, 132.

85 Canadian Mental Health Association, et al., *Proceedings of a Conference on Student Mental Health*, 125–33. For more on this conference and the role of students in promoting services devoted to mental health, see Jasen, "Student Activism, Mental Health, and English-Canadian Universities in the 1960s," 455–80.

86 Schwartz, "Report on Health and Psychiatric Services on Canadian Campuses," 7.

87 Pitsula, *As One Who Serves*, 295.

88 In 1939 UBC became the first university to offer psychiatric services. The University of Toronto followed suit in 1947. See Schwarz, "Report on Health and Psychiatric Services on Canadian Campuses," 17; UTA, University

Historian, A83-0036, Box 34, file University Health Service, G.E. Wode-house, "University Health Service, University of Toronto," 1976.

89 "Report of the Director of the University Health Service," in University of Toronto, *President's Report*, 1948–9.

90 UAA, "Student Services," http://www.ualberta.ca/ARCHIVES/guide/5SERVICE/129.htm, accessed 18 October 2004.

91 In 1954, of the 1,181 results administered, 321 received counselling. See "Personnel and Student Services," UBC, *President's Report*, 1952–3, 25. See also Mackay, "Psychology at British Columbia," 225–6.

92 "Report of the Student Counsellor," Acadia University, *Report of the President*, 1966–7.

93 Peter Rempel, quoted in Canadian Mental Health Association et al., *Proceedings of a Conference on Student Mental Health*, 68. In 1967–8, the president of St. Francis Xavier noted the need for "… co-ordination of Guidance, Counselling, Psychological, Psychiatric and Athletic Services under the Student Health Service." See St. F.X. Archives, RG 18/1/6631-6650, President's Report, 1966–8, 45.

94 Schwartz, "Report on Health and Psychiatric Services on Canadian Campuses," 17. The level of service differed by campus. UBC provided one part-time consultant and two full-time resident psychiatrists, while the University of Toronto employed three full-time and two part-time psychiatrists. See Schwartz, ibid., 23, 27.

95 Quoted in Canadian Mental Health Association et al. *Proceedings of a Conference on Student Mental Health*, 54.

96 "Personnel and Student Services," UBC, *President's Report*, 1952–3, 25.

97 Starr, *The Social Transformation of American Medicine*, 193.

98 Ibid., 191–2.

8. From Character to Personality: Changing Visions of Citizenship, 1940s to 1960s

1 DUA, President's Office, UA3, 39-9, S.A. Korning, "Communication from the Physical Education Department about Physical Activities at Dalhousie," 1938–9.

2 Falconer, "The Place of the University in National Life," 421–35. See also Kirkwood, *For College Women … and Men*.

3 "Address of Principal" in McGill University, *Annual Report*, 1935–6. Similarly, see Ryerson, "Hygeialogy: The Art and Science of Personal Health," 303–11.

4 UCA/VUA, SCM, Box 84-53, file: First Hazen Conference, 1941, "The influence of the University in Canada on the life of the Student," 9–11.

5 Ibid., 10.

6 Ibid., 11.

7 Ibid., 7.

8 MUA, RG 42, 2-133, Physical Education Reorganization, "Memorandum Re Required Programme of Physical Activity," 21 February 1940.

9 M.L. Vliet, "University Sport During Wartime," *The Gateway*, 1 December 1942, 4, cited in Kate Lamont, *'We Can Achieve': A History of Women in Sport at the University of Alberta*, 38–9.

10 UCA/VUA, SCM, Box 84-53, file: First Hazen Conference, 1941, "The influence of the University in Canada on the life of the Student," 16.

11 Ibid., 13; italics in original.

12 Ibid., 14.

13 MUA, RG 30, Faculty of Education, 65-175, Minutes of Senate Committee on Physical Education, 5 June 1944.

14 "Report of the Physical Education Department for Men," in Dalhousie University, *President's Report*, 1950–4.

15 "Report of the Director of Athletics and Physical Education for Men," in University of Toronto, *President's Report*, 1952–3.

16 "Report of the Director of Physical Education for Women," in University of Toronto, *President's Report*, 1952–3.

17 Slack, "Here's What Physical Education Means to You," 18–19, 31.

18 UTA, School of Physical and Health Education, A83-0046, Box 3, File: Presidential Committee, Report of the Presidential Committee on Athletic Programs, 1962.

19 Dana L. Farnsworth, "The College Mental Health Programme as an Aid to Learning," 5, and Graham B. Blaine, Jr., "The Prevention and Treatment of Emotional Problems Among University Students," 39-40, in Canadian Mental Health Association et al., *Proceedings of a Conference on Student Mental Health*.

20 Dana L. Farnsworth, "The College Mental Health Programme as an Aid to Learning," in Canadian Mental Health Association et al., *Proceedings of a Conference on Student Mental Health*, 5–6.

21 Ibid., 28.

22 Graham B. Blaine, Jr., "The Prevention and Treatment of Emotional Problems among University Students," in Canadian Mental Health Association et al., *Proceedings of a Conference on Student Mental Health*, 50.

23 M. Jean-Charles Bouffard, quoted in Canadian Mental Health Association et al., *Proceedings of a Conference on Student Mental Health*, 56.

24 Dr J. Wendell Macleod, "The Responsibility of Canadian Universities for Student Mental Health," in Canadian Mental Health Association et al., *Proceedings of a Conference on Student Mental Health*, 103.

25 See chap. 3, 61–2.
26 For this slippage, see Christie and Gauvreau, *A Full-Orbed Christianity*, and Gidney, "Under the President's Gaze," 48. On the continued ethical grounding of, and social democratic impulse within, British psychology in the first half of the twentieth century, see Thomson, *Psychological Subjects*.
27 Warren, "The Shift from Character to Personality," 540.
28 Nicholson, *Inventing Personality*, 39.
29 Ibid., 189.
30 Nicholson, "Gordon Allport, Character, and the 'Culture of Personality,' 1897–1937," 54.
31 Ibid., 64.
32 Graham B. Blaine, Jr., "Summary and Remarks," in Canadian Mental Health Association et al., *Proceedings of a Conference on Student Mental Health*, 117.
33 UCA/VUA, SCM, Box 84-53, file: First Hazen Conference, 1941, "The influence of the University in Canada on the life of the Student," 14; italics in original. While the report used the term "Christian," given the composition of conference participants, the term likely referred more narrowly to Protestants. Mid-century was a period in which liberal Protestants made attempts at reconciliation with Catholics and Jews and voiced recognition of diversity within Christianity. The report thus reflected the spirit of the times in acknowledging the importance of diversity of faith, though that diversity was still generally assumed to fall within the Judeo-Christian traditions.
34 Graham B. Blaine, Jr., "Summary and Remarks," in Canadian Mental Health Association et al., *Proceedings of a Conference on Student Mental Health*, 117.
35 "Physical Education," St. Francis Xavier University, *Calendar*, 1957–8 and 1966–7.
36 In Ontario, for example, reform initiatives promoted, though were not fully able to implement, the disestablishment of Christianity within schools. See Gidney and Millar, "The Christian Recessional in Ontario's Public Schools," 281–5.
37 Quoted in Canadian Mental Health Association et al., *Proceedings of a Conference on Student Mental Health*, 54.
38 Graham B. Blaine, "The Prevention and Treatment of Emotional Problems among University Students," in Canadian Mental Health Association et al., *Proceedings of a Conference on Student Mental Health*, 50.
39 Pierre Dansereau, "Introductory Remarks," in Canadian Mental Health Association et al., *Proceedings of a Conference on Student Mental Health*, 3.
40 Cooper, "Writing the History of Development," 14–15. For this process in Canada, see, for example, Campbell, *Respectable Citizens*, 8; Fahrni, *Household Politics*, 16–21; Tillotson, *The Public at Play*, 27–8.

41 Campbell, *Respectable Citizens*, 9. Similarly, Theresa Richardson notes that in the United States the 1940 White House Conference on Children in a Democracy "moved child mental and physical health, educational opportunity and social welfare within the realm of entitlement, rather than moral obligation extended by benevolent reformers." See *The Mental Hygiene Movement and Social Policy in the United States and Canada*, 154.

42 Ignatieff, *The Rights Revolution*; Clément, *Canada's Rights Revolution*.

43 Ignatieff, *The Rights Revolution*, 24.

44 Ibid., 90.

45 Davies and Guppy, *The Schooled Society*, 232. For this process within history and social studies curricula, see von Heyking, *Creating Citizens*.

46 UCA/VUA, SCM, Box 84-53, file: First Hazen Conference, 1941, "The influence of the University in Canada on the life of the Student," 4–6.

47 Neil Morrison, quoted in Canadian Mental Health Association et al., *Proceedings of a Conference on Student Mental Health*, 18.

48 Quoted in Canadian Mental Health Association et al., *Proceedings of a Conference on Student Mental Health*, 90.

49 Gidney, "The Canadian Association of University Teachers and the Rise of Faculty Power, 1951–70."

50 Queen's University, *Report of the Principal's Committee on Teaching and Learning*, 6, 36, 54.

51 Lexier, "The Community of Scholars," 125–44. For an emphasis on the early role of faculty in helping to produce demand for a fundamental reshaping of the nature of the university, see Gidney, "The Canadian Association of University Teachers and the Rise of Faculty Power, 1951–70." For the radicalization of some students and faculty, see, for example, Adelman and Lee, *The University Game*, and McGuigan, *Student Protest*.

52 Lexier, "'The Backdrop Against Which Everything Happened,'" 1–18; Gidney, "War and the Concept of Generation."

53 For the idea of personality as a more gender-neutral category, I am indebted to Ian Nicholson, *Inventing Personality*, 80.

54 Historians have shown this in particular in relation to the discourse of psychologists regarding the family. See for example, Gleason, *Normalizing the Ideal*, and Mary Louise Adams, *The Trouble with Normal: Postwar Youth and the Making of Heterosexuality*.

55 Gidney, *A Long Eclipse*, chap. 7.

56 Hébert, "Carabines, poutchinettes co-eds ou freschettes sont-elles des étudiantes?" 622.

57 Davies, "The Paradox of Progressive Education," 279.

58 Horowitz, "The 1960s and the Transformation of Campus Cultures," 14; Gidney, *A Long Eclipse*, 113.

59 "Report of the Director of the University Health Service," in University of Toronto, *President's Report*, 1962–3.

60 Jasen, "The English Canadian Liberal Arts Curriculum," 250.

61 Ibid., 247–8, 251. See also Jasen, "Student Activism, Mental Health, and English-Canadian Universities," 475; Westhues, "Inter-Generational Conflict in the Sixties," 400–1; Reid, "Education for What?" 1–16; Zirnhelt, "A Student Manifesto," 53–61.

62 Westhues, "Inter-Generational Conflict in the Sixties," 394.

63 Ibid., 395.

64 Rossinow, *The Politics of Authenticity*.

65 Westhues, "Inter-Generational Conflict in the Sixties," 400. See also Owram, *Born at the Right Time*, 204.

66 For this literature see, for example, Lears, "From Salvation to Self-Realization," 3–38; Susman, "'Personality' and the Making of Twentieth-Century Culture," 212–26. For this line of interpretation in Canada, see, for example, von Heyking, *Creating Citizens*, 153, and Cook, "From 'Evil Influence' to Social Facilitator," 1–32. Examining the context of Canadian elementary and high schools, Jack Martin and Ann-Marie McLellan argue that psychology has fundamentally transformed schooling so that education now places "as much or more emphasis on the personal development, interests, and entitlements of students ... as on their intellectual development or transformation into productive citizens and members of their communities." See *The Education of Selves*, 2. For critiques of Susman's and others' arguments, see Fox, "The Culture of Liberal Protestant Progressivism, 1875–1925," 647; Brown, "Being Present, Owning the Past, and Growing into the Future," 174–6. For a more positive view see Hunt, *Governing Morals*, 4, and White and Hunt, "Citizenship: Care of the Self, Character and Personality," 97.

67 Susman, "'Personality' and the Making of Twentieth-Century Culture," 217. For the reference to individual distinctiveness, see page 218.

68 Brown, "Being Present, Owning the Past, and Growing into the Future," 182.

69 Ibid., 177.

70 Wright, "Theorizing Therapeutic Culture," 329.

71 Ibid., 333.

72 Thomson, "Constituting Citizenship," 242. See also, Thomson, *Psychological Subjects*, 278–87.

73 Rossinow, *The Politics of Authenticity*, 6–7.

74 Leinberger and Tucker, *The New Individualists*, 12.

75 Rose, *Inventing Our Selves*, 98.

76 Ibid., 114.
77 Ibid., 72.
78 Ibid., 32.
79 Ibid., 87.
80 Ibid., 17.
81 Ibid., 151. For Rose, this is not a progressive movement, from repression
   to freedom. Rather, he understands that freedom as potentially coercive,
   choices made "within a narrow range of possibilities whose restrictions are
   hard to discern because they form the horizon of what is thinkable" (17).
   On the shift from character to personality as heralding "changes in the
   practices and values of citizenship," see also White and Hunt, "Citizenship:
   Care of the Self, Character and Personality," 93–116. For the quote, see
   page 101.

Conclusion

1 For final references to compulsory physical training see, for example, Mc-
  Master University, *Calendar*, 1968–9; University of Saskatchewan, *Calendar*,
  1972–3; Mount Allison, *Calendar*, 1972–3; "Physical Education," St. Francis
  Xavier University, *Calendar*, 1972–3.
2 The men's program was terminated due to lack of facilities. See Gurney, *A
  Century to Remember*, 50; Kidd, "Athletics," 121.
3 The last reference to UWOs compulsory program seems to appear in 1960–1.
  The University of Manitoba cancelled its program in 1964. At Dalhousie
  University, physical education was mandatory up until 1953–4, after which
  its *Calendar* advised rather than required students to take such a course.
  See "Physical, Health and Recreation Education," UWO, *Announcement*,
  1960–1; UMA, UPC PROP 94, Hilary Findlay, "Physical Education at the
  University of Manitoba: An Historical Overview," unpublished paper, 1978;
  "Health and Physical Education," Dalhousie University, *Calendar*, 1953–4
  and 1954–5.
4 In the 1930s, St. Francis Xavier University required first- and second-year
  male students to engage in three hours a week of physical exercise. This
  was reduced to one hour a week by the late 1950s and, by the late 1960s,
  to a one-year program to be completed prior to graduation. In 1962, the
  required program at the University of Toronto was reduced from two years
  to one. In addition, students had a choice of completing physical education
  sometime in the first or second year or else paying a fine of fifty dollars.
  See "Physical Education," St. Francis Xavier University, *Calendar*, 1957–8,
  1966–7; UTA, School of Physical and Health Education, A83-0046, Box 3,

File: Presidential Committee, "Report of President's Committee on Athletic Programs, 1962," and, File: Program-Required, "Report on Compulsory Physical Education for 1st Year Women," 1969.

5 See, for example, "Report of Acting Director of Student Health Services," in University of Alberta, *Report of the Board of Governors*, 1960–1; "University Health Service," UBC *Calendar*, 1965–6; University of Toronto, *Calendar*, 1972–3.

6 Bender, "Inspecting Workers," 51–75.

7 Krywulak, "Inventing Labour Problems and Solutions," 78.

8 Stephen, *Pick One Intelligent Girl*, 5, 211.

9 Schwartz, "How Deans of Women Became Men," 424–7; Bailey, "From Panty Raid to Revolution," 191.

10 Comacchio, "'The Rising Generation,'" 142–3.

11 Starr, *The Social Transformation of American Medicine*, 13.

12 Ibid., 14.

13 Ibid., 14–15.

14 Ibid., 134–40.

15 See chapter 8, note 40.

16 Christie and Gauvreau, *A Full-Orbed Christianity*.

17 Gleason, *Normalizing the Ideal*; Adams, *The Trouble With Normal*.

18 Ignatieff, *The Rights Revolution*.

Bibliography

Primary Sources

Barton, Jas. W. "What Physical Examination of Students Shows." *University of Toronto Monthly* (November 1919): 51–2.

Blaine, Graham B. "The Problems of Adolescence." *Student Medicine* 7, 4 (1958): 253–67.

Canadian Mental Health Association, Canadian Union of Students, World University Service of Canada. *Proceedings of a Conference on Student Mental Health Held at Queen's University, Kingston, Ontario, May 10th to 13th, 1963.* Toronto: University of Toronto Press, 1963.

Cartwright, E.M. "Athletics and Physical Education for Girls." In Ontario Educational Association, *Yearbook and Proceedings* (1923): 274–81.

Congress of the Universities of the British Empire. *Report of Proceedings*, 1936. London: Bell and Sons, 1936.

– *Report of Proceedings*, 1926. London, Bell and Sons, 1926.

Falconer, Roy. "The Place of the University in National Life." *University of Toronto Quarterly* 4, 3(1934–5): 421–35.

Fraser, Roy. "What Can the University Contribute to Public Health Education?" *Canadian Public Health Journal* 30 (1939): 424–30.

Gordon, Edith H. "The Need of Physical Training in Schools." In Ontario Educational Association, *Yearbook and Proceedings* (1924): 131–6.

Graham, E.E. "Health Work in a Junior College." *Canadian Public Health Journal* (June 1932): 288–9.

Grant, H.G. "Students' Health Service of Dalhousie University." *Canadian Public Health Journal* 24 (1933): 485–90.

Guest, Edna. "Problems of Girlhood and Motherhood." *The Public Health Journal* 13, 5 (1922): 193–8.

Hawgood, Barbara Excell. "Go East, Young Woman." In *Still Running: Personal Stories by Queen's Women Celebrating the Fiftieth Anniversary of the Marty Scholarship*, edited by Joy Parr, 88–94. Kingston: Queen's University Alumnae Association, 1987.

Kirkwood, M.M. *For College Women … and Men.* Toronto: Oxford University Press, 1938.

Lamb, Arthur S. "Physical Education." In Ontario Educational Association, *Yearbook and Proceedings* (1923): 159–68.

Legge, Robert T. "The Relation of Mental Hygiene to a University Administrative Hygiene Program." In American Student Health Association, *Proceedings* (December 1927): 90–1.

Macdonald, Bruce. "The Relation of Play to the Education of the Child." *The Public Health Journal* 15, 8 (1924): 341–7.

MacMurchy, Helen. "The Woman in the Medical Profession." *Acta Victoriana* 47, 5 (1923): 28.

McHenry, E.W., Ruth Crawford, and Lillian Barber. "The Heights and Weights of a Canadian Group." *Canadian Journal of Public Health* 38, 9 (1947): 437–41.

Porter, George D. "Preserving the Health of the Student Body." *University of Toronto Monthly* 22, 7 (1922): 289.

– "Exercise and Health." In Ontario Educational Association, *Yearbook and Proceedings* (1926): 223–6.

Ryerson, Stanley E. "Hygeialogy: The Art and Science of Personal Health." *Canadian Journal of Public Health* 37, 8 (1946): 303–11.

Schwarz, Conrad J. *Report on Health and Psychiatric Services on Canadian Campuses.* Ottawa: Canadian Union of Students, 1967.

Slack, Zerada. "Here's What Physical Education Means to You." *Health* (January–February 1957): 18–19, 31.

Stevens, Warren. "Why Athletics?" *Health* (March 1935): 14.

Thompson, L.J. "Organization in a University for Instruction in Mental Hygiene and for Safeguarding the Mental Health of Students." In American Student Health Association, *Proceedings* (December 1927): 85–90.

Secondary Sources

Adams, Annmarie. "'Rooms of Their Own: The Nurses' Residences at Montreal's Royal Victoria Hospital." *Material History Review* 40 (1994), 29–41.

Adams, Mary Louise. *The Trouble with Normal: Postwar Youth and the Making of Heterosexuality.* Toronto: University of Toronto Press, 1997.

Adelman, Howard, and Dennis Lee, eds. *The University Game.* Toronto: Anansi, 1968.

Ainley, Marianne Gosztonyi. "Last in the Field? Canadian Women Natural Scientists, 1815–1965." In *Despite the Odds: Essays on Canadian Women and Science*, edited by Marianne Gosztonyi Ainley, 25–62. Montreal: Véhicule Press, 1990.

Ainsworth, Dorothy S. *The History of Physical Education in Colleges for Women*. New York: A.S. Barnes, 1930.

– "A History of Physical Education in Colleges for Women (U.S.A.)." In *A History of Physical Education and Sport in the United States and Canada*, edited by Earle F. Zeigler, 167–80. Champaign, IL: Stipes, 1975.

Allen, Richard. *The Social Passion: Religion and Social Reform in Canada, 1914–28*. Toronto: University of Toronto Press, 1971.

Andrews, Margaret W. "Epidemic and Public Health: Influenza in Vancouver, 1918–1919." *BC Studies* 34 (1977): 21–44.

Armstrong, David. *Political Anatomy of the Body: Medical Knowledge in Britain in the Twentieth Century*. Cambridge, MA: Cambridge University Press, 1983.

Arnup, Katherine. "'Victims of Vaccination?': Opposition to Compulsory Immunization in Ontario, 1900–90." *Canadian Bulletin of Medical History* 9 (1992): 159–76.

– *Education for Motherhood: Advice for Mothers in Twentieth-Century Canada*. Toronto: University of Toronto Press, 1994.

Atkinson, Paul. "Fitness, Feminism and Schooling." In *The Nineteenth-Century Woman: Her Cultural and Physical World*, edited by Sara Delamont and Lorna Duffin, 92–133. London: Croom Helm, 1978.

Axelrod, Paul. *Making a Middle Class: Student Life in English Canada during the Thirties*. Montreal: McGill-Queen's University Press, 1990.

– *The Promise of Schooling: Education in Canada, 1800–1914*. Toronto: University of Toronto Press, 1997.

Bailey, Beth. "Scientific Truth ... And Love: The Marriage Education Movement in the United States." *Journal of Social History* 20, 4 (1987): 711–32.

– "From Panty Raids to Revolution: Youth and Authority, 1950–1970." In *Generations of Youth: Youth Cultures and History in Twentieth-Century America*, edited by Joe Austin and Michael Nevin Willard, 187–204. New York: New York University Press, 1998.

Baltutis, Peter E. "'To Enlarge Our Hearts and To Widen Our Horizon': Archbishop Neil McNeil and the Origins of Social Catholicism in the Roman Catholic Archdiocese of Toronto, 1912–1934." *Canadian Catholic Historical Association Historical Studies* 74 (2008): 29–50.

Barman, Jean. *Growing Up British in British Columbia: Boys in Private School, 1900–1950*. Vancouver: University of British Columbia Press, 1984.

Barry, John M. *The Great Influenza: The Epic Story of the Deadliest Plague in History*. New York: Viking, 2004.

Bashaw, Carolyn Terry. *"Stalwart Women": A Historical Analysis of Deans of Women in the South.* New York: Teachers College Press, 1999.

Bashaw, Carolyn Terry. "'Reassessment and Redefinition'" The NAWDC and Higher Education for Women." In *Women Administrators in Higher Education: Historical and Contemporary Perspectives,* edited by Jana Nidiffer and Carolyn Terry Bashaw, 157–82. Albany, NY: SUNY Press, 2001.

Baskerville, Peter. *A Silent Revolution? Gender and Wealth in English Canada 1860–1930.* Montreal: McGill-Queen's University Press, 2008.

Bederman, Gail. *Manliness and Civilization: A Cultural History of Gender and Race in the United States, 1880–1917.* Chicago: University of Chicago Press, 1995.

Bender, Daniel E. "Inspecting Workers: Medical Examination, Labor Organizing, and the Evidence of Sexual Difference." *Radical History Review* 80 (2001): 51–75.

Bennett, Bruce L. "Dr. Dudley A. Sargent and the Harvard Summer School of Physical Education." In *A History of Physical Education and Sport in the United States and Canada,* edited by Earle F. Ziegler, 129–37. Champaign, IL: Stipes, 1975.

Bliss, Michael. "'Pure Books on Avoided Subjects': Pre-Freudian Sexual Ideas in Canada." In *Medicine in Canadian Society: Historical Perspectives,* edited by S.E.D. Shortt, 255–83. Montreal: McGill-Queen's University Press, 1981.

Bonde, Hans. "Globalization Before Globalization: Niels Bukh and the American Connection." *International Journal of the History of Sport* 26, 13 (2009): 2000–14.

Bothwell, Robert S., and John R. English. "Pragmatic Physicians: Canadian Medicine and Health Care Insurance, 1910–1945." In *Medicine in Canadian Society: Historical Perspectives,* edited by S.E.D. Shortt, 479–93. Montreal: McGill-Queen's University Press, 1981.

Bouchier, Nancy B., and Ken Cruikshank. "Abandoning Nature: Swimming Pools and Clean, Healthy Recreation in Hamilton, Ontario, c. 1930s–1950s." *Canadian Bulletin of Medical History* 28, 2 (2011): 315–37.

Brandt, Allan M. *No Magic Bullet: A Social History of Venereal Disease in the United States since 1880.* New York: Oxford University Press, 1985.

Brown, Jeffrey Scott. "Being Present, Owning the Past, and Growing into the Future: Temporality, Revelation and the Therapeutic Culture." In *The River of History: Trans-national and Trans-disciplinary Perspectives on the Immanence of the Past,* edited by Peter Farrugia, 173–94. Calgary: University of Calgary Press, 2005.

Bryans, Helen. "Secondary School Curriculum for Girls." In *Physical Education in Canada,* edited by M.L. Van Vliet, 124–39. Scarborough, ON: Prentice-Hall, 1965.

Burke, Sara Z. "'Being Unlike Man': Challenges to Co-education at the University of Toronto, 1884–1909." *Ontario History* 93, 1 (2001): 11–31.

– "Women of Newfangle: Co-Education, Racial Discourse and Women's Rights in Victorian Ontario." *Historical Studies in Education* 19, 1 (2007): 111–33.

Byl, John. "The Margaret Eaton School, 1901–1942: Women's Education in Elocution, Drama and Physical Education." PhD dissertation, State University of New York at Buffalo, 1992.

Cahn, Susan K. *Coming on Strong: Gender and Sexuality in Twentieth-Century Women's Sport.* Cambridge, MA: Harvard University Press, 1994.

Cameron, James D. *For the People: A History of St. Francis Xavier University.* Montreal: McGill-Queen's University Press, 1996.

Cameron, Ross D. "Tom Thomson, Antimodernism, and the Ideal of Manhood." *Journal of the Canadian Historical Association* 10 (1999): 185–208.

Campbell, Lara. *Respectable Citizens: Gender, Family, and Unemployment in Ontario's Great Depression.* Toronto: University of Toronto Press, 2009.

Carr, Ian, and Robert Beamish. *Manitoba Medicine: A Brief History.* Winnipeg: University of Manitoba Press, 1999.

Cassel, Jay. *The Secret Plague: Venereal Disease in Canada 1838–1939.* Toronto: University of Toronto Press, 1987.

Chenier, Elise. *Strangers in Our Midst: Sexual Deviancy in Postwar Ontario.* Toronto: University of Toronto Press, 2008.

Christie, Nancy, and Michael Gauvreau. *A Full-Orbed Christianity: The Protestant Churches and Social Welfare in Canada, 1900–1940.* Montreal: McGill-Queen's University Press, 1996.

Christou, Theodore Michael. *Progressive Education: Revisioning and Reforming Ontario's Public Schools, 1919–1942.* Toronto: University of Toronto Press, 2012.

Churchill, David S. "Making Broad Shoulders: Body-Building and Physical Culture in Chicago, 1890–1920." *History of Education Quarterly* 48, 3 (2008): 341–70.

Clément, Dominique. *Canada's Rights Revolution: Social Movements and Social Change, 1937–82.* Vancouver: University of British Columbia Press, 2008.

Cleveland, Janne, and Margaret Conrad. "Mary Dulhanty (1909–1999)." In *The Small Details of Life: 20 Diaries by Women in Canada, 1830–1996,* edited by Kathryn Carter, 323–50. Toronto: University of Toronto Press, 2002.

Coburn, Kathleen. *In Pursuit of Coleridge.* London: Bodley Head, 1977.

Cohen, Sol. "The Mental Hygiene Movement, the Development of Personality and the School: The Medicalization of American Education." *History of Education Quarterly* 23, 2 (1983): 123–49.

– *Challenging Orthodoxies: Toward a New Cultural History of Education.* New York: Peter Lang, 1999.

Comacchio, Cynthia. *"Nations are Built of Babies": Saving Ontario's Mothers and Children, 1900–1940.* Montreal: McGill-Queen's University Press, 1993.

– "'The Rising Generation': Laying Claim to the Health of Adolescents in English Canada, 1920–70." *Canadian Bulletin of Medical History* 19, 1 (2002): 139–78.

– *Dominion of Youth: Adolescence and the Making of Modern Canada, 1920 to 1950.* Waterloo, ON: Wilfrid Laurier University Press, 2006.

Cook, Sharon Anne. "From 'Evil Influence' to Social Facilitator: Representations of Youth Smoking, Drinking, and Citizenship in Canadian Health Textbooks, 1890–1960." *Journal of Curriculum Studies* (2008): 1–32.

Cooper, Frederick. "Writing the History of Development." *Journal of Modern European History* 8, 1 (2010): 5–23.

Copp, Terry. *Battle Exhaustion: Soldiers and Psychiatrists in the Canadian Army, 1939–1945.* Montreal: McGill-Queen's University Press, 1990.

Cosentino, Frank, and Maxwell L. Howell. *A History of Physical Education in Canada.* Toronto: General Publishing, 1971.

Curtis, Bruce. *The Politics of Population: State Formation, Statistics, and the Census of Canada, 1840–1875.* Toronto: University of Toronto Press, 2001.

Daley, Caroline. *Leisure and Pleasure: Reshaping and Revealing the New Zealand Body, 1900–1960.* Auckland: Auckland University Press, 2003.

Danziger, Kurt. *Naming the Mind: How Psychology Found Its Language.* London: Sage Publication, 1997.

Davies, Scott. "The Paradox of Progressive Education: A Frame Analysis." *Sociology of Education* 75, 4 (2002): 269–86.

Davies, Scott, and Neil Guppy. *The Schooled Society: An Introduction to the Sociology of Education.* 2nd ed. Don Mills, ON: Oxford University Press, 2010.

Dehli, Kari. "'Health Scouts' for the State? Schools and Public Health Nurses in Early Twentieth-Century Toronto." *Historical Studies in Education* 2, 2 (1990): 247–64.

Demerson, Velma. *Incorrigible.* Waterloo, ON: Wilfrid Laurier University Press, 2004.

Denham, Robert D. *The Correspondence of Northrup Frye and Helen Kemp 1932–1939.* Vol. 1, *1932–1935.* Toronto: University of Toronto Press, 1996.

Dennis, Robert H. "Beginning to Restructure the Institutional Church: Canadian Social Catholics and the CCF, 1931–1944." *Canadian Catholic Historical Association Historical Studies* 74 (2008): 51–71.

Dodd, Dianne. "Helen MacMurchy, M.D.: Gender and Professional Conflict in the Medical Inspection of Toronto Schools, 1910–11." *Ontario History* 93, 2 (2001): 127–49.

Dowbiggin, Ian Robert. *Keeping America Sane: Psychiatry and Eugenics in the United States and Canada, 1880–1940.* Ithaca, NY: Cornell University Press, 1997.

Drover, Victoria Lamb. "A Place for Everyone, But Everyone in Their Place: The Inclusion of Female Students, Staff, and Faculty at the University of Saskatchewan, 1907–1922." MA thesis, University of Saskatchewan, 2009.

Duder, Cameron. "'Two Middle-Aged and Very Good-Looking Females That Spend All Their Week-Ends Together': Female Professors and Same-Sex Relationships in Canada, 1910–1950." In *Historical Identities: The Professoriate in Canada,* edited by Paul Stortz and E. Lisa Panayotidis, 332–50. Toronto: University of Toronto Press, 2006.

Duffin, Jacalyn. *Lovers and Livers: Disease Concepts in History.* Toronto: University of Toronto Press, 2005.

Duffy, John. *The Sanitarians: A History of American Public Health.* Urbana: University of Illinois Press, 1990.

Dyreson, Mark. "Regulating the Body and the Body Politic: American Sport, Bourgeois Culture, and the Language of Progress, 1880–1920." In *The New American Sport History: Recent Approaches and Perspectives,* edited by S.W. Pope, 121–44. Urbana: University of Illinois Press, 1997.

Ellis, Jason A. "'Backward and Brilliant Children': A Social and Policy History of Disability, Childhood, and Education in Toronto's Special Education Classes, 1910 to 1945." PhD dissertation, York University, 2011.

Emery, George. *Facts of Life: The Social Construction of Vital Statistics, Ontario 1869–1952.* Montreal: McGill-Queen's University Press, 1993.

Fahrni, Magda. "'Elles sont partout...': Les femmes et la ville en temps d'épidémie Montréal, 1918–1920." *Revue d'Histoire de L'Amérique Française* 58, 1 (2004): 67–85.

– *Household Politics: Montreal Families and Postwar Reconstruction.* Toronto: University of Toronto Press, 2005.

Fass, Paula S. *The Damned and the Beautiful: American Youth in the 1920s.* New York: Oxford University Press, 1977.

Feldberg, Georgina D. *Disease and Class: Tuberculosis and the Shaping of Modern North American Society.* New Brunswick, NJ: Rutgers University Press, 1995.

Fingard, Judith. "Gender and Inequality at Dalhousie: Faculty Women Before 1950." *Dalhousie Review* 64, 4 (1984–85): 687–703.

Fingard, Judith, and John Rutherford. "Social Disintegration, Problem Pregnancies, Civilian Disasters: Psychiatric Research in Nova Scotia in the 1950s." In *Mental Health and Canadian Society: Historical Perspectives,* edited by James E. Moran and David Wright, 193–220. Montreal: McGill-Queen's University Press, 2006.

Fletcher, Sheila. *Women First: The Female Tradition in English Physical Education, 1880–1980.* London: Athlone Press, 1984.

Ford, Anne Rochon. *A Path Not Strewn With Roses: One Hundred Years of Women at the University of Toronto, 1884–1984.* Toronto: University of Toronto Press, 1985.

Fox, Richard Wightman. "The Culture of Liberal Protestant Progressivism, 1875–1925." *Journal of Interdisciplinary History* 23, 3 (1993): 639–60.

Frager, Ruth A., and Carmela Patrias. *Discounted Labour: Women Workers in Canada, 1870–1939.* Toronto: University of Toronto Press, 2005.

Gaffield, Chad, Lynne Marks, and Susan Laskin. "Student Populations and Graduate Careers: Queen's University, 1895–1900." In *Youth, University, and Canadian Society: Essays in the Social History of Higher Education,* edited by Paul Axelrod and John G. Reid, 3–25. Montreal: McGill-Queen's University Press, 1989.

Gauvreau, Michael. "The Emergence of Personalist Feminism: Catholicism and the Marriage Preparation Movement in Quebec, 1940–1960." In *Households of Faith: Family, Gender, and Community in Canada, 1760–1969,* edited by Nancy Christie, 319–47. Montreal: McGill-Queen's University Press, 2002.

Gauvreau, Michael. *The Catholic Origins of Quebec's Quiet Revolution, 1931–1970.* Montreal: McGill-Queen's University Press, 2005.

Gerber, Ellen W. *Innovators and Institutions in Physical Education.* Philadelphia: Lea and Febiger, 1971.

Gidney, Catherine. "Under the President's Gaze: Sexuality and Morality at a Canadian University during the Second World War." *Canadian Historical Review* 82, 1 (2001): 36–54.

– *A Long Eclipse: The Liberal Protestant Establishment and the Canadian University, 1920–1970.* Montreal: McGill-Queen's University Press, 2004.

– "The Athletics-Physical Education Dichotomy Revisited: The Case of the University of Toronto, 1900–1940." *Sport History Review* 37 (2006): 130–49.

– "Institutional Responses to Communicable Diseases at Victoria College, University of Toronto, 1900–1940." *Canadian Bulletin of Medical History* 24, 2 (2007): 265–90.

– "The Canadian Association of University Teachers and the Rise of Faculty Power, 1951–70." In *Debating Dissent: Canada and the Sixties,* edited by Lara Campbell, Dominique Clément, and Greg Kealey, 67–79. Toronto: University of Toronto Press, 2012.

– "War and the Concept of Generation: The International Teach-Ins at the University of Toronto, 1965–1968." In *Cultures, Communities, and Conflict: Histories of Canadian Universities and War,* edited by Paul Stortz and Lisa Panayotidis. Toronto: University of Toronto Press, 2012.

- "'Less Inefficiency, More Milk': The Politics of Food and the Culture of the English-Canadian University, 1900–1950." In *Edible Histories, Cultural Politics: Towards a Canadian Food History*, edited by Franca Iacovetta, Valerie Korinek, and Marlene Epp, 286–304. Toronto: University of Toronto Press, 2012.
- "Feminist Ideals and Everyday Life: Professional Women's Feminism at Victoria College, University of Toronto, 1900–1940." In *Feminist History in Canada: New Essays on Women, Gender, Work, and Nation*, edited by Catherine Carstairs and Nancy Janovicek, 96–117. Vancouver: UBC Press, 2013.
Gidney, Catherine, and R.D. Gidney. "Branding the Classroom: Commercialism in Canadian Schools, 1920–1960." *Histoire sociale/Social History* 41, 82 (2008): 345–79.
Gidney, R.D., and W.P.J. Millar. *Professional Gentlemen: The Professions in Nineteenth-Century Ontario.* Toronto: University of Toronto Press, 1994.
- "The Christian Recessional in Ontario's Public Schools." In *Religion and Public Life in Canada: Historical and Comparative Perspectives*, edited by Marguerite Van Die, 275–93. Toronto: University of Toronto Press, 2001.
- "The Salaries of Teachers in English Canada, 1900–1940: A Reappraisal." *Historical Studies in Education* 22, 1 (2010): 1–38.
Gillett, Margaret. *We Walked Very Warily: A History of Women at McGill.* Montreal: Eden Press Women's Publications, 1981.
- "The Heart of the Matter: Maude Abbott, M.D., 1869–1940." In *Despite the Odds: Essays on Canadian Women and Science*, edited by Marianne Gosztonyi Ainley, 179–94. Montreal: Véhicule Press, 1990.
Glazer, Penina Migdal, and Miriam Slater. *Unequal Colleagues: The Entrance of Women into the Professions, 1890–1940.* New Brunswick, NJ: Rutgers University Press, 1987.
Gleason, Mona. *Normalizing the Ideal: Psychology, Schooling, and the Family in Postwar Canada.* Toronto: University of Toronto Press, 1999.
- "Race, Class, and Health: School Medical Inspection and 'Healthy' Children in British Columbia, 1890 to 1930." *Canadian Bulletin of Medical History* 19 (2002): 95–112.
- "'Lost Voices, Lost Bodies'? Doctors and the Embodiment of Children and Youth in English Canada from 1900 to the 1940s." In *Lost Kids: Vulnerable Children and Youth in Twentieth Century Canada and the United States*, edited by Mona Gleason, Tamara Myers, Leslie Paris, and Veronica Strong-Boag, 136–53. Vancouver: UBC Press, 2010.
- *Small Matters: Canadian Children in Sickness and Health, 1900–1940.* Montreal: McGill-Queen's University Press, 2013.
Graham, Patricia Albjerg. "Expansion and Exclusion: A History of Women in American Higher Education." *Signs* 3, 4 (1978): 759–73.

Griffiths, N.E.S. *The Splendid Vision: Centennial History of the National Council of Women of Canada, 1893–1993.* Ottawa: Carleton University Press, 1993.

Griswold, Robert L. "The 'Flabby American,' the Body, and the Cold War." In *A Shared Experience: Men, Women and the History of Gender*, edited by Laura McCall and Donald Yacovone, 323–48. New York: New York University Press, 1998.

Gurney, Helen. *Girls' Sports: A Century of Progress in Ontario High Schools.* Don Mills, ON: Ontario Federation of School Athletic Associations, 1979.

– *A Century to Remember 1893–1993: Women's Sports at the University of Toronto.* Toronto: University of Toronto Women's T-Holders' Association, 1993.

Hacker, Carlotta. *The Indomitable Lady Doctors.* Toronto: Clark, Irwin and Co., 1974.

Hall, M. Ann. *Feminism and Sporting Bodies: Essays on Theory and Practice.* Champaign, IL: Human Kinetics, 1996.

– *The Girl and the Game: A History of Women's Sport in Canada.* Peterborough, ON: Broadview Press, 2002.

Hallman, Dianne M., and Anna H. Lathrop. "Sustaining the Fire of 'Scholarly Passion': Mary G. Hamilton (1883–1972) and Irene Poelzer (1926–)." In *Women Teaching, Women Learning: Historical Perspectives*, edited by Elizabeth M. Smyth and Paula Bourne, 45–64. Toronto: Inanna, 2006.

Harley, David. "Rhetoric and the Social Construction of Sickness and Healing." *Social History of Medicine* 12, 3 (1999): 407–35.

Harrigan, Patrick J. *Finding Their Place: The History of the Canadian Council of University Physical Education and Kinesiology Administrators (CCUPEKA).* Toronto: CCUPEKA, Patrick J. Harrigan, and the Faculty of Physical Education and Health, University of Toronto, 2004.

– "Women's Agency and the Development of Women's Intercollegiate Athletics, 1961–2001." *Historical Studies in Education* 15, 1 (2003): 37–76.

Harrison, Helen E. "In the Picture of Health: Portraits of Health, Disease and Citizenship in Canada's Public Health Advice Literature, 1920–1960." PhD dissertation, Queen's University, 2001.

Harrison, Mark. *Disease and the Modern World: 1500 to the Present Day.* Cambridge, MA: Polity, 2004.

Heap, Ruby. "From the Science of Housekeeping to the Science of Nutrition: Pioneers in Canadian Nutrition and Dietetics at the University of Toronto's Faculty of Household Science, 1900–1950." In *Challenging Professions: Historical and Contemporary Perspectives on Women's Professional Work*, edited by Elizabeth Smyth, Sandra Acker, Paula Bourne, and Alison Prentice, 141–70. Toronto: University of Toronto Press, 1999.

Hébert, Karine. "Between the Future and the Present: Montreal University Student Youth and the Post-war Years, 1945–1960." In *Cultures of Citizenship in Post-war Canada, 1940–1955*, edited by Nancy Christie and Michael Gauvreau, 163–200. Montreal: McGill-Queen's University Press, 2003.

– "Carabines, poutchinettes co-eds ou freschettes sont-elles des étudiantes? Les filles à l'Université McGill et à l'Université de Montréal (1900–1960)." *Revue d'Histoire de L'Amérique Française* 57, 2 (2004): 593–625.

Horowitz, Helen Lefkowitz. *Alma Mater: Design and Experience in the Women's College from their Nineteenth-Century Beginnings to the 1930s.* Amherst: University of Massachusetts Press, 1984.

– "The 1960s and the Transformation of Campus Cultures." *History of Education Quarterly* 26, 1 (1986): 1–38.

Houston, C. Stuart. *Steps on the Road to Medicare. Why Saskatchewan Led the Way.* Montreal: McGill-Queen's University Press, 2002.

Howell, Colin. *Blood, Sweat, and Cheers: Sport and the Making of Modern Canada.* Toronto: University of Toronto Press, 2001.

– *Northern Sandlots: A Social History of Maritime Baseball.* Toronto: University of Toronto Press, 1995.

Howell, David, and Peter Lindsay. "Social Gospel and the Young Boy Problem, 1895–1925." *Canadian Journal of History of Sport* 17, 1 (1986): 75–87.

Hoy, Suellen. *Chasing Dirt: The American Pursuit of Cleanliness.* New York: Oxford University Press, 1995.

Hudon, Christine. "'Le Muscle et le Vouloir': Les sports dans les colleges classiques masculins au Québec, 1870–1940." *Historical Studies in Education* 17, 2 (2005): 243–63.

Humphries, Mark Osborne. "The Horror at Home: The Canadian Military and the 'Great' Influenza Pandemic of 1918." *Journal of the Canadian Historical Association* 16, 1 (2005): 235–60.

Hunt, Alan. *Governing Morals: A Social History of Moral Regulation.* Cambridge, MA: Cambridge University Press, 1999.

Iacovetta, Franca. *Gatekeepers: Reshaping Immigrant Lives in Cold War Canada.* Toronto: Between the Lines, 2006.

Ignatieff, Michael. *The Rights Revolution.* Toronto: Anansi, 2007.

James, Cathy. "A Passion for Service: Edith Elwood and the Social Character of Reform." In *Women Teaching, Women Learning: Historical Perspectives*, edited by Elizabeth M. Smyth and Paula Bourne, 105–30. Toronto: Inanna, 2006.

Jasen, Patricia. "The English Canadian Liberal Arts Curriculum: An Intellectual History, 1880–1950." PhD dissertation, University of Manitoba, 1987.

– "Student Activism, Mental Health, and English-Canadian Universities in the 1960s." *Canadian Historical Review* 92, 3 (2011): 455–80.

Johnson, Niall P.A.S., and Juergen Mueller. "Updating the Accounts: Global Mortality of the 1918–1920 'Spanish' Influenza Pandemic." *Bulletin of the History of Medicine* 76 (2002): 105–15.

Jones, Esyllt W. "Contact across a Diseased Boundary: Urban Space and Social Interaction During Winnipeg's Influenza Epidemic, 1918–19." *Journal of the Canadian Historical Association* 13, 1 (2002): 119–39.

Kealey, Linda. "Historical Perspectives on Health Care in Canada." In *Health Care in Canada: Demographic and Fiscal Issues*, edited by Joe Ruggeri and Weiqiu Yu, 131–51. Fredericton: Policy Studies Centre, University of New Brunswick, 2003.

Kendrick, Martin, and Krista Slade. *Spirit of Life: The Story of Women's College Hospital*. Toronto: Women's College Hospital, 1993.

Keyes, Mary Eleanor. "John Howard Crocker LL.D., 1870–1959." MA thesis, University of Western Ontario, 1964.

Keys, Barbara J. *Globalizing Sport: National Rivalry and International Community in the 1930s*. Cambridge, MA: Harvard University Press, 2006.

Kidd, Bruce. *The Struggle for Canadian Sport*. Toronto: University of Toronto Press, 1996.

– "Athletics: Transforming Amateurism." In *A Strange Elation. Hart House: The First Eighty Years*, edited by David Kilgour, 115–25. Toronto: Hart House, 1999.

Kiefer, Nancy, and Ruth Roach Pierson. "The War Effort and Women Students at the University of Toronto, 1939–45." In *Youth, University and Canadian Society: Essays in the Social History of Higher Education*, edited by Paul Axelrod and John G. Reid, 161–83. Montreal: McGill-Queen's University Press, 1989.

King, Alyson E. "The Experience of the Second Generation of Women Students at Ontario Universities, 1900–1930." PhD dissertation, OISE, University of Toronto, 1999.

– "Centres of 'Home-Like Influence': Residences for Women at the University of Toronto." *Material History Review* 49 (1999): 39–59.

Kinnear, Mary. *In Subordination: Professional Women, 1870–1970*. Montreal: McGill-Queen's University Press, 1995.

Kirk, David. *Schooling Bodies: School Practice and Public Discourse, 1880–1950*. London: Leicester University Press, 1998.

Kirkconnell, Watson. *The Fifth Quarter-Century: Acadia University, 1938–1963*. Wolfville, NS: Governors of Acadia University, 1968.

Kline, Wendy. *Building a Better Race: Gender, Sexuality, and Eugenics from the Turn of the Century to the Baby Boom*. Berkeley: University of California Press, 2001.

Kraut, Alan M. *Silent Travelers: Germs, Genes, and the "Immigrant Menace."* New York: Basic Books, 1994.

Krywulak, Tim. "Inventing Labour Problems and Solutions: The Emergence of Human Resources Management in Canada, 1900–1945." *Journal of the Canadian Historical Association* 15, 1 (2004): 71–95.

Kuhlberg, Mark. "An Acute Yet Brief Bout of 'returned-soldier-itis': The University of Toronto's Faculty of Forestry after the First World War." In *Cultures, Communities, and Conflict: Histories of Canadian Universities and War*, edited by Paul Stortz and E. Lisa Panayotidis, 51–69. Toronto: University of Toronto Press, 2012.

Lamont, Kate. *"We Can Achieve": A History of Women in Sport at the University of Alberta*. Edmonton: Academic Printing and Publishing, 1988.

LaPierre, Paula J.S. "The First Generation: The Experience of Women University Students in Central Canada." PhD dissertation, OISE, University of Toronto, 1993.

Lathrop, Anna H. "Elegance and Expression, Sweat and Strength: Body Training, Physical Culture and Female Embodiment in Women's Education at the Margaret Eaton Schools, 1901–1941." PhD dissertation, University of Toronto, 1997.

– "Contested Terrain: Gender and 'Movement' in Ontario Elementary Physical Education, 1940–70." *Ontario History* 94, 2 (2002): 165–82.

Lears, T.J. Jackson. "From Salvation to Self-Realization: Advertising and the Therapeutic Roots of the Consumer Culture, 1880–1930." In *The Culture of Consumption: Critical Essays in American History, 1880–1980*, edited by R.W. Fox and T.J. Jackson Lears, 3–38. New York: Pantheon Books, 1983.

Leavitt, Judith Walzer. "Gendered Expectations: Women and Early Twentieth-Century Public Health." In *U.S. History as Women's History: New Feminist Essays*, edited by Linda K. Kerber, Alice Kessler-Harris, and Kathryn Kish Sklar, 147–69. Chapel Hill: University of North Carolina Press, 1995.

Leinberger, Paul, and Bruce Tucker. *The New Individualists: The Generation After The Organization Man*. New York: HarperCollins, 1991.

Lenskyj, Helen. "Femininity First: Sport and Physical Education for Ontario Girls, 1890–1930." *Canadian Journal of the History of Sport* 13, 2 (1982): 4–17.

– "The Role of Physical Education in the Socialization of Girls in Ontario, 1890–1930." PhD dissertation, University of Toronto, 1983.

– *Out of Bounds: Women, Sport and Sexuality*. Toronto: Women's Press, 1986.

Levenstein, Harvey. *Revolution at the Table: The Transformation of the American Diet*. New York: Oxford University Press, 1988.

Lewis, Jane. "The Prevention of Diphtheria in Canada and Britain, 1914–1945." *Journal of Social History* 20, 1 (1986): 163–76.

Lewis, Norah. "Physical Perfection for Spiritual Welfare: Health Care for the Urban Child, 1900–1939." In *Studies in Childhood History: A Canadian*

Perspective, edited by Patricia T. Rooke and R.L. Schnell, 135–66. Calgary: Detselig, 1982.

Lexier, Roberta. "'The Backdrop Against Which Everything Happened': English-Canadian Student Movements and Off-Campus Movements for Change." *History of Intellectual Culture* 7, 1 (2007): 1–18.

– "The Community of Scholars: The English-Canadian Student Movement and University Governance." In *Mobilizations, Protests and Engagements: Canadian Perspectives on Social Movements*, edited by Marie Hammond Callaghan and Matthew Hayday, 125–44. Halifax: Fernwood, 2008.

Light, Beth, and Ruth Roach Pierson, eds. *No Easy Road: Women in Canada 1920s to 1960s*. Toronto: New Hogtown Press, 1990.

Logan, Harry T. *Tuum Est: A History of the University of British Columbia*. Vancouver: University of British Columbia, 1958.

Lowe, Margaret A. *Looking Good: College Women and Body Image, 1875–1930*. Baltimore: Johns Hopkins University Press, 2003.

Macdonald, Charlotte. *Strong, Beautiful and Modern: National Fitness in Britain, New Zealand, Australia and Canada, 1935–1960*. Vancouver: University of British Columbia Press, 2011.

MacDougall, Heather. *Activists and Advocates: Toronto's Health Department 1883–1983*. Toronto: Dundurn Press, 1990.

Mackay, Donald C.G. "Psychology at British Columbia." In *History of Academic Psychology*, edited by Mary J. Wright and C. Roger Myers, 220–32. Toronto: C.J. Hogrefe, 1982.

Mackinnon, Alison. *Love and Freedom: Professional Women and the Reshaping of Personal Life*. Cambridge, MA: Cambridge University Press, 1997.

Macleod, David. *Building Character in the American Boy: The Boy Scouts, YMCA, and their Forerunners, 1870–1920*. Madison: University of Wisconsin Press, 1983.

Macleod, Malcolm. *A Bridge Built Halfway: A History of Memorial University College, 1925–1950*. Montreal: McGill-Queen's University Press, 1990.

Mangan, J.A. *Athleticism in the Victorian and Edwardian Public School: The Emergence and Consolidation of an Educational Ideology*. Cambridge, MA: Cambridge University Press, 1981.

– "Discipline in the Dominion: The 'Canuck' and the Cult of Manliness." In *The Games Ethic and Imperialism: Aspects of the Diffusion of an Ideal*, edited by J.A. Mangan, 142–67. Harmondsworth, UK: Viking, 1986.

Mann, Andrea, and Sue Inglis. "The Early Years: Women's Athletics at McMaster University." *Canadian Association for Health, Physical Education and Recreation* 60, 4 (1994): 9–13.

Markham, Susan E. "The Indelible Mark of Springfield College: Its Role In Developing Recreation Leadership in Canada, 1915 to 1935." Paper

resented to the North American Society of Sport History Conference, May
1997.

Marks, Lynne. "'A Fragment of Heaven on Earth'? Religion, Gender, and Family in Turn-of-the-Century Canadian Church Periodicals." *Journal of Family History* 26, 2 (2001): 251–71.

Marsh, Leonard C. *Canadians In and Out of Work: A Survey of Economic Classes and their Relation to the Labour Market.* Toronto: Oxford University Press, 1940.

Martin, Jack, and Ann-Marie McLellan. *The Education of Selves: How Psychology Transformed Students.* New York: Oxford University Press, 2013.

McCarthy, Doris. *A Fool in Paradise: An Artist's Early Life.* Toronto: Macfarlane Walter and Ross, 1990.

McCrone, Kathleen E. *Playing the Game: Sport and the Physical Emancipation of English Women, 1870–1914.* Lexington: University Press of Kentucky, 1988.

McCuaig, Katherine. "Tuberculosis: The Changing Concepts of the Disease in Canada 1900–1950." In *Health, Disease and Medicine: Essays in Canadian History,* edited by Charles C. Roland, 296–307. McMaster University: The Hannah Institute for the History of Medicine, 1984.

– *The Weariness, the Fever, and the Fret: The Campaign against Tuberculosis in Canada 1900–1950.* Montreal: McGill-Queen's University Press, 1999.

McGinnis, Janice P. Dickin. "The Impact of Epidemic Influenza: Canada, 1918–1919." *Canadian History Association Historical Papers* (1977): 121–40.

McGowan, Mark G. "The Maritimes' Region and the Building of a Canadian Church: The Case of the Diocese of Antigonish after Confederation." *CCHA Historical Studies* 70 (2004): 48–70.

McGuigan, Gerald F., with George Payerle and Patricia Horrobin, eds. *Student Protest.* Toronto: Methuen, 1968.

McKillop, A.B. "Marching As to War: Elements of Ontario Undergraduate Culture, 1880–1914." In *Youth, University and Canadian Society: Essays in the Social History of Higher Education,* edited by Paul Axelrod and John G. Reid, 75–93. Montreal: McGill-Queen's University Press, 1989.

– *Matters of Mind: The University in Ontario, 1791–1951.* Toronto: University of Toronto Press, 1994.

McLaren, Angus. *Our Own Master Race: Eugenics in Canada, 1885–1945.* Toronto: McClelland and Stewart, 1990.

McLaren, Angus, and Arlene Tigar McLaren. *The Bedroom and the State: The Changing Practices and Politics of Contraception and Abortion in Canada, 1880–1997.* 2nd ed. Don Mills, ON: Oxford University Press, 1997.

McMurray, Gordon A. "Psychology at Saskatchewan." In *History of Academic Psychology,* edited by Mary J. Wright and C. Roger Myers, 178–91. Toronto: C.J. Hogrefe, 1982.

McPherson, Kathryn. *Bedside Matters: The Transformation of Canadian Nursing, 1900–1990.* Toronto: University of Toronto Press, 1996.

Meagher, John. "Professional Preparation." In *Physical Education in Canada,* edited by M.L. Van Vliet, 64–81. Scarborough, ON: Prentice-Hall, 1965.

Meckel, Richard. "Going to School, Getting Sick: The Social and Medical Construction of School Disease in the Late Nineteenth Century." In *Formative Years: Children's Health in the United States, 1880–2000,* edited by Alexandra Minna Stern and Howard Markel, 185–207. Ann Arbor: University of Michigan Press, 2002.

Metcalfe, Alan. *Canada Learns to Play: The Emergence of Organized Sport, 1807–1914.* Toronto: Oxford University Press, 1987.

Miedema, Gary. *For Canada's Sake: Public Religion, Centennial Celebrations, and the Remaking of Canada in the 1960s.* Montreal: McGill-Queen's University Press, 2005.

Millar, W.P.J., and R.D. Gidney. "'Medettes': Thriving or Just Surviving? Women Students in the Faculty of Medicine, University of Toronto, 1910–1951." In *Challenging Professions: Historical and Contemporary Perspectives on Women's Professional Work,* edited by Elizabeth Smyth, Sandra Acker, Paula Bourne, and Alison Prentice, 215–33. Toronto: University of Toronto Press, 1999.

Miller, Ian Hugh Maclean. *Our Glory and Our Grief: Torontonians and the Great War.* Toronto: University of Toronto Press, 2002.

Mitchinson, Wendy. "Marion Hilliard: 'Raring to Go All the Time'." In *Great Dames,* edited by Elspeth Cameron and Janice Dickin, 227–44. Toronto: University of Toronto Press, 1997.

– *Giving Birth in Canada, 1900–1950.* Toronto: University of Toronto Press, 2002.

– "'All Matter Peculiar to Woman and Womanhood': The Medical Context for Women's Education in Canada in the First Half of the Twentieth Century." In *Women Teaching, Women Learning: Historical Perspectives,* edited by Elizabeth M. Smyth and Paula Bourne, 158–73. Toronto: Inanna, 2006.

Moody, Barry M. "Esther Clark Goes to College." *Atlantis* 20, 1 (1995): 39–48.

Moran, James E., and David Wright. *Mental Health and Canadian Society: Historical Perspectives.* Montreal: McGill-Queen's University Press, 2006.

Moran, Jeffrey P. *Teaching Sex: The Shaping of Adolescence in the Twentieth Century.* Cambridge, MA: Harvard University Press, 2000.

Moriarty, R.J. "The Organizational History of the Canadian Intercollegiate Athletic Union Central (C.I.A.U.C.) 1906–1955." PhD dissertation, Ohio State University, 1971.

Morrow, Don. "The Strathcona Trust in Ontario, 1911–1939." *Canadian Journal of the History of Sport and Physical Education* 8, 1 (1977): 72–90.

Moss, Mark. *Manliness and Militarism: Educating Young Boys in Ontario for War.* Don Mills, ON: Oxford University Press, 2001.

Mott, Morris. "Confronting 'Modern' Problems through Play: The Beginning of Physical Education in Manitoba's Public Schools, 1900–1915." In *Schools in the West: Essays in Canadian Educational History,* edited by Nancy M. Sheehan, J. Donald Wilson, and David C. Jones, 57–71. Calgary: Detselig, 1986.

Mrozek, Donald J. "Sport in American Life: From National Health to Personal Fulfillment, 1890–1940." In *Fitness in American Culture: Images of Health, Sport, and the Body, 1830–1940,* edited by Kathryn Grover, 18–46. Amherst: University of Massachusetts Press, 1989.

Murray, Heather. "Making the Modern: Twenty-Five Years of the Margaret Eaton School of Literature and Expression." *Essays in Theatre/Études theatrales* 10, 1 (1991): 39–57.

Myers, C. Roger. "Psychology at Toronto." In *History of Academic Psychology,* edited by Mary J. Wright and C. Roger Myers, 68–99. Toronto: C.J. Hogrefe, 1982.

Naylor, C. David. *Private Practice, Public Payment: Canadian Medicine and the Politics of Health Insurance, 1911–1966.* Montreal: McGill-Queen's University Press, 1986.

Neary, Peter. "Canadian Universities and Canadian Veterans of World War II." In *The Veterans Charter and Post–World War II Canada,* edited by Peter Neary and J.L. Granatstein, 110–48. Montreal: McGill-Queen's University Press, 1998.

Nicholson, Ian A.M. "Gordon Allport, Character, and the 'Culture of Personality,' 1897–1937." *History of Psychology* 1, 1 (1998): 52–68.

– *Inventing Personality: Gordon Allport and the Science of Selfhood.* Washington, DC: American Psychological Association, 2003.

O'Bryan, Maureen H. "Physical Education – A Study of Professional Education in Ontario Universities." PhD dissertation, University of Toronto, 1973.

O'Grady, Jean. *Margaret Addison: A Biography.* Montreal: McGill-Queen's University Press, 2001.

Owram, Doug. *The Government Generation: Canadian Intellectuals and the State, 1900–1945.* Toronto: University of Toronto Press, 1986.

– *Born at the Right Time: A History of the Baby Boom Generation.* Toronto: University of Toronto Press, 1996.

Palmieri, Patricia Ann. *In Adamless Eden: The Community of Women Faculty at Wellesley.* New Haven, CT: Yale University Press, 1997.

Park, Roberta J. "Muscles, Symmetry and Action: 'Do You Measure Up?' Defining Masculinity in Britain and America from the 1860s to the early 1900s." *International Journal of the History of Sport* 22, 3 (2005): 365–95.

– "'Taking Their Measure' in Play, Games, and Physical Training: The
American Scene, 1870s to World War I." *Journal of Sport History* 33, 2 (2006):
193–217.

Parkes, A.E. Marie. *The Development of Women's Athletics at the University of Toronto.*
Toronto: The Women's Athletic Association, University of Toronto, 1961.

Patterson, K. David, and Gerald F. Pyle. "The Geography and Mortality of the
1918 Influenza Pandemic." *Bulletin of the History of Medicine* 65, 1 (1991):
4–21.

Patterson, Robert S. "Society and Education during the Wars and Their In-
terlude, 1914–1945." In *Canadian Education: A History*, edited by J. Donald
Wilson, Robert M. Stamp, and Louis-Philippe Audet, 360–84. Scarborough,
ON: Prentice-Hall, 1970.

– "Progressive Education: Impetus to Educational Change in Alberta and
Saskatchewan." In *Education in Canada: An Interpretation*, edited by E. Brian
Titley and Peter J. Miller, 169–92. Calgary: Detselig, 1982.

Petrina, Stephen. "The Medicalization of Education: A Historiographical
Synthesis." *History of Education Quarterly* 46, 4 (2006): 503–31.

Pettigrew, Eileen. *The Silent Enemy: Canada and the Deadly Flu of 1918.* Saskatoon,
SK: Western Producer Prairie Books, 1983.

Pickles, Katie. "Colonial Counterparts: The First Academic Women in Anglo-
Canada, New Zealand and Australia." *Women's History Review* 10, 2 (2001):
273–97.

Pitsula, James M. *As One Who Serves: The Making of the University of Regina.* Montreal: McGill-Queen's University Press, 2006.

– "Manly Heroes: The University of Saskatchewan and the First World War." In
Cultures, Communities, and Conflict: Histories of Canadian Universities and War,
edited by Paul Stortz and E. Lisa Panayotidis, 121–45. Toronto: University of
Toronto Press, 2012.

Porter, John. *The Vertical Mosaic.* Toronto: University of Toronto Press, 1965.

Porter, Theodore M. *The Rise of Statistical Thinking, 1820–1900.* Princeton, NJ:
Princeton University Press, 1988.

Poutanen, Mary Anne. "Containing and Preventing Contagious Disease:
Montreal's Protestant School Board and Tuberculosis, 1900–1947." *Canadian
Bulletin of Medical History* 23, 2 (2006): 401–28.

Prentice, Alison. "Bluestockings, Feminists, or Women Workers? A Preliminary
Look at Women's Early Employment at the University of Toronto." *Journal of
the Canadian Historical Association* (1991): 231–61.

– "Scholarly Passion: Two Persons Who Caught It." In *Women Who Taught:
Perspectives on the History of Women and Teaching*, edited by Alison Prentice and
Marjorie R. Theobald, 258–83. Toronto: University of Toronto Press, 1991.

– "Three Women in Physics." In *Challenging Professions: Historical and Contemporary Perspectives on Women's Professional Work*, edited by Elizabeth Smyth, Sandra Acker, Paula Bourne, and Alison Prentice, 119–40. Toronto: University of Toronto Press, 1999.

Prescott, Heather Munro. "Sending Their Sons Into Danger: Cornell University and the Ithaca Typhoid Epidemic of 1903." *New York History* 78, 3 (1997): 273–308.

– "The White Plague Goes to College: Tuberculosis Prevention Programs in Colleges and Universities, 1920–1960." *Bulletin of the History of Medicine* 74 (2000): 735–72.

– "Using the Student Body: College and University Students as Research Subjects in the United States during the Twentieth Century." *Journal of the History of Medicine and Allied Sciences* 57 (2002): 3–38.

– *Student Bodies: The Influence of Student Health Services in American Society and Medicine*. Ann Arbor: University of Michigan Press, 2007.

Quiney, Linda J. "'Filling the Gaps': Canadian Voluntary Nurses, the 1917 Halifax Explosion, and the Influenza Epidemic of 1918." *Canadian Bulletin of Medical History* 19, 2 (2002): 351–74.

Reed, T.A. *The Blue and White: A Record of Fifty Years of Athletic Endeavour at the University of Toronto*. Toronto: University of Toronto Press, 1944.

Reese, William J. "The Origins of Progressive Education." *History of Education Quarterly* 41, 1 (2001): 1–24.

Reid, Julyan. "Education for What?" In *Student Power and the Canadian Campus*, edited by Tim and Julyan Reid, 1–16. Toronto: Peter Martin, 1969.

Reiss, Steven A. "Sport and the Redefinition of Middle-Class Masculinity in Victorian America." In *The New American Sport History: Recent Approaches and Perspectives*, edited by S.W. Pope, 173–97. Urbana: University of Illinois Press, 1997.

Richardson, Theresa R. *The Century of the Child: The Mental Hygiene Movement and Social Policy in the United States and Canada*. Albany, NY: SUNY Press, 1989.

Robinson, Marion O. *Give My Heart: The Dr. Marion Hilliard Story*. New York: Doubleday, 1964.

Rose, Nikolas. *Governing the Soul: The Shaping of the Private Self*. London: Routledge, 1990.

– *Inventing Our Selves: Psychology, Power, and Personhood*. Cambridge, MA: Cambridge University Press, 1998.

Rosenberg, Charles. "Introduction – Framing Disease: Illness, Society, and History." In *Framing Disease: Studies in Cultural History*, edited by Charles E. Rosenberg and Janet Golden, xiii–xxvi. New Brunswick, NJ: Rutgers University Press, 1992.

Rossinow, Doug. *The Politics of Authenticity: Liberalism, Christianity, and the New Left in America*. New York: Columbia University Press, 1998.

Rossiter, Margaret W. *Women Scientists in America: Struggles and Strategies to 1940*. Baltimore: Johns Hopkins University Press, 1982.

Rotundo, E. Anthony. *American Manhood: Transformations in Masculinity from the Revolution to the Modern Era*. New York: Basic Books, 1993.

Rupp, Leila J. *Worlds of Women: The Making of an International Women's Movement*. Princeton, NJ: Princeton University Press, 1997.

Ruyter, Nancy Lee Chalfa. "American Delsartism: Precursor of an American Dance Art." *International Journal of the History of Sport* 26, 13 (2009): 2015–30.

Sangster, Joan. *Regulating Girls and Women: Sexuality, Family, and the Law in Ontario, 1920–1960*. Don Mills, ON: Oxford University Press, 2001.

Schwartz, Robert A. "How Deans of Women Became Men." *The Review of Higher Education* 20, 4 (1997): 419–36.

Scott, Anne Firor. *Natural Allies: Women's Associations in American History*. Urbana: University of Illinois Press, 1993.

Scraton, Sheila. *Shaping Up to Womanhood: Gender and Girls' Physical Education*. Buckingham, UK: Open University Press, 1992.

Selles, Joanna. *Methodists and Women's Education in Ontario, 1836–1925*. Montreal: McGill-Queen's University Press, 1996.

Smith, Michael. "Graceful Athleticism or Robust Womanhood: The Sporting Culture of Women in Victorian Nova Scotia, 1870–1914." *Journal of Canadian Studies* 23, 1&2 (1988): 120–37.

– "Dampness, Darkness, Dirt, Disease: Physicians and the Promotion of Sanitary Science in Public Schools." In *Profiles of Science and Society in the Maritimes Prior to 1914*, edited by Paul A. Bogaard, 195–218. Fredericton, NB: Acadiensis Press, 1990.

Smith, Ronald. *Sports and Freedom: The Rise of Big-Time College Athletics*. New York: Oxford University Press, 1988.

Smyth, Elizabeth, Sandra Acker, Paula Bourne, and Alison Prentice, eds. *Challenging Professions: Historical and Contemporary Perspectives on Women's Professional Work*. Toronto: University of Toronto Press, 1999.

Starr, Paul. *The Social Transformation of American Medicine*. New York: Basic Books, 1982.

Stephen, Jennifer A. *Pick One Intelligent Girl: Employability, Domesticity, and the Gendering of Canada's Welfare State, 1939–1947*. Toronto: University of Toronto Press, 2007.

Stewart, John. "John Ryle, the Institute of Social Medicine and the Health of Oxford Students." *Family and Community History* 7, 1 (2004): 59–71.

Stewart, Lee. *"It's Up to You": Women at UBC in the Early Years.* Vancouver: UBC Press, 1990.

Strange, Carolyn. *Toronto's Girl Problem: The Perils and Pleasures of the City, 1880–1930.* Toronto: University of Toronto Press, 1995.

Strange, Carolyn, and Tina Loo. *Making Good: Law and Moral Regulation in Canada, 1867–1939.* Toronto: University of Toronto Press, 1997.

Strong-Boag, Veronica. "Canada's Women Doctors: Feminism Constrained." In *A Not Unreasonable Claim: Women and Reform in Canada, 1880s–1920s,* edited by Linda Kealey, 109–29. Toronto: Women's Press, 1979.

– *The New Day Recalled: Lives of Girls and Women in English Canada, 1919–1939.* Toronto: Copp Clark Pitman, 1988.

Stuart, Meryn. "War and Peace: Professional Identities and Nurses' Training, 1914–1930." In *Challenging Professions: Historical and Contemporary Perspectives on Women's Professional Work,* edited by Elizabeth Smyth, Sandra Acker, Paula Bourne, and Alison Prentice, 171–93. Toronto: University of Toronto Press, 1999.

Susman, Warren I. "'Personality' and the Making of Twentieth-Century Culture." In *New Directions in American Intellectual History,* edited by John Higham and Paul K. Conkin, 212–26. Baltimore: Johns Hopkins University Press, 1979.

Sutherland, Neil. *Children in English-Canadian Society: Framing the Twentieth-Century Consensus.* Toronto: University of Toronto, 1976.

– *Growing Up: Childhood in English Canada From the Great War to the Age of Television.* Toronto: University of Toronto Press, 1997.

Szasz, Ferenc. "The Stress on 'Character and Service' in Progressive America." *Mid-America: An Historical Review* 63, 3 (1981): 145–56.

Tanner, J.M. *A History of the Study of Human Growth.* Cambridge, MA: Cambridge University Press, 1981.

Thomson, Mathew. "Constituting Citizenship: Mental Deficiency, Mental Health and Human Rights in Inter-war Britain." In *Regenerating England: Science, Medicine and Culture in Inter-war Britain,* ed. Christopher Lawrence and Anna-K Mayer, 231–50. Amsterdam: Rodopi, 2000.

– *Psychological Subjects: Identity, Culture, and Health in Twentieth-Century Britain.* Oxford: Oxford University Press, 2006.

Tillotson, Shirley. *The Public at Play: Gender and the Politics of Recreation in Post-War Ontario.* Toronto: University of Toronto Press, 2000.

– *Contributing Citizens: Modern Charitable Fundraising and the Making of the Welfare State, 1920–66.* Vancouver: UBC Press, 2008.

Todd, Jan. *Physical Culture and the Body Beautiful: Purposive Exercise in the Lives of American Women, 1800–1870.* Macon, GA: Mercer University Press, 1998.

Tomes, Nancy. *The Gospel of Germs: Men, Women, and the Microbe in American Life.*
    Cambridge, MA: Harvard University Press, 1998.
Twohig, Peter L. "'Local Girls' and 'Lab Boys': Gender, Skill and Medical Labo-
    ratories in Nova Scotia in the 1920s and 1930s." *Acadiensis* 31, 1
    (Autumn 2001): 55–75.
Urla, Jacqueline, and Alan C. Swedlund. "The Anthropometry of Barbie: Unset-
    tling Ideals of the Feminine Body in Popular Culture." In *Deviant Bodies: Criti-
    cal Perspectives on Difference in Science and Popular Culture,* edited by Jennifer
    Terry and Jacqueline Urla, 277–313. Bloomington: Indiana University Press,
    1995.
Verbrugge, Martha H. "Recreating the Body: Women's Physical Education and
    the Science of Sex Differences in America, 1900–1940." *Bulletin of the History
    of Medicine* 71 (1997): 273–304.
– *Active Bodies: A History of Women's Physical Education in Twentieth-Century
    America.* New York: Oxford University Press, 2012.
Vernon, Keith. "A Healthy Society for Future Intellectuals: Developing Student
    Life at Civic Universities." In *Regenerating England: Science, Medicine and Cul-
    ture in Inter-War Britain,* edited by Christopher Lawrence and Anna-K. Mayer,
    179–202. Atlanta, GA: Rodopi, 2000.
– "The Health and Welfare of University Students in Britain, 1920–1939." *His-
    tory of Education* 37, 2 (2008): 227–52.
Vertinsky, Patricia A. *The Eternally Wounded Woman: Women, Doctors, and Exercise
    in the Late Nineteenth Century.* Manchester: Manchester University Press, 1990.
– "Embodying Normalcy: Anthropometry and the Long Arm of William H.
    Sheldon's Somatotyping Project." *Journal of Sport History* 29, 1 (2002): 95–133.
– "Memory and Monument: The Gymnasium as War Memorial." In *Disciplin-
    ing Bodies in the Gymnasium: Memory, Monument, Modernism,* edited by Patricia
    Vertinsky and Sherry McKay, 13–31. London: Routledge, 2004.
– "'Power Geometries': Disciplining the Gendered Body in the Spaces of the
    War Memorial Gymnasium." In *Disciplining Bodies in the Gymnasium: Memory,
    Monument, Modernism,* edited by Patricia Vertinsky and Sherry McKay, 48–73.
    London: Routledge, 2004.
– "Transatlantic Traffic in Expressive Movement: From Delsarte and Dalcroze to
    Margaret H'Doubler and Rudolf Laban." *International Journal of the History of
    Sport* 26, 13 (2009): 2031–51.
von Heyking, Amy. *Creating Citizens: History and Identity in Alberta's Schools, 1905
    to 1980.* Calgary: University of Calgary Press, 2006.
Wall, Sharon. *The Nurture of Nature: Childhood, Antimodernism, and Ontario Sum-
    mer Camps, 1920–55.* Vancouver: University of British Columbia Press, 2009.

Walton, Yvette Margaret. "The Life and Professional Contributions of Ethel
   Mary Cartwright, 1880–1955." MA thesis, University of Western Ontario,
   1976.
Warren, Heather A. "The Shift from Character to Personality in Mainline Prot-
   estant Thought, 1935–1945." *Church History: Studies in Christianity and Culture*
   67, 3 (1998): 537–55.
Way, Howard Paul. "A Survey of Small College Health Service Programs." MA
   thesis, Springfield College, 1935.
Weatherall, Miles. "Drug Treatment and the Rise of Pharmacology." In *Cam-
   bridge Illustrated History of Medicine*, edited by Roy Porter, 246–77. Cambridge,
   MA: Cambridge University Press, 2001.
Weindling, Paul. "The Immunological Tradition." In *Companion Encyclopedia of
   the History of Medicine*, vol. 1, edited by W.F. Bynum and Roy Porter, 192–204.
   London: Routledge, 1993.
Welch, Paula D. *History of American Physical Education and Sport.* Springfield, IL:
   C.C. Thomas, 1996.
Welshman, John. "Physical Education and the School Medical Services in Eng-
   land and Wales, 1907–1939." *Social History of Medicine* 9, 1 (1999): 31–48.
Westhues, Kenneth. "Inter-Generational Conflict in the Sixties." In *Prophecy
   and Protest: Social Movements in Twentieth-Century Canada*, edited by Samuel D.
   Clark, J. Paul Grayson, and Linda M. Grayson, 387–408. Toronto: Gage, 1975.
Wherrett, George Jasper. *The Miracle of the Empty Beds: A History of Tuberculosis in
   Canada.* Toronto: University of Toronto Press, 1977.
White, Melanie, and Alan Hunt. "Citizenship: Care of the Self, Character and
   Personality." *Citizenship Studies* 4, 2 (2000): 93–116.
Whitson, David. "The Embodiment of Gender: Discipline, Domination, and
   Empowerment." In *Women, Sport and Culture*, ed. Susan Birrell and Cheryl L.
   Cole, 353–71. Champaign, IL: Human Kinetics, 1994.
Whorton, James C. *Crusaders for Fitness: The History of American Health Reformers.*
   Princeton, NJ: Princeton University Press, 1982.
Wipper, Kirk A.W. *Retrospect and Prospect: A Record of the School of Physical and
   Health Education, University of Toronto, 1940–1965. Presented in the Twenty-fifth
   Anniversary Year.* Toronto: n.p., 1965.
Wright, Katie. "Theorizing Therapeutic Culture: Past Influences, Future Direc-
   tions." *Journal of Sociology* 44, 4 (2008): 321–36.
Wright, Mary J., and C. Robert Myers, eds. *History of Academic Psychology in
   Canada.* Toronto: C.J. Hogrefe, 1982.
Yosifon, David, and Peter N. Stearns. "The Rise and Fall of American Posture."
   American Historical Review 103, 4 (1998): 1057–95.

Zirnhelt, David. "A Student Manifest: In Search of a Real and Human Edu-
    cational Alternative." In *Student Protest*, edited by Gerald F. McGuigan, with
    George Payerle and Patricia Horrobin, 53–61. Toronto: Methuen, 1968.
Zweiniger-Bargielowska, Ina. "Building a British Superman: Physical Culture in
    Interwar Britain." *Journal of Contemporary History* 41, 4 (2006): 595–610.

Index

Victoria College, 13, 162; disease at,
35–8, 40–45, 47–50; health care,
183; living conditions, 78–9, 80–1,
183; medical examinations, 3,
16, 21–2, 24, 39, 78, 86, 88, 150,
216n1; mental health, 150–1;
physical training, 55–6, 57, 71–3,
90–1, 140, 201n6; residence dons,
111–12; women's health, 3, 16.
See also health services, cost
of; infirmary; physicians: and
opposition to health services;
professional women

Warren, Heather, 171
Wasserman test, 23, 48, 96–7, 187
Watson, Dr. Melville, 32
Weekes, Edith A., 71
Westhues, Kenneth, 178
Wright, Katie, 180
Wodehouse, Dr G.E., 161, 172–3
women. *See* professional women
Women's Amateur Athletic
Federation of Canada, 68, 114

Yosifon, David, 84, 138
Yuhasz, M.S., 139